W.B. SAUNDERS COMPANY

A Division of Elsevier Inc.

Elsevier Inc. • 1600 John F. Kennedy Blvd., Suite 1800 • Philadelphia, Pennsylvania 19103-2899

http://www.theclinics.com

GASTROENTEROLOGY CLINICS OF NORTH AMERICA Volume 37, Number 3
September 2008 ISSN 0889-8553, ISBN-13: 978-1-4160-6297-4, ISBN-10: 1-4160-6297-1

Editor: Kerry Holland

Gastroenterology Clinics of North America (ISSN 0889-8553) is published quarterly by Elsevier Inc., 360 Park Avenue South, New York, NY 10010-1710. Months of issue are March, June, September, and December. Business and Editorial Offices: 1600 John F. Kennedy Blvd., Suite 1800, Philadelphia, PA 19103-2899. Customer Service Office: 6277 Sea Harbor Drive, Orlando, FL 32887-4800. Periodicals postage paid at New York, NY and additional mailing offices. Subscription prices are $237.00 per year (US individuals), $121.00 per year (US students), $344.00 per year (US institutions), $261.00 per year (Canadian individuals), $410.00 per year (Canadian institutions), $309.00 per year (international individuals), $157.00 per year (international students), and $426.00 per year (international institutions). Foreign air speed delivery is included in all *Clinics* subscription prices. All prices are subject to change without notice. **POSTMASTER**: Send address changes to *Gastroenterology Clinics of North America*, Elsevier Periodicals Customer Service 6277 Sea Harbor Drive, Orlando, FL 32887-4800. **Customer Service: 1-800-654-2452 (US). From outside the United States, call 1-407-563-6020. Fax: 1-407-563-8521. E-mail: JournalsCustomerService-usa@elsevier.com.**

Reprints. For copies of 100 or more, of articles in this publication, please contact the Commercial Reprints Department, Elsevier Inc., 360 Part Avenue South, New York, New York 10010-1710. Tel. (212) 633-3813, Fax: (212) 462-1935, e-mail: reprints@elsevier.com.

Gastroenterology Clinics of North America is also published in Italian by Il Pensiero Scientifico Editore, Rome, Italy; and in Portuguese by Interlivros Edicoes Ltda., Rua Commandante Coelho 1085, 21250 Cordovil, Rio de Janeiro, Brazil.

Gastroenterology Clinics of North America is covered in *MEDLINE/PubMed (Index Medicus), Excerpta Medica, Current Contents/Clinical Medicine, Science Citation Index, ISI/BIOMED*, and *BIOSIS*.

Printed in the United States of America.

Contributors

GUEST EDITOR

SATISH S.C. RAO, MD, PhD, FRCP (LON)
Director, Section of Neurogastroenterology & GI Motility, and Professor, Department of Internal Medicine, University of Iowa Carver College of Medicine, University of Iowa Hospitals, Iowa City, Iowa

AUTHORS

DAVID C.C. BARTOLO, MBChB, BSc (Hons), FRCS
Department of Colorectal Surgery, Western General Hospital, Edinburgh, United Kingdom

ADIL E. BHARUCHA, MBBS, MD
Professor of Medicine, Division of Gastroenterology and Hepatology, College of Medicine, Mayo Clinic, Rochester, Minnesota

CATHERINE S. BRADLEY, MD, MSCE
Associate Professor, Departments of Obstetrics and Gynecology and Epidemiology, University of Iowa Carver College of Medicine and College of Public Health, University of Iowa Hospitals and Clinics, Iowa City, Iowa

PETER S. CHONG, MB, MS, FRCS, FRCSE
Department of Colorectal Surgery, Western General Hospital, Edinburgh; and Consultant Colorectal Surgeon, Department of Surgery, Gartnavel General Hospital, Glasgow, United Kingdom

MIGUEL A. CUESTA, MD, PhD
Surgeon, Department of Surgery, University Hospital "Vrije Universiteit," Amsterdam, The Netherlands

JEAN-NICOLAS DACHER, MD, PhD
Department of Radiology, Rouen University Hospital Charles Nicolle; and University of Rouen, Rouen, France

RICHELLE J.F. FELT-BERSMA, MD, PhD
Gastroenterologist, Department of Gastroenterology, University Hospital "Vrije Universiteit," Amsterdam, The Netherlands

MARC A. GLADMAN, MBBS, PhD, MRCOG, FRCS (Gen Surg)
Clinical Lecturer in Surgery, Centre for Academic Surgery, Institute of Cell and Molecular Science, Barts and The London School of Medicine and Dentistry, Whitechapel, London, United Kingdom

CHARLES H. KNOWLES, MBBChir, PhD, FRCS (Gen Surg)
Senior Lecturer in Colorectal Surgery, Honorary Consultant Surgeon, Center for Academic Surgery, Institute of Cell and Molecular Science, Barts and The London School of Medicine and Dentistry, Whitechapel, London, United Kingdom

EDITH KONING, MD
Department of Radiology, Rouen University Hospital Charles Nicolle; and University of Rouen, Rouen, France

KARL J. KREDER, MD, MBA
Professor and Vice Chair, Department of Urology, University of Iowa Carver College of Medicine, University of Iowa Hospitals and Clinics, Iowa City, Iowa

FELIX W. LEUNG, MD
Professor of Medicine, David Geffen School of Medicine at University of California, Los Angeles, Los Angeles; and Chief of Gastroenterology, Sepulveda Ambulatory Care Center, VA Greater Los Angeles Healthcare System, North Hills, California

PAOLA MASI, MD
Department of Pediatrics, University of Naples "Federico II", Via Pansini, Italy

ERASMO MIELE, MD
Department of Pediatrics, University of Naples "Federico II", Via Pansini, Italy

RAVINDER K. MITTAL, MD
Pelvic Floor Function and Disorder Group, Division of Gastroenterology, University of California, San Diego VA Health Care Center, San Diego, California

R. JOHN NICHOLLS, MD, FRCS
Professor of Colorectal Surgery, Department of Biosurgery and Surgical Technology, St Mary's Hospital, Division of Surgery, Oncology, Reproductive Biology and Anaesthetics, Imperial College, London; and Emeritus Consultant Colorectal Surgeon, Department of Surgery, St Mark's Hospital, Harrow, United Kingdom

RIEN J.M. NIJMAN, MD, PhD
Professor, Chair, Department of Urology, University Medical Centre Groningen, Groningen, The Netherlands

CHRISTINE NORTON, PhD, MA, RN
Associate Dean (Research), King's College London, Florence Nightingale School of Nursing and Midwifery; and Professor of Gastrointestinal Nursing, Burdett Institute of Gastrointestinal Nursing, St. Mark's Hospital, Harrow, United Kingdom

VARUNA RAIZADA, MD
Pelvic Floor Function and Disorder Group, Division of Gastroenterology, University of California, San Diego VA Health Care Center, San Diego, California

SATISH S.C. RAO, MD, PhD, FRCP (LON)
Director, Section of Neurogastroenterology & GI Motility, and Professor, Department of Internal Medicine, University of Iowa Carver College of Medicine, University of Iowa Hospitals, Iowa City, Iowa

CELINE SAVOYE-COLLET, MD, PhD
Department of Radiology, Rouen University Hospital Charles Nicolle; and University of Rouen, Rouen, France

JOHN F. SCHNELLE, PhD
Hamilton Chair Professor, Center for Quality Aging, Director, Department of Medicine, Vanderbilt University Medical Center, Nashville, Tennessee

S. MARK SCOTT, PhD
Senior Clinical Scientist, GI Physiology Unit and Neurogastroenterology Group (Centre for Academic Surgery), Institute of Cell and Molecular Science, Barts and The London School of Medicine and Dentistry, The Royal London Hospital, Whitechapel, London, United Kingdom

KAREN E. SMITH, MD
Major, US Army (Active Duty), Fellow Associate, Department of Urology, University of Iowa Carver College of Medicine, University of Iowa Hospitals and Clinics, Iowa City, Iowa

ANNAMARIA STAIANO, MD
Department of Pediatrics, University of Naples "Federico II", Via Pansini, Italy

PARIS P. TEKKIS, MD, FRCS
Reader in Surgery & Consultant Colorectal Surgeon, Department of Academic Surgery, Chelsea and Westminster Hospital, Division of Surgery, Oncology, Reproductive Biology, and Anaesthetics, Imperial College, London, United Kingdom

M. TIERSMA E. STELLA, MD, PhD
Gynecologist, Department of Gynecology, University Hospital "Vrije Universiteit," Amsterdam, The Netherlands

EMANUEL TRABUCO, MD
Instructor, Department of Obstetrics and Gynecology, College of Medicine, Mayo Clinic, Rochester, Minnesota

Contents

Preface xiii

Satish S.C. Rao

Pelvic Floor Anatomy and Applied Physiology 493

Varuna Raizada and Ravinder K. Mittal

Pelvic floor muscles have two major functions: they provide support or act as a floor for the abdominal viscera including the rectum; and they provide a constrictor or continence mechanism to the urethral, anal, and vaginal orifices (in females). This article discusses the relevance of pelvic floor to the anal opening and closure function, and discusses new findings with regards to the role of these muscles in the vaginal and urethra closure mechanisms.

Manometric, Sensorimotor, and Neurophysiologic Evaluation of Anorectal Function 511

S. Mark Scott and Marc A. Gladman

With advances in diagnostic technology, it is now accepted that in the field of functional bowel disorders, symptom-based assessment is unsatisfactory as the sole means of directing therapy. A robust taxonomy based on underlying pathophysiology has been suggested, highlighting a crucial role for physiologic testing in clinical practice. A wide number of complementary investigations currently exist for the assessment of anorectal structure and function, some of which have a clinical impact in patients with functional disorders of evacuation and continence by markedly improving diagnostic yield and altering management. The techniques, limitations, measurements, and clinical use of manometric, sensorimotor, and neurophysiologic tests of anorectal function are presented.

Urodynamic Evaluation of the Bladder and Pelvic Floor 539

Catherine S. Bradley, Karen E. Smith, and Karl J. Kreder

Pelvic floor disorders including lower urinary tract dysfunction are common, and may be evaluated by urodynamic tests, such as cystometry, uroflowmetry, pressure flow studies, electromyography, and video-urodynamics. These urodynamic tests provide objective information regarding the normal and abnormal function of the urinary tract and pelvic floor, and provide a better understanding of the pathophysiologic processes that cause lower urinary tract symptoms. This article describes typical urodynamic studies and their roles in the evaluation of common pelvic floor disorders, including stress urinary incontinence, overactive bladder, and pelvic organ prolapse.

Radiologic Evaluation of Pelvic Floor Disorders 553

Celine Savoye-Collet, Edith Koning, and Jean-Nicolas Dacher

Several imaging modalities are available ranging from fluoroscopic techniques to ultrasonography and MRI for the evaluation of patients with pelvic floors disorders. High-resolution ultrasonography and MRI not only provide superior delineation of the pelvic floor anatomy but also reveal pathology and functional changes. This article focuses on standard imaging procedures including defecography, ultrasonography, and MRI and discusses its use in clinical practice by illustrating both normal and abnormal patterns.

Dyssynergic Defecation and Biofeedback Therapy 569

Satish S.C. Rao

Constipation caused by dyssynergic defecation is common and affects up to one half of patients with this disorder. It is possible to diagnose this problem through history, prospective stool diaries, and anorectal physiologic tests. Randomized controlled trials have now established that biofeedback therapy is not only efficacious but superior to other modalities and that the symptom improvement is caused by a change in underlying pathophysiology. Development of userfriendly approaches to biofeedback therapy and use of home biofeedback programs will significantly enhance the adoption of this treatment by gastroenterologists and colorectal surgeons.

Fecal Incontinence and Biofeedback Therapy 587

Christine Norton

Biofeedback as delivered in most clinical settings in Western medicine has been consistently reported to improve symptoms of fecal incontinence. Closer scrutiny of the elements of the intervention and controlled studies, however, have consistently failed to find any benefit of the biofeedback element of this complex package of care; nor has any superiority been found for one modality over another. There is a need for further well-designed and adequately powered randomized controlled trials. Meanwhile, there can be little doubt that conservative interventions improve many patients with fecal incontinence to the point where most report satisfaction with treatment and do not wish to consider more invasive options, such as surgery.

Surgical Treatment of Patients with Constipation and Fecal Incontinence 605

Marc A. Gladman and Charles H. Knowles

Patients with constipation and fecal incontinence usually come to the attention of the surgeon when conservative measures have failed to alleviate sufficiently severe symptoms. Following detailed clinical and physiologic assessment, the surgeon should tailor the procedure to specific underlying physiologic abnormalities to restore function. This article describes the rationale, indications (including patient selection), results, and current position controversies of surgical procedures for constipation and fecal incontinence, dividing these into those regarded as historical, contemporary, or evolving. Reported surgical outcome data must be interpreted with caution because for most studies the evidence is of low quality, making comparison of different procedures problematic and emphasizing the need for better designed and conducted clinical trials.

Hemorrhoids and Fissure in Ano **627**

Peter S. Chong and David C.C. Bartolo

Hemorrhoids and anal fissures are common benign anorectal conditions that form a significant part of a colorectal surgeon's workload. This review summarizes and evaluates the current techniques available in their management.

Rectal Prolapse, Rectal Intussusception, Rectocele, Solitary Rectal Ulcer Syndrome, and Enterocele **645**

Richelle J.F. Felt-Bersma, M. Tiersma E. Stella, and Miguel A. Cuesta

Rectal prolapse is best diagnosed by physical examination and by having the patient strain as if to defecate; a laparoscopic rectopexy is the preferred treatment approach. Intussusception is more an epiphenomena than a defecatory disorder and should be managed conservatively. Solitary rectal ulcer syndrome is a consequence of chronic straining and therapy should be aimed at restoring a normal bowel habit with behavioral approaches including biofeedback therapy. Rectocele correction may be considered if it can be definitively established that it is a cause of defecation disorder and only after conservative measures have failed. An enterocele should only be operated when pain and heaviness are predominant symptoms and it is refractory to conservative therapy.

Ileal Pouch Dysfunction: Diagnosis and Management **669**

Paris P. Tekkis and R. John Nicholls

Restorative proctocol ectomy is the elective surgical procedure of choice for most patients who have ulcerative colitis or familial adenomatous polyposis. This major advance has offered an alternative to permanent ileostomy in these patients.

Functional and Chronic Anorectal and Pelvic Pain Disorders **685**

Adil E. Bharucha and Emanuel Trabuco

Several organic and functional disorders of the urinary bladder, reproductive tract, anorectum, and the pelvic floor musculature cause pelvic pain. This article describes functional disorders in which chronic pelvic and anorectal pain cannot be explained by a structural or other specified pathology. Currently, these functional disorders are classified into urogynecologic conditions or cystitis and painful bladder syndrome, anorectal disorders, and the levator ani syndrome. Although nomenclature suggests that these conditions are distinct, there is considerable overlap of their symptoms and these disorders have much in common.

Urinary and Fecal Incontinence in Nursing Home Residents 697

Felix W. Leung and John F. Schnelle

Urinary and fecal incontinence are comorbid conditions affecting over 50% of nursing home residents. Management should focus on identifying and treating underlying causes. Despite appropriate management, residents may remain incontinent because of dementia and health- or restraint-related immobility. This article reviews the results of studies that have documented how prompted voiding programs can significantly reduce urinary and fecal incontinence, particularly if the intervention includes dietary and exercise components. Documentation of noninvasive and efficacious interventions by randomized, controlled trials and the labor costs of implementing these measures can lead to changes in how nursing home care is provided and funded.

Pediatric Anorectal Disorders 709

Paola Masi, Erasmo Miele, and Annamaria Staiano

This article reports the clinical, physiopathologic, diagnostic, and therapeutic aspects of the most common anorectal disorders in children. In particular, it focuses on the differential diagnosis between organic and functional constipation. In addition, the authors separately examine some of the clinical conditions such as atopy, neurologic diseases, and anorectal malformations, in which chronic constipation may be an important clinical manifestation.

Diagnosis and Management of Urinary Incontinence and Functional Fecal Incontinence (Encopresis) in Children 731

Rien J.M. Nijman

The ability to maintain normal continence for urine and stools is not achievable in all children by a certain age. Gaining control of urinary and fecal continence is a complex process, and not all steps and factors involved are fully understood. While normal development of anatomy and physiology are prerequisites to becoming fully continent, anatomic abnormalities, such as bladder exstrophy, epispadias, ectopic ureters, and neurogenic disturbances that can usually be recognized at birth and cause incontinence, will require specialist treatment, not only to restore continence but also to preserve renal function. Most forms of urinary incontinence are not caused by an anatomic or physiologic abnormality and, hence, are more difficult to diagnose and their management requires a sound knowledge of bladder and bowel function.

Index 749

FORTHCOMING ISSUES

December 2008

Gastroesophageal Reflux Disease
Gary W. Falk, MD, MS,
Guest Editor

March 2009

Esophageal Cancer
Guy Eslick, MD, *Guest Editor*

RECENT ISSUES

June 2008

Eosinophilic and Autoimmune Gastrointestinal Disease: New Insights and New Entities
Nicholas J. Talley, MD, PhD,
Guest Editor

March 2008

Colon Cancer Screening, Surveillance, Prevention, and Therapy
Mitchell S. Cappell, MD, PhD,
Guest Editor

December 2007

Pathology and Clinical Relevance of Neoplastic Precursor Lesions of the Gastrointestinal Tract, Liver, and Pancreaticobiliary System
Robert D. Odze, MD, FRCPc,
Guest Editor

Pelvic Floor Anatomy and Applied Physiology

Varuna Raizada, MD, Ravinder K. Mittal, MD*

KEYWORDS

- Levator ani • External anal canal • Internal anal canal
- Function

Pelvic floor muscles have two major functions: they provide support or act as a floor for the abdominal viscera including the rectum; and they provide constrictor or continence mechanism to the urethral, anal, and vaginal orifices (in females). This article discusses the relevance of pelvic floor to the anal opening and closure function, and discusses new findings with regards to the role of these muscles in the vaginal closure mechanisms.

The bony pelvis is composed of sacrum, ileum, ischium, and pubis. It is divided into the false (greater) and true (lesser) pelvis by the pelvic brim. The sacral promontory, the anterior ala of the sacrum, the arcuate line of the ilium, the pectineal line of the pubis, and the pubic crest that culminates in the symphysis pubis, mark the pelvic brim. The shape of the female bony pelvis can be classified into four broad categories: (1) gynecoid, (2) anthropoid, (3) android, and (4) platypelloid. The pelvic diaphragm is a wide but thin muscular layer of tissue that forms the inferior border of the abdominopelvic cavity. Composed of a broad, funnel-shaped sling of fascia and muscle, it extends from the symphysis pubis to the coccyx and from one lateral sidewall to the other. The urogenital diaphragm, also called the "triangular ligament," is a strong, muscular membrane that occupies the area between the symphysis pubis and ischial tuberosities and stretches across the triangular anterior portion of the pelvic outlet. The pelvic ligaments are not classic ligaments but are thickenings of retroperitoneal fascia and consist primarily of blood and lymphatic vessels, nerves, and fatty connective tissue. Anatomists call the retroperitoneal fascia "subserous fascia," whereas surgeons refer to this fascial layer as "endopelvic fascia." The connective tissue is denser immediately adjacent to the lateral walls of the cervix and the vagina. The broad ligaments are a thin, mesenteric-like double reflection of peritoneum stretching from the lateral pelvic sidewalls to the uterus. The cardinal, or Mackenrodt's, ligaments extend from the lateral aspects of the upper part of the cervix and the vagina to the pelvic wall.

Supported by National Institutes of Health grant RO1-DK60733
Pelvic Floor Function and Disorder Group, Division of Gastroenterology, University of California, GI-111D, San Diego VA Health Care Center, 3350 La Jolla Village Drive, San Diego, CA 92161, USA
* Corresponding author.
E-mail address: rmittal@ucsd.edu (R.K. Mittal).

Gastroenterol Clin N Am 37 (2008) 493–509
doi:10.1016/j.gtc.2008.06.003 gastro.theclinics.com
0889-8553/08/$ – see front matter. Published by Elsevier Inc.

The uterosacral ligaments extend from the upper portion of the cervix posteriorly to the third sacral vertebra.

The pelvic floor is comprised of a number of muscles and they are organized into superficial and deep muscle layers. There is significant controversy with regards to the nomenclature, but generally speaking the superficial muscle layer and the muscles relevant to the anal canal function are the external anal sphincter (EAS), perineal body, and possibly the puboperineal (or transverse perinei) muscles (**Fig. 1**). The deep pelvic floor muscles consist of pubococcygeus, ileococcygeus, coccygeus, and puborectalis muscles. Puborectalis muscle is located in between the superficial and deep muscle layers, and it is better to view this as the middle muscle layer of the pelvic floor. In addition to the skeletal muscles of the pelvic floor, caudal extension of the circular and longitudinal smooth muscles from the rectum into the anal canal constitutes the internal anal sphincter (IAS) and EAS of the anal canal, respectively. Discussed are the salient and the controversial aspects of anatomy of the pelvic floor and anal sphincter muscles, followed by a discussion of the function of each component of the pelvic floor muscles and their role in anal sphincter closure and opening.

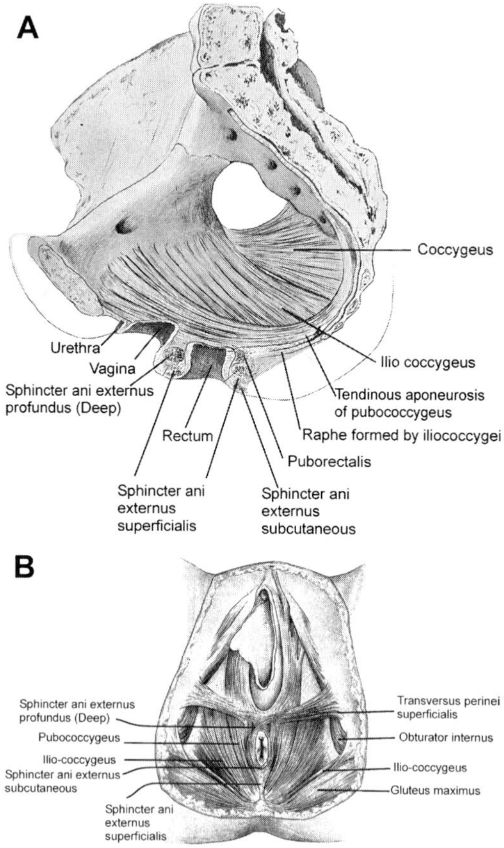

Fig. 1. (*A*) Pelvic floor muscles seen in the sagittal section of pelvis. (*B*) Pelvic floor muscles as seen from the perineal surface. (*Adapted from* Thompson P. The myology of the pelvic floor. Newton (MA): McCorquoddale; 1899; with permission.)

ANATOMIC CONSIDERATIONS

Internal Anal Sphincter

Circular muscle layer of the rectum expands caudally into the anal canal and becomes the IAS. The circular muscles in the sphincteric region are thicker than those of the rectal circular smooth muscle with discrete septa in between the muscle bundles. Similarly, the longitudinal muscles of the rectum extend into the anal canal and end up as thin septa that penetrate into the puborectalis and EAS muscles. Longitudinal muscle of the anal canal is also referred to as the "conjoined tendon" (muscle) because some authors believe that skeletal muscles of the pelvic floor (puboanalis) join the smooth muscles of the rectum to form a conjoint tendon. Immunostaining for the smooth and skeletal muscles in this region shows, however, that the smooth muscles make up the entire longitudinal muscle layer of the anal canal.[1,2]

The autonomic nerves, sympathetic (spinal nerves) and parasympathetic (pelvic nerves), supply the IAS.[3] Sympathetic fibers originate from the lower thoracic ganglia to form the superior hypogastric plexus. Parasympathetic fibers originate from the 2nd, 3rd, and 4th sacral nerves to form the inferior hypogastric plexus, which in turn gives rise to superior, middle, and inferior rectal nerves that ultimately supply the rectum and anal canal. These nerves synapse with the myenteric plexus of the rectum and anal canal. Most of the tone of the IAS is myogenic (ie, caused by unique properties of the smooth muscle itself). Angiotensin 2 and prostaglandin $F_{2\alpha}$ play modulatory roles. Sympathetic nerves mediate IAS contraction through the stimulation of α and relaxation through β_1, β_2, and β_3 adrenergic receptors. Recent studies show a predominance of low affinity β_3 receptors in the IAS. Stimulation of parasympathetic or pelvic nerves causes IAS relaxation through nitric oxide–containing neurons located in the myenteric plexus.[4] Vasointestinal intestinal peptide and carbon monoxide are other potential inhibitory neurotransmitters of the inhibitory motor neurons but most likely play limited roles. There are also excitatory motor neurons in the myenteric plexus of IAS and the effects of these neurons are mediated through acetylcholine and substance P. Some investigators believe that the excitatory and inhibitory effects of myenteric neurons on the smooth muscles of IAS are mediated through the Interstitial cells of Cajal (ICC), but other investigators do not necessarily confirm these findings.[4] Degeneration of myenteric neurons resulting in impaired IAS relaxation is the hallmark of Hirschsprung's disease.[5]

External Anal Sphincter

In his original description of 1769, Santorini[6] stated that EAS has three separate muscle bundles: (1) subcutaneous, (2) superficial, and (3) deep. Large numbers of publications continue to show EAS to be made up of these three components. Several investigators have found, however, that the subcutaneous and superficial muscle bundles only constitute the EAS.[7–10] The subcutaneous portion of the EAS is located caudal to the IAS and the superficial portion surrounds the distal part of IAS. The deep portion of the EAS is either very small and merges imperceptibly with the puborectalis muscle, or in the authors' opinion has been confused with the puborectalis muscle. In several schematics published in the literature,[11] including the one by Netter (**Fig. 2**), the EAS is made of three components. A close inspection of these schematics reveals that the puborectalis muscle is entirely missing from these drawings. Based on three-dimensional ultrasound (US) and MRI, the authors believe that the puborectalis muscle is actually the deepest part of the EAS. Shafik[9] described that the EAS consists of three loops; the puborectalis muscle forms the top loop in his drawing (**Fig. 3**). Histologic studies by Fritsch and coworkers[1] and the MRI imaging study of Stoker and

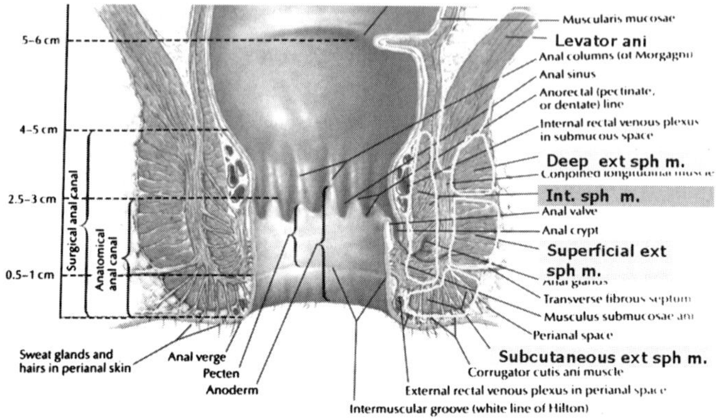

Fig. 2. This schematic shows that the external anal sphincter is made up of a subcutaneous, superficial, and deep part. It is believed that deep external anal sphincter is actually the puborectalis muscle. (*Reprinted from* Netter Anatomy Illustration Collection, © Elsevier Inc. All Rights Reserved. The image has been cropped from its original format to show relevant portion.)

colleagues[12] (**Fig. 4**) are quite convincing that the EAS muscle is composed of only the subcutaneous and superficial portions.[1] Anteriorly, the EAS is attached to the perineal body and transverse perinei muscle, and posteriorly to the anococcygeal raphae. EAS, however, is not a circular muscle in its entirety; rather, it is attached to the transverse perinei (also called "puboperineal") muscle on either side.[8] The posterior wall of the EAS is shorter in its craniocaudal extent than the anterior wall. This should not be misconstrued as a muscle defect in the axial US and MRIs of the lower anal canal. Another implication of this peculiar anatomy is when the anal canal pressure is measured using circumferential side holes; the posterior side holes exit first from the anal canal,[13] thereby causing apparent circumferential asymmetry of the anal canal pressures. The muscle fibers of EAS are composed of fast and slow twitch types, which allow it to maintain sustained tonic contraction at rest and also to contract rapidly with voluntary squeeze. Motor neurons in Onuf's nucleus (located in the sacral spinal cord) innervate EAS muscle through the inferior rectal branches of the right and left pudendal nerves.[11]

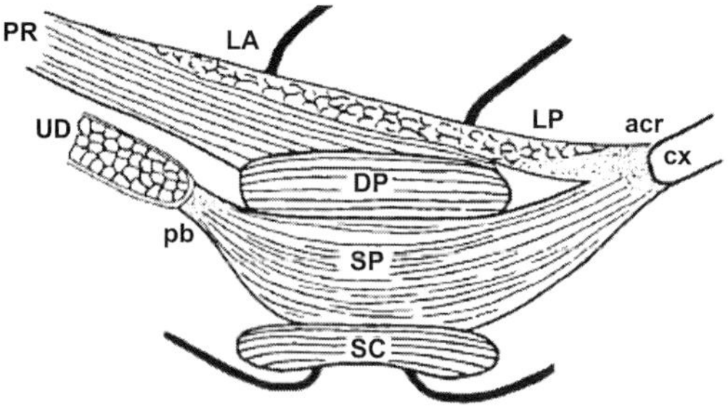

Fig. 3. A sketch of the external anal sphincter from a lateral view, as described by Shafik. External anal sphincter is described as made of three loops: basal loop (BL), intermediate loop (IL), and deep loop (DP). Note the relationship between the puborectalis muscle (PR) and DP. It is believed that DP is actually the posterior part of the puborectalis muscle. LA, levator ani; LP, levator plate; DP, deep portion; SP, superficial portion; SC, subcutaneous portion; cx, coccyx; UD, urogenital diaphragm. (*Adapted from* Bogduk N. Issues in anatomy: the external anal sphincter revisited. Aust N Z J Surg 1996;66:626–9; with permission.)

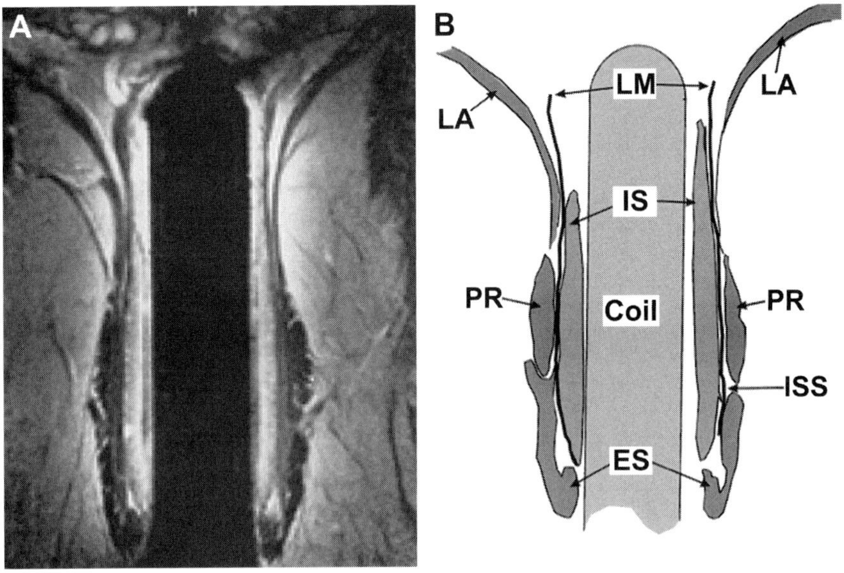

Fig. 4. Anatomy based on MRI. (*A*) Coronal mid anal T2-weighted fast-spin-echo (2500/100) MRI obtained with an endoanal coil. (*B*) Corresponding drawing demonstrates the internal sphincter (IS), intersphincteric space (ISS), longitudinal muscle (LM), external sphincter (ES), puborectalis muscle (PR), and levator ani muscle (LA). These MRIs show that a part of the external anal sphincter is located below and a small portion surrounds the internal anal sphincter. Puborectalis muscle surrounds the upper part of the internal anal sphincter. Based on MRI it is quite clear that external anal sphincter consists of only two parts: subcutaneous (below the internal anal sphincter) and superficial (around the internal anal sphincter). (*Adapted from* Stoker J, Halligan S, Bartram CI. Pelvic floor imaging. Radiology 2001; 218:621–41; with permission.)

PUBORECTALIS AND DEEP PELVIC FLOOR MUSCLES

In 1555, Vesalius[14] wrote an account of the pelvic floor muscles, which he named "musculus sedem attollens." This was later replaced by the more definitive name of "levator ani" by Von Behr and coworkers.[15] The pelvic diaphragm, first so named in 1861 by Meyer,[16] included primitive flexors and abductors of the caudal part of the vertebral column. These muscles included coccygeus (also referred to as "ischiococcygeus"), ileococcygeus, and pubococcygeus and these three muscles were believed to constitute the levator ani muscle. They originate from the pectinate line of the pubic bone and the fascia of the obturator internus muscle and are inserted into the coccyx. Holl,[17] a German anatomist, in 1897 described that some of the pubococcygeus muscle fibers, instead of inserting into the coccyx, looped around the rectum and to these fibers he assigned the name "puborectalis" or "sphincter recti." It seems that the puborectalis muscle originates from the middle of inferior pubic rami rather than from the pubic symphysis. The puborectalis muscle is now included in the levator ani muscle group and the term "levator ani" is used synonymously with pelvic diaphragm muscles. Thompson[18] in a classic text on this subject, quoted Sappey,[19] writing that "the levator ani is one of those muscle which has been studied the most, and at the same time one about which we know the least." Sappey also stated that the "The doctrine of continuity of fibers between two or more muscles of independent actions has been applied to the levator ani at various scientific epochs, and this ancient error, renewed without ceasing, has singularly contributed to complicate its study." It is interesting that to this date the nomenclature, anatomy, neural innervation, and functions of the levator ani and pelvic diaphragm are still veiled in deep mystery. Based on anatomic dissection studies, the pubococcygeus, puborectalis, and puboperineal muscles originate from the pubic bone and are difficult to differentiate from each other. These muscles have also been collectively called the "pubovisceralis muscle," a concept originally championed by Lawson[20] and currently supported by Delancey[21,22] in most of his writings. The term pubovisceral muscle is well accepted in the urogynecologic texts; however, it is rarely mentioned in the anatomic textbooks or gastroenterology literature. Lawson[20] believed that the portions of the pubovisceral muscle are inserted into the urethra, vagina, perineal body, and anal canal and to those portions he assigned the names pubouretheralis, pubovaginalis, puboperinealis, and puboanalis muscles, respectively. According to Lawson, the major function of these muscles is to provide physical support to the visceral organs.

Branches from the sacral nerve roots of S2, S3, and S4 innervate the pelvic floor muscles. There is considerable controversy, however, as to whether the pudendal nerves actually innervate the levator ani muscles. An electrophysiologic study by Percy and colleagues[23] found the electrical stimulation of the pudendal nerve did not activate the puborectalis muscle. It is possible, however, that in their study the electrodes may not have been precisely located in the puborectalis portion of the levator ani muscle. The authors' opinion is that the puborectalis muscle (middle layer of pelvic floor muscle) is actually innervated by the pudendal nerve[24] (from below) and the deep muscles (pubococcygeus, ileococcygeus, and coccygeus) are innervated by the direct branches of sacral nerve roots S3 and S4.[3] The significance is that pudendal nerve damage may cause dysfunction of puborectalis muscle and EAS muscles (both constrictor muscles) and this in turn may cause fecal incontinence.

PELVIC FLOOR IMAGING

Advances in MRI, CT scanning, and three-dimensional US imaging have provided novel insights into the anatomy and function of the pelvic floor muscles. Ultrafast CT scanning can image dynamic changes in the pelvic floor muscle during contraction and defecation.[25] These studies reveal that the levator hiatus becomes smaller during pelvic floor contraction and larger during the act of defecation (**Fig. 5**). The changes in the pelvic floor hiatus size are predominantly related to the puborectalis muscle and

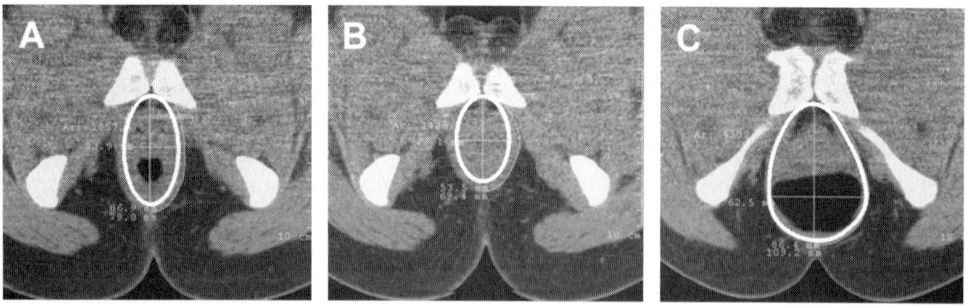

Fig. 5. Seated CT defecography. Axial images of puborectalis at rest (*A*), squeeze (*B*), and defecation (*C*). Note that the pelvic floor hiatus becomes smaller during squeeze and larger during defection. (*Adapted from* Li D, Guo M. Morphology of the levator ani muscle. Dis Colon Rectum 2007;50:1831–9; with permission.)

they reflect the constrictor function of pelvic floor. The ascent (elevation) and descent of the pelvic floor, however, including the levator plate, is mostly likely related to the contraction and relaxation of the pubococcygeus, ileococcygeus, and ischiococcygeus muscles.

MRI studies have outlined the anatomy of pelvic floor muscles much more clearly than was possible with anatomic dissection studies. Hoyle and colleagues[26] developed imaging programs to outline the details of pelvic floor muscle. Their studies reveal physiologic gaps in the ileococcygeus muscle, which one may perceive as defects in the pelvic floor muscles. Elegant studies by Bharucha and colleagues,[27–29] using dynamic MRI technique, have demonstrated changes in the anorectal angle during squeeze and during the act of defecation. Changes in the anorectal angle reflect the constrictor function of pelvic diaphragm muscle, and it is believed that these changes in the anorectal angle are caused by the contraction and relaxation of the puborectalis muscle (**Figs. 6** and **7**). It is likely, however, that craniocaudal movements of the anorectal angle are predominantly related to the pubococcygeus, ileococcygeus, and ischiococcygeus muscles. During pelvic floor contraction, the anorectal angle becomes acute and it moves cephalad. During relaxation and defecation, however, the anorectal angle becomes obtuse and moves caudad.

Two-dimensional and three-dimensional endoanal US are used widely to detect defects in the anal sphincter complex. More recently, three-dimensional US using cutaneous (transperineal) approach provided novel insights into the anatomy and function of the anal sphincter muscles and pelvic floor muscles. The major advantages of three-dimensional transperineal US are that (1) it is subject friendly (no insertion of the transducer into the anal canal is required); (2) it can be performed in the physician's office; and (3) it is relatively inexpensive. Dietz and coworkers[30–32] have used this technique quite effectively to study the physiology and pathophysiology of pelvic floor muscles under various conditions. This technique is relatively simple; it requires placement of

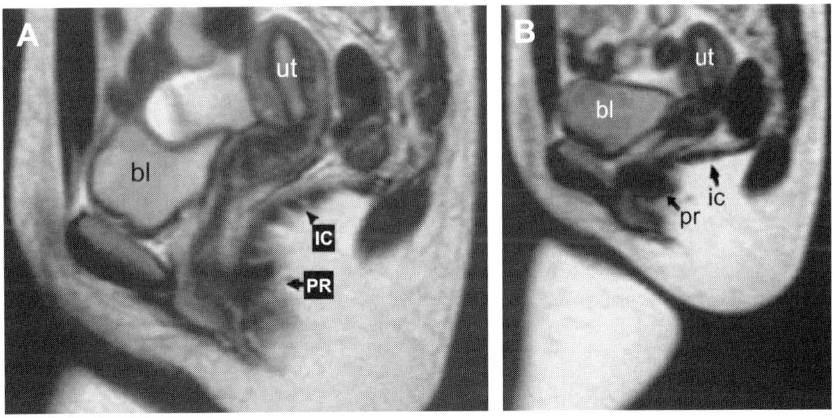

Fig. 6. MRIs at rest and squeeze in the mid sagittal plane. These images show movements of the anorectal angle and levator plate (formed by the ileococcygeus muscle). Sagittal at rest (*A*) and straining (*B*) showing the changes in the different components of the levator ani. On straining, the resting convex shape of the IC becomes flattened, and the genital hiatus reduces in size because of ventral movement of the puborectalis. bl, bladder; ut, uterus; IC, ileococcygeus; PR, puborectalis. (*Adapted from* Singh K, Jakab M, Reid WM, et al. Three-dimensional magnetic resonance imaging assessment of levator ani morphologic features in different grades of prolapse. Am J Obstet Gynecol 2003;188:910–5; with permission.)

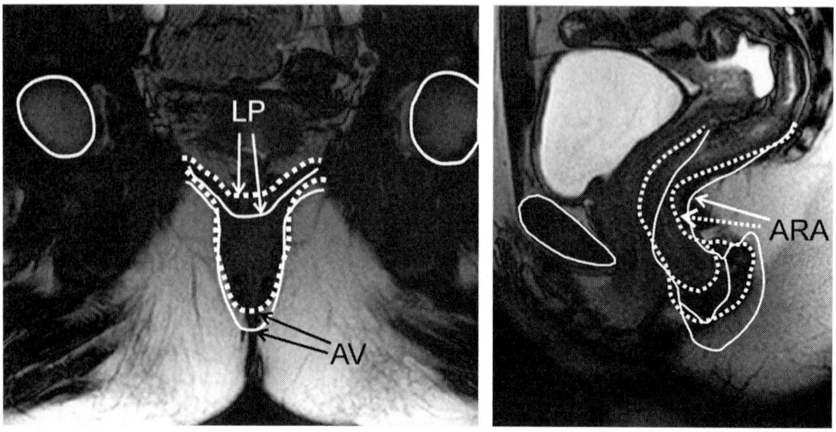

Fig. 7. Magnetic resonance images (MRI) in the mid sagittal and coronal planes; these images were obtained at rest (solid) and squeeze (dotted) and then the images were overlapped to show the movement of various anatomical structures during squeeze. Note the cranial and ventral movements of the anal canal and change in the anorectal angle with squeeze. In the coronal images, note the vertical movement of the anus, and flattening of the levator plate with squeeze. Obtained from author.

the US transducer on the skin of the perineum. A three-dimensional US volume is acquired over a period of 6 to 8 seconds and US images can be analyzed off-line in the coronal, sagittal, transverse, or any other plane. This technique also allows capturing of dynamic or cine images in two or three planes and makes it possible to study the motion of various pelvic floor structures in real time. In addition, the software program can slice these image volumes at every 1 mm or any desired distance to provide the two-dimensional tomographic images at close distances (**Fig. 8**). The authors have extended the use of three-dimensional US imaging to study the anal canal closure mechanism,[33] vaginal high-pressure zone,[34] and the role of puborectalis muscle in the genesis of anal canal and vaginal canal pressures. Defects in the anal sphincter and puborectalis muscles can be detected relatively easily using the three-dimensional US imaging technique.[35]

SENSORY FUNCTION OF THE RECTUM AND ANAL CANAL

Similar to other viscera, colonic distention results in nondescript discomfort and at higher degrees of distention one feels pain that is poorly localized. Rectal distention, however, is perceived as rectal fullness that is more localized and somewhat defined (ie, as a desire to defecate). In addition to mucosal nerve endings, there are also low threshold, slowly adapting mechanoreceptors in the muscularis propria of the rectum. These intraganglionic laminar endings detect mechanical deformation of the myenteric ganglia and are most likely involved in detecting tension in the circular and longitudinal muscles of the rectum. The anal canal responds to distention and mechanical shearing stimuli. It is lined by numerous free and organized nerve endings (ie, Meissner's corpuscles, Krause's end-bulbs, Golgi-Mazzoni bodies, and genital corpuscles). The nerve ending are exquisitely sensitive to light touch, pain, and temperature. Sensory traffic from the rectum and anal canal is conveyed to the spinal cord by unmyelinated small C fibers and larger A fibers.[11]

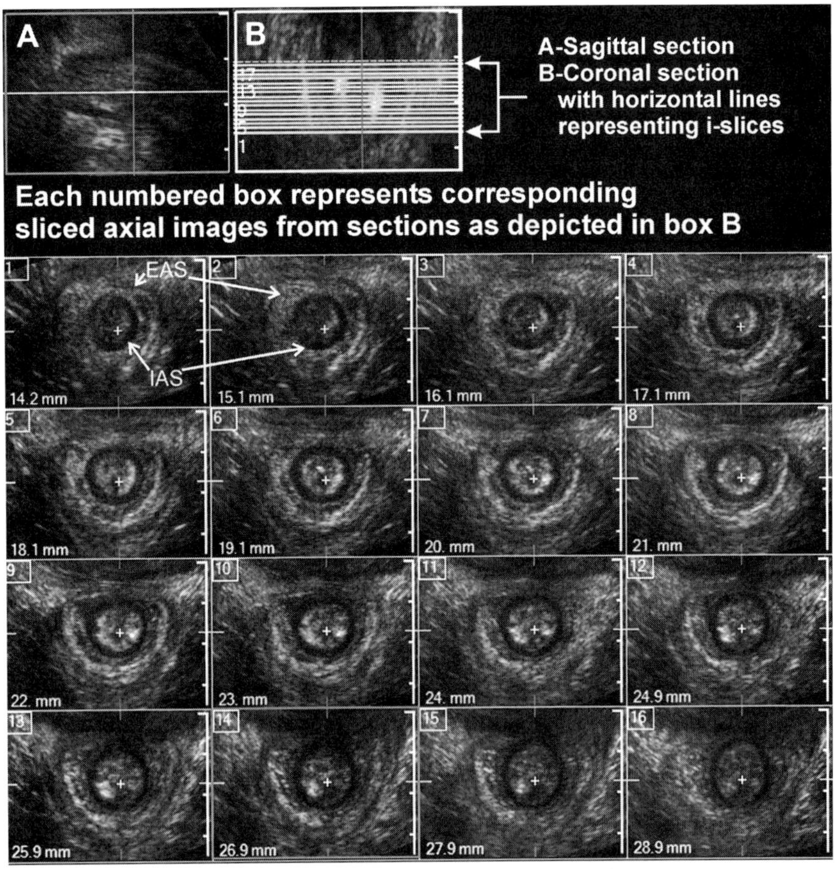

Fig. 8. Ultrasound images of the anal canal obtained from the 3D-US volume: cross-sectional (axial) images along the length of anal canal in a nulliparous subject. In this example the anal sphincter complex is shown at every 1 mm distance using I-Slice function of HD-11 (Philips). Marked in the figure are the IAS (black circle) and the EAS (white outer ring) are smooth, uniform and symmetrical. Obtained from author.

APPLIED PHYSIOLOGY

Ideally speaking, one should describe the function of each component of the pelvic floor muscle individually; however, no such information is available. Broadly, the pelvic floor muscles can be considered to have two important functions. They provide support or "floor" to the pelvic viscera; and they provide constrictor functions to the urethra, vagina, and anal canal. Described next is the role of the pelvic floor muscles on the rectum and anal canal, touching on their role in the closure function of the vagina. Furthermore, it is quite likely that the puborectalis muscle plays an important role in the urethral closure mechanism; however, more studies are needed in this area. In cadavers, the pelvic floor is shaped like a basin but in living individuals it is shaped like a dome.[36,37] Why is that the case? Muscles in general have relatively simple function; they shorten as they contract. Generally, the insertion point of the muscle moves toward the point of the origin (sphincter muscles being an exception). In the case of pubococcygeus, ileococcygeus, and ischiococcygeus, such an action results in the movement of coccyx anteriorly (ventrally) toward the pubic bone.[38] During pelvic floor contraction the coccyx moves ventrally and cranially. The change in the shape of the pelvic floor during contraction, from a basin to dome, is caused by the shortening of the pubococcygeus, ileococcygeus, and ischiococcygeus muscles. At the same time, conversion from basin to the dome lifts the pelvic viscera (including the rectum) in the cranial direction and provides mechanical support or floor to the rectum and other pelvic floor viscera. It is likely that the weakness of these muscles results in perineal descent. Decent of the pelvic visceral organs (including rectum) can be measured in radiologic studies (MRI or barium defecography) by determining the location of the anorectal angle in relationship with the pubococcygeus line.[39,40] The latter is an imaginary line connecting the lower edge of pubic symphysis and the tip of coccyx. In normal individuals, the anorectal angle is located either cranial or very close to the pubococcygeal line and it moves below the pubococcygeal line with the descending perineal syndrome or weakness of the pelvic floor muscle. There is general consensus that the IAS and EAS are the major constrictors of anal canal. The puborectalis muscle is generally believed to be important in maintenance of the anorectal angle.[27,41] Contraction of puborectalis muscle results in an acute anorectal angle and relaxation (during defecation) causes this angle to become obtuse. The anorectal angle can be measured with barium defecography[42] or MRI.[27] As described in the following paragraphs, however, recent studies show that the puborectalis muscle is actually involved in the anal canal closure mechanism (ie, in the genesis of anal canal pressure).[33,43]

ANAL CANAL PRESSURE

Anal canal pressure is a major determinant of the strength of anal continence mechanism and its brief discussion is extremely relevant. Anal canal pressure can be measured with perfusion manometry (using either side hole or sleeve sensor); solid-state transducers; or more recently with a large number of closely spaced array of pressure sensors (high-resolution manometry).[29] Furthermore, the pressures can be displayed in the form of colored topographic (contour) plots, which are convenient to visualize. Classical studies by Duthie and Watts[44] have shown that most of the resting pressure (70%–80%) in the anal canal is related to the IAS and the remainder to the EAS. With voluntary anal squeeze, the increase in the anal canal pressure is mostly caused by the EAS. Anatomic and functional studies, using simultaneous three-dimensional US imaging and side hole perfusion manometry, have provided novel insights into the genesis of anal canal pressure.[43] Based on the three-dimensional US images one can determine the precise length and the anatomic relationship of the IAS, EAS, and puborectalis muscle and then locate the anal canal pressures in relationship with these anatomic structures. These studies reveal that in the proximal part of the anal canal the closure pressures are related to the contraction of IAS and puborectalis muscle, in the middle to the contraction of the EAS, and in the distal part to the contraction of only the EAS (**Figs. 9** and **10**).

VAGINAL HIGH-PRESSURE ZONE

How does puborectalis, a U-shaped muscle, increase the anal canal pressure? The two anterior limbs of puborectalis muscle are attached to the two pubic rami and posteriorly they join each other behind the anal canal. Contraction of the puborectalis muscle lifts up the anal canal in the ventral or anterior direction and in so doing causes compression of the anal canal, vagina, and urethra against the back of pubic symphysis (**Fig. 11**). It then follows that there would be a high-pressure zone in the vagina,

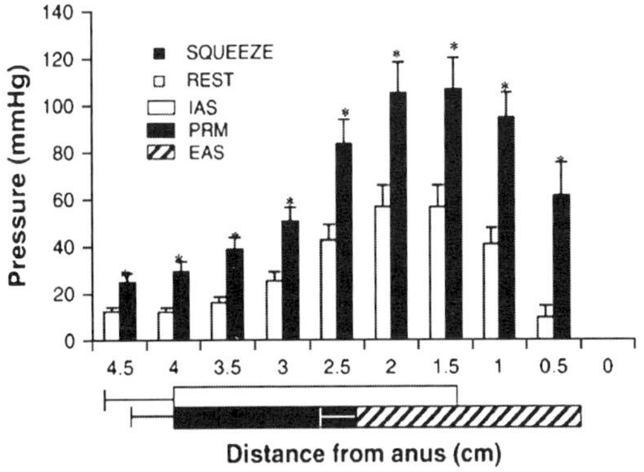

Fig. 9. Anal canal pressures along the length of the canal and its relationship with anatomical structures: Anal canal pressure was measured using the station pull through technique. Each bar represents mean+SE from the 17 subjects. Note the baseline pressure and the squeeze pressures at each station. The pressures during squeeze at all stations are significantly higher than at rest ($p < 0.005$). Also note, the location of Internal anal sphincter (IAS), puborectalis (PRM) and external anal sphincter (EAS) along the length of the anal canal. Obtained from author.

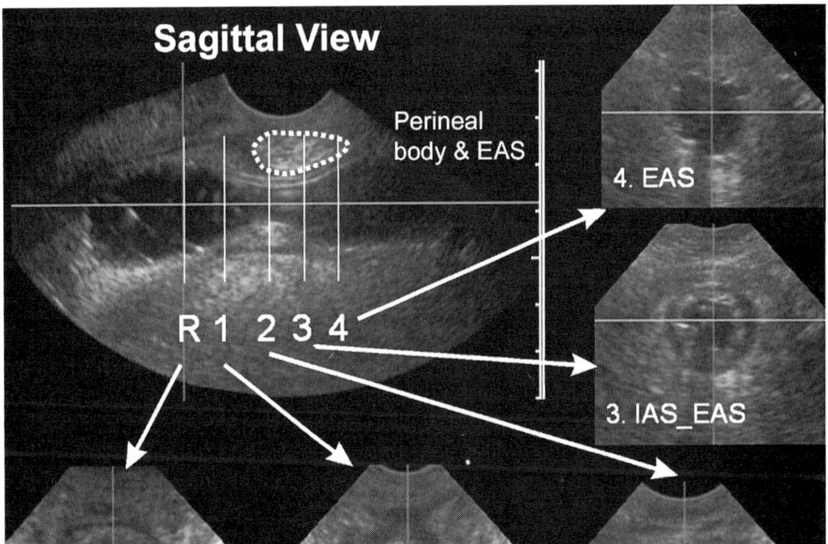

Fig. 10. Ultrasound images of the anal canal in the sagittal and axial planes with a water filled bag placed in the anal canal: the sagittal image shows the anal canal along its entire length. Axial images at various locations along the length of anal canal allow visualization of various components of the anal closure mechanism. Axial images at R=rectum, 1=Puborectalis (PRM) & Internal sphincter (IAS), 2 = PRM, IAS, and external anal sphincter (EAS), 3 = IAS & EAS, 4 = EAS only. Obtained from author.

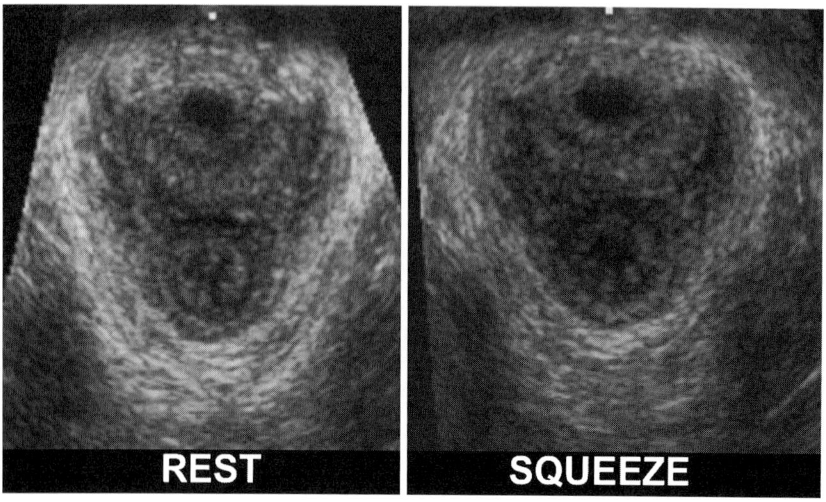

Fig. 11. Pelvic Floor Hiatus Captured from the 3D ultrasound images at rest and during a pelvic floor contraction: Note that with contraction the hiatus becomes smaller and the puborectalis muscle moves towards the pubic symphsis. The anterior motion of the puborectalis muscle compresses, anal canal, vagina and urethra against the back of pubic symphsis, which constitutes the constrictor function of pelvic diaphragm. Obtained from author.

which is indeed true.[45] Pressure characteristics of the vaginal high-pressure zone reveal that the anterior and posterior pressure in the vagina are higher than the lateral pressure, which suggests that vagina is compressed in the anteroposterior direction by the puborectalis muscle. Three-dimensional US images show that the pelvic floor hiatus becomes smaller and larger with the contraction and relaxation of the puborectalis muscle, respectively.[24,46] Pudendal nerve block increases dimensions of the pelvic floor hiatus and decreases vaginal pressure.[24] Distention of the vagina increases the anteroposterior length of the puborectalis muscle and allows it to contract stronger (based on the length tension principle). Anal canal pressure in the proximal part of the anal canal (part surrounded by the puborectalis muscle) and not the distal part (surrounded by the EAS) increases with vaginal distention.[47]

Because the vagina does not possess any intrinsic sphincter mechanism, the vaginal high-pressure zone is entirely related to the puborectalis muscle. The significance of the latter finding is that one can easily assess the puborectalis muscle function using vaginal manometry. It is likely that future studies will use this important understanding further to define the role of puborectalis muscle in fecal continence, incontinence, and other pelvic floor disorders.

Pelvic Floor Muscles and Fecal Incontinence

The etiology of fecal incontinence is multifactorial and can be broadly divided into problems related to (1) diarrhea or excessive amount of liquid stools, (2) reservoir or rectal dysfunction, and (3) anal canal closure dysfunction. It is quite clear that the three separate and distinct anatomic structures (IAS, EAS, and puborectalis muscle) guard the anal canal opening (triple security). Does this represent redundancy or is it rather that a fine orchestration of these three structures is crucial in keeping continence under different circumstances and for different rectal contents (air, liquid, and solids)? Further studies are needed to prove or disprove these points. Read and colleagues[48] in the 1980s, based on anal canal pressure studies, found that the dysfunction of EAS is the most common cause of fecal incontinence. A small subset of patients was also found to have a defective IAS.[49] Endoanal US imaging studies of Sultan and colleagues[50] found anatomic defects in the EAS muscle of 35% of women following vaginal delivery. The latter also suggests that anatomic defects of the EAS are one of the most common causes of fecal incontinence. More recent studies suggest, however, a "multihit hypothesis" in the genesis of fecal incontinence. Fernandez-Fraga and coworkers[51] used a novel instrument (perineal dynamometer) to study the pelvic floor function in patients with fecal incontinence. They found that patients have functional defect in more than one muscle of anal continence and the severity of fecal incontinence was related to the composite effect of damage to the three continence muscles. Biofeedback therapy resulted in improvement of fecal incontinence symptoms and the improvement correlated best with the improvement in levator ani function, rather than with the improvement in the IAS, EAS pressure. A study by Bharucha and colleagues[28] confirmed findings of Fernandez-Fraga and coworkers[51] and their study lends further credence to the "multihit hypothesis" of fecal incontinence.

Studies by Delancey and coworkers[52] and Dietz and Lanzarone[53] show that anatomic disruptions of the puborectalis muscle are quite common following childbirth (20%–35%). It is clear, however, that all these subjects do not have symptoms of fecal incontinence. The authors' studies in asymptomatic multiparous women confirm findings of Jung and colleagues.[33] Further studies are required to determine the relationship between anatomic disruptions as seen on the imaging studies and functional impairment of puborectalis muscle function. It is clear, however, that patients with fecal incontinence have defects in more than one muscle of continence and the symptoms are more severe in patients with defects in the multiple muscles.

Pelvic Floor Muscles and Constipation

Constipation affects 20% to 30% of the adult population in the United States[54] and its etiology, similar to that of fecal incontinence, is multifactorial. Broadly, there are two major types of constipation: slow transit type, in which the movement of fecal material through the colon is slow; and outlet obstruction type, in which the patient has trouble evacuating rectal contents. Hirschsprung's disease, characterized by failure of caudal migration of myenteric plexus, may be considered as a cause of outlet obstruction type of constipation. Hirschsprung's disease is uncommon, however, in adults. Outlet obstruction, secondary to pelvic floor dysfunction, accounts for 50% or more cases of constipation in adults.[55] Originally described by Preston and Lennard-Jones[56] in 1985 as anismus, the entity has received several names (ie, pelvic floor dyssynergia, paradoxical puborectalis muscle contraction, paradoxical sphincter contraction, and dyssynergic defecation).[55] Normally, during the act of defecation or Valsalva maneuver the respiratory diaphragm and abdominal wall contract together, which results in an increase in intra-abdominal and rectal pressure. Simultaneously, there is relaxation of the pelvic floor muscles and anal sphincter muscles during defecation. Based on the rectal and anal sphincter pressure recordings, Olsen and Rao[55] categorized dyssynergic defecation disorders into three different types: type 1, increase in the rectal pressure and anal sphincter contraction; type 2, no increase in the rectal pressure and sphincter contraction; and type 3, increase in the rectal pressure but either absent or incomplete sphincter relaxation. Dyssynergic defecation is usually acquired but in some cases the symptoms are present from childhood, which suggests that the individual never "learned the defecation process" correctly.

Paradoxical pelvic floor contraction can be recognized on the anal sphincter recording; electromyographic recordings (using anal plug electrodes or cutaneous electrodes); and imaging studies. The latter can be performed using radiograph fluoroscopy (barium defecography); CT fluoroscopy; and MRI. During the act of defecation two events occur in the pelvic floor muscles: pelvic floor descends and pelvic floor hiatus becomes larger. The descent of pelvic floor muscles is seen as a drop in the anorectal angle to below the pubococcygeal line (an imaginary line connecting the lower end of pubic symphysis and coccyx) and widening of the pelvic floor hiatus (also seen as increase in the anorectal angle). With pelvic floor contraction, the anorectal angle moves cranially and ventrally. The reverse occurs during defecation. In patients with constipation, MRI defecography studies show heterogeneity of abnormalities of the abdominal wall contraction, pelvic floor descent, and puborectalis muscle relaxation.[40] The most important finding in these studies is that the puborectalis muscle either does not relax or it does so incompletely. The latter results in either no change or in a slight decrease in the anorectal angle. The advantage of MRI defecography is that it allows clear visualization of the pelvic viscera and various other anatomic abnormalities associated with pelvic floor disorders (eg, rectocele, cystocele, rectal intussusception, and prolapse). Recent studies show that biofeedback treatment for constipation is quite effective in treating constipation related to the pelvic floor muscle dysfunction and results in amelioration of the physiologic muscle abnormalities.[54,57]

SUMMARY

Pelvic floor muscles have two important functions: they provide physical support to the pelvic viscera; and they provide constrictor mechanism to the anal canal, vagina, and urethra. Newer imaging and physiologic studies strongly suggest that these two functions of the pelvic floor are quite distinct and are likely related to different components of the pelvic floor muscles. The pubococcygeus, ileococcygeus, and ischiococcygeus most likely provide the physical support or act as a floor for the pelvic viscera. The puborectalis muscle provides the constrictor function to the anal canal, vagina, and urethra.

The urethra and anal canal each have two constrictors or sphincters of their own. In the case of anal canal these are the IAS and EAS, and in the case of urethra they are the smooth muscle sphincter (located at the bladder neck) and rhabdosphincter (external urethral sphincter). Based on physiologic studies, it seems that the puborectalis muscle is the third constrictor or the sphincter of anal canal. Future studies are likely to reveal that puborectalis muscle also serves as a constrictor for the urethra. Vagina, however, has only one constrictor mechanism, which is solely provided by the puborectalis portion or the pelvic floor muscle. The authors believe that puborectalis muscle is the common link between gastroenterologist, colorectal surgeon, urologist, and urogynecologist, the specialties of medicine caring for patients with pelvic floor disorders.

Pelvic floor disorders are many and are generally lumped together. It may be possible, however, broadly to subclassify them into disorders of pelvic floor support (prolapse, descending perineal syndrome) and constrictor function (urinary and fecal incontinence). Furthermore, these disorders may be further divided into dysfunctions of pelvic floor contraction (fecal and urinary incontinence) and relaxation (constipation and urinary retention). As a clear picture of functional anatomy of pelvic floor muscles emerges, it is imminent that different components of the pelvic floor muscles will be implicated in different pelvic floor disorders. With such a functional classification "splitter approach" it may be possible to target specific therapeutic strategies to treat specific pelvic floor muscle disorders more effectively.

REFERENCES

1. Fritsch H, Brenner E, Lienemann A, et al. Anal sphincter complex: reinterpreted morphology and its clinical relevance. Dis Colon Rectum 2002;45(2):188–94.
2. Fritsch H, Aigner F, Ludwikowski B, et al. Epithelial and muscular regionalization of the human developing anorectum. Anat Rec (Hoboken) 2007;290(11):1449–58.
3. Dyck PJ, Thomas PK. Autonomic and somatic systems to the anorectum and pelvic floor. 4th edition. Philadelphia: Elsevier Saunders; 2005.
4. Rattan S. The internal anal sphincter: regulation of smooth muscle tone and relaxation. Neurogastroenterol Motil 2005;17(Suppl 1):50–9.
5. Goyal RK, Hirano I. The enteric nervous system. N Engl J Med 1996;334:1106–15.
6. Santorini J. Septemdecim tabulae; 1715.
7. Bogduk N. Issues in anatomy: the external anal sphincter revisited. Aust N Z J Surg 1996;66:626–9.
8. Ayoub SF. Anatomy of the external anal sphincter in man. Acta Anat (Basel) 1979; 105:25–36.
9. Shafik A. A new concept of the anatomy of the anal sphincter mechanism and the physiology of defecation. The external anal sphincter: a triple-loop system. Invest Urol 1975;12:412–9.
10. Peschers UM, DeLancey JO, Fritsch H, et al. Cross-sectional imaging anatomy of the anal sphincters. Obstet Gynecol 1997;90(5):839–44.
11. Bharucha AE. Pelvic floor: anatomy and function. Neurogastroenterol Motil 2006; 18(7):507–19.
12. Stoker J, Halligan S, Bartram CI. Pelvic floor imaging. Radiology 2001;218:621–41.
13. Taylor BM, Beart RW Jr, Phillips SF. Longitudinal and radial variations of pressure in the human anal sphincter. Gastroenterology 1984;86:693–7.
14. Vesalius A. De humnai corporis fabrica libri septum. 2nd edition; 1555.
15. Von Behr A. Handbook of human anatomy. Philadelphia: Lindsay & Blakiston; 1847.
16. Meyer G. Lehrbuch der Anatomie des Menschem; 1861.
17. Holl M. Handbuch des anatomie. Jena (Germany): Fischer; 1897 [in German].
18. Thompson P. The myology of the pelvic floor. Newton (MA): McCorquoddale; 1899.
19. Sappey P. Traite d, Anatomie Descriptive. 2nd edition; 1739.
20. Lawson JO. Pelvic anatomy. I. Pelvic floor muscles. Ann R Coll Surg Engl 1974; 54:244–52.
21. DeLancey JO, Delmas V. Groos anatomy and functional anatomy of the pelvic floor. Philadelphia: Elsevier Saunders; 2004.
22. Kearney R, Sawhney R, DeLancey JO. Levator ani muscle anatomy evaluated by origin-insertion pairs. Obstet Gynecol 2004;104:168–73.
23. Percy JP, Neill ME, Swash M, et al. Electrophysiological study of motor nerve supply of pelvic floor. Lancet 1981;1:16–7.
24. Guaderrama NM, Liu J, Nager CW, et al. Evidence for the innervation of pelvic floor muscles by the pudendal nerve. Obstet Gynecol 2005;106:774–81.
25. Li D, Guo M. Morphology of the levator ani muscle. Dis Colon Rectum 2007;50:1831–9.
26. Hoyte L, Jakab M, Warfield SK, et al. Levator ani thickness variations in symptomatic and asymptomatic women using magnetic resonance-based 3-dimensional color mapping. Am J Obstet Gynecol 2004;191:856–61.
27. Fletcher JG, Busse RF, Riederer SJ, et al. Magnetic resonance imaging of anatomic and dynamic defects of the pelvic floor in defecatory disorders. Am J Gastroenterol 2003;98:399–411.

28. Bharucha AE, Fletcher JG, Harper CM, et al. Relationship between symptoms and disordered continence mechanisms in women with idiopathic faecal incontinence. Gut 2005;54:546–55.
29. Bharucha AE, Fletcher JG. Recent advances in assessing anorectal structure and functions. Gastroenterology 2007;133:1069–74.
30. Dietz HP. Ultrasound imaging of the pelvic floor. Part II: three-dimensional or volume imaging. Ultrasound Obstet Gynecol 2004;23:615–25.
31. Dietz HP. Ultrasound imaging of the pelvic floor. Part I: two-dimensional aspects. Ultrasound Obstet Gynecol 2004;23:80–92.
32. Dietz HP, Shek C, Clarke B. Biometry of the pubovisceral muscle and levator hiatus by three-dimensional pelvic floor ultrasound. Ultrasound Obstet Gynecol 2005;25:580–5.
33. Jung SA, Pretorius DH, Weinstein M, et al. Closure mechanism of the anal canal in women: assessed by three-dimensional ultrasound imaging. Dis Colon Rectum 2008;51:932–9.
34. Jung SA, Pretorius DH, Padda BS, et al. Vaginal high-pressure zone assessed by dynamic 3-dimensional ultrasound images of the pelvic floor. Am J Obstet Gynecol 2007;197:52 e51–7.
35. Weinstein MM, Pretorius DH, Jung S-A, et-al. Transcutaneous 3-dimensional ultrasound imaging: a novel technique to detect anatomical defects in the muscles of anal sphincter complex. Clinical Gastroenterology and Hepatology, in press.
36. Guo M, Li D. Pelvic floor images: anatomy of the levator ani muscle. Dis Colon Rectum 2007;50:1647–55.
37. Hjartardottir S, Nilsson J, Petersen C, et al. The female pelvic floor: a dome–not a basin. Acta Obstet Gynecol Scand 1997;76:567–71.
38. Bo K, Lilleas F, Talseth T, et al. Dynamic MRI of the pelvic floor muscles in an upright sitting position. Neurourol Urodyn 2001;20:167–74.
39. Singh K, Jakab M, Reid WM, et al. Three-dimensional magnetic resonance imaging assessment of levator ani morphologic features in different grades of prolapse. Am J Obstet Gynecol 2003;188:910–5.
40. Bharucha AE, Fletcher JG, Seide B, et al. Phenotypic variation in functional disorders of defecation. Gastroenterology 2005;128:1199–210.
41. Locke III GR, Pemberton JH, Phillips SF. AGA technical review on constipation. American Gastroenterological Association. Gastroenterology 2000;119:1766–78.
42. Shorvon PJ, McHugh S, Diamant NE, et al. Defecography in normal volunteers: results and implications. Gut 1989;30:1737–49.
43. Liu J, Guaderrama N, Nager CW, et al. Functional correlates of anal canal anatomy: puborectalis muscle and anal canal pressure. Am J Gastroenterol 2006;101:1092–7.
44. Duthie HL, Watts JM. Contribution of the external anal sphincter to the pressure zone in the anal canal. Gut 1965;6:64–8.
45. Guaderrama NM, Nager CW, Liu J, et al. The vaginal pressure profile. Neurourol Urodyn 2005;24:243–7.
46. Weinstein MM, Jung SA, Pretorius DH, et al. The reliability of puborectalis muscle measurements with 3-dimensional ultrasound imaging. Am J Obstet Gynecol 2007;197:68 e61–6.
47. Padda BS, Jung SA, Pretorius D, et al. Effects of pelvic floor muscle contraction on anal canal pressure. Am J Physiol Gastrointest Liver Physiol 2007;292:G565–71.

48. Read NW, Haynes WG, Bartolo DC, et al. Use of anorectal manometry during rectal infusion of saline to investigate sphincter function in incontinent patients. Gastroenterology 1983;85:105–13.
49. Sun WM, Read NW, Donnelly TC. Impaired internal anal sphincter in a subgroup of patients with idiopathic fecal incontinence. Gastroenterology 1989;97:130–5.
50. Sultan AH, Kamm MA, Hudson CN, et al. Anal-sphincter disruption during vaginal delivery. 23. N Engl J Med 1993;329:1905–11.
51. Fernandez-Fraga X, Azpiroz F, Malagelada JR. Significance of pelvic floor muscles in anal incontinence. Gastroenterology 2002;123:1441–50.
52. DeLancey JO, Kearney R, Chou Q, et al. The appearance of levator ani muscle abnormalities in magnetic resonance images after vaginal delivery. Obstet Gynecol 2003;101:46–53.
53. Dietz HP, Lanzarone V. Levator trauma after vaginal delivery. Obstet Gynecol 2005;106:707–12.
54. Chiarioni G, Whitehead WE, Pezza V, et al. Biofeedback is superior to laxatives for normal transit constipation due to pelvic floor dyssynergia. Gastroenterology 2006;130:657–64.
55. Olsen AL, Rao SS. Clinical neurophysiology and electrodiagnostic testing of the pelvic floor. Gastroenterol Clin North Am 2001;30:33–54, v-vi.
56. Preston DM, Lennard-Jones JE. Anismus in chronic constipation. Dig Dis Sci 1985;30:413–8.
57. Chiarioni G, Salandini L, Whitehead WE. Biofeedback benefits only patients with outlet dysfunction, not patients with isolated slow transit constipation. Gastroenterology 2005;129:86–97.

Manometric, Sensorimotor, and Neurophysiologic Evaluation of Anorectal Function

S. Mark Scott, PhD*, Marc A. Gladman, MBBS, PhD, MRCOG, FRCS (Gen Surg)

KEYWORDS

• Anorectal • Manometry • Sensorimotor • Neurophysiologic
• Pathophysiology

The two major functions of the anorectum are preservation of continence and regulation of defecation. Multiple factors are involved in the control of these processes, involving both physiologic and psychobehavioral mechanisms. Investigation of the anorectum should be performed in the context of a global pelvic floor evaluation, aimed at both morphology and anatomy, and function. With advances in diagnostic technology, it is now accepted that in the field of functional bowel disorders, symptom-based assessment, although important, is unsatisfactory as the sole means of directing therapy. The symptom repertoire of the gut is limited and relatively nonspecific, such that similar symptom profiles may reside in differing pathoetiologies and pathophysiologies.[1] In a field of practice in which normal physiologic function is so complex, reliance on clinical symptoms alone as a basis for taxonomy is now obsolete. A robust taxonomy based on underlying pathophysiology must be paramount.[1]

A wide number of complementary investigations currently exist for the assessment of anorectal structure and function (**Table 1**). Ideally, a comprehensive assessment of all understood and measurable components that contribute toward continence or defecation should be performed, although in clinical practice only a limited number of factors are routinely assessed. Nevertheless, the diagnostic yield undoubtedly improves the broader the series of tests performed,[2] and all patients should undergo as thorough an assessment as is available, performed in a structured and systematic manner. This article focuses on contemporary tests of motor and sensory function of

GI Physiology Unit and Neurogastroenterology Group (Centre for Academic Surgery), Institute of Cell and Molecular Science, Barts and The London School of Medicine and Dentistry, The Royal London Hospital, 3rd Floor Alexandra Wing, Whitechapel, London E1 1BB, UK
* Corresponding author.
E-mail address: m.scott@qmul.ac.uk (S.M. Scott).

Gastroenterol Clin N Am 37 (2008) 511–538
doi:10.1016/j.gtc.2008.06.010
gastro.theclinics.com

Table 1
Diagnostic tests available

Investigation	Modality Assessed	Clinical Use
Anorectal manometry	(1) Anal sphincter function	Established, limited value
Traditional	(2) Rectoanal reflexes	Established, limited value
	(3) Rectal sensation (balloon)	Established
	(4) Rectal compliance	Established, limited value
	(5) Defecatory maneuvers	Established
	(6) Saline continence test	Obsolete
High resolution	See (1, 2, and 5 above)	Research
Vector volume	Anal sphincter function, pressure profile	Obsolete
Prolonged ambulatory	Anorectal/rectosigmoid motility	Research
Perineometer	Pelvic floor descent	Obsolete
Perineal dynamometer	Puborectalis function	Research
Barostat studies	(1) Rectal sensation	Established
	(2) Rectal compliance	Established
	(3) Rectal tone, tension	Research
	(4) Rectal capacity	Research
	(5) Rectal motility	Research
Impedance planimetry	Rectal biomechanical properties	Research
Endoanal ultrasound	Two-dimensional imaging of the anal sphincters	Established
	Three-dimensional imaging of the anal sphincters	Research
Endoanal MRI	Imaging of the anal sphincters	Research
Neurophysiologic		
Nerve conduction	Pudendal nerve terminal motor latency	Established, limited value
Electromyography	(1) Motor unit action potentials	Established, limited value
	(2) Fiber density	Established, limited value
	(3) Jitter	Research
Evoked potentials	(1) Motor	Research
	(2) Somatosensory	Research
Other	Anocutaneous reflex	Established, limited value
	Strength-duration test	Research
Anorectal sensation		
Electrostimulation	(1) Mucosal electrosensitivity	Established, limited value
Thermal stimulation	(2) Mucosal thermosensitivity	Research
Rectal evacuation		
Balloon expulsion test	Rectal evacuatory function	Established
Evacuation proctography	Rectal evacuatory function	Established
Scintigraphic proctography	Rectal evacuatory function	Obsolete
Dynamic MRI proctography	Rectal evacuatory function, pelvic organ movement	Research
Colonic transit studies		
Radiopaque markers	Global colonic transit	Established
Scintigraphy	Segmental colonic transit	Established, limited value

the anorectum, and neurophysiologic assessment of the pelvic floor, with an aim to highlight their presently accepted clinical use.

MANOMETRIC EVALUATION

Anorectal Manometry

This is the most established and widely available investigative tool, and provides a means of evaluating various parameters of both anal and rectal function, and rectoanal coordinated activity. It is best performed in a laboratory with the necessary technical and interpretative expertise.[3] A manometric evaluation commonly encompasses a series of measurements designed to test for (1) deficits in anal sphincter function; (2) presence or absence of rectoanal reflexes; and (3) rectal sensory function and compliance (see the section on sensorimotor evaluation). In addition, a manometric assessment may also include components designed to assess defecatory function, namely rectoanal pressure relationships during bearing down and straining maneuvers, and expulsion of a rectal balloon.

The selection (and order) of measurements to be performed depends on a number of issues, including the presenting symptoms and reason for referral.[4] The principal indications are fecal incontinence and constipation, and certain components of a manometric investigation may be considered more useful in the former (eg, evaluation of sphincter function), whereas others may be more valuable in the latter (eg, defecatory maneuvers); however, these disorders frequently coexist[5] and there is an increasing body of literature supporting the concept that fecal (often overflow) incontinence is frequently secondary to incomplete rectal evacuation or fecal impaction caused by disordered defecation.[6,7] Consequently, a comprehensive manometric assessment incorporating all components should often be performed. Anorectal manometry may also be useful to (1) facilitate biofeedback training; (2) assess patients before surgery (eg, as a prognostic indicator of continence prior to pouch construction); (3) allow an objective assessment of therapeutic efficacy; and (4) assess patients with functional anorectal pain, particularly if this is suspected to be secondary to pelvic floor dysfunction.[4,8]

Equipment

This consists of four major components: (1) a thin, flexible intraluminal pressure-sensing catheter; (2) pressure transducers; (3) a balloon for inflation within the rectum (either integral to the catheter assembly or fixed to an independent catheter); and (4) the amplification-recording-display system. Currently, a six-sensor catheter (be it either water-perfused or solid-state) of less than 5 mm diameter, configured to enable recordings from both the longitudinal and radial axis is recommended.[4] A balloon (preferably nonlatex) of not less than 4 cm should ideally be tied to the end. One pressure sensor, and a lumen opening to allow for inflation, should be located inside the balloon. The remaining five sensors should be arranged radially and spaced 1 cm apart.[4] Various computerized amplification and recording systems are commercially available, complete with dedicated online display, review, and analysis software. All allow large-volume data storage, with database functionality. Small, portable recorders are also available, which enable ambulatory measurements. Calibration of the manometric system is essential to yield accurate, reliable, and clinically helpful manometric data. This should be done in accordance with the manufacturer's recommended guidelines.

Limitations

Recorded pressures depend on the technique used to measure them, and are influenced by a number of factors, including the pressure sensor itself; the recording technique; catheter diameter; orientation of the recording ports and sensors; perfusion rate (for perfused-tube catheters); patient posture; and patient compliance. All of these factors must be borne in mind when both performing and interpreting these tests.

Unfortunately, the biggest pitfall with anorectal manometry is the lack of uniformity regarding equipment and technique,[9] consequently, large[10] and robust normative reference data sets, obtained in age- and gender-matched subjects, are generally lacking from the literature. Although several working party or position papers have been published,[4,11–14] they fail to reach consensus opinion as to the optimal method for performing a manometric assessment. As a consequence, comparison of results between centers is problematic. Each individual institution is encouraged to develop its own control values (preferably gender and age stratified) or, if using normative data from the literature, adopt similar methodology, such that a particular result may be compared with the appropriate normal range.[4,11,14]

Patient preparation

Because of the minimal risks associated with manometry, written consent is considered optional.[14] The patient should be fully informed about the details of the procedure, however, which enhances subject cooperation and comfort. Bowel preparation is also optional, and should only be required if fecal loading is detected on digital rectal examination; either a 500-mL tap water enema or phosphate enema have been advocated.[4] Tests should be performed with the patient in the left-lateral position with knees and hips flexed.[4]

Anal Sphincter Function

Technique

The objectives of assessment are to (1) identify the functional anal canal length; (2) record maximum resting anal canal tone, which predominantly reflects internal anal sphincter (IAS) function; and (3) record voluntary anal squeeze pressures, which reflects external anal sphincter (EAS) function.

Two methods can be used: station or manual pull-through[15] of the catheter, or stationary.[16] The former is recommended,[14,17] and the most commonly used technique. The manometry catheter is advanced into the rectum, and then withdrawn manually by 0.5- or 1-cm increments, or "stations." For each station, the pressure should be allowed to stabilize. When the recording sensors pass into the high-pressure zone, there is an increase in pressure. The maximal resting anal pressures at each station should be recorded, as should the longitudinal position of the peak resting pressure. For evaluation of anal squeeze pressures, the procedure should be repeated; once the pressure has stabilized at each station, the patient is instructed to squeeze their anus as hard as possible. It is important to limit gluteal muscle involvement. The squeeze should be sustained for 30 seconds, which gives a measure of fatigability of the EAS.[4] The maximal pressure obtained at each station during the squeeze maneuver and longitudinal position of the peak squeeze pressure are recorded.

Others advocate the use of a stationary technique,[4,13,16] which is more time-efficient. Basal anal pressures are measured along the anal canal by averaging recordings at each longitudinal recording site over a 1-minute segment at rest. Squeeze pressures are evaluated by asking the patient to squeeze their anal canal two or three times, as above.[4]

Measurements and clinical use

Functional anal canal length This is defined as the length of the anal canal over which resting pressure exceeds that of the rectum by greater than 5 mm Hg,[16,18] or alternatively, as the length of the anal canal over which pressures are greater than half of the maximal pressure at rest.[19] The length of the functional anal canal is usually shorter in incontinent patients than normal control subjects,[20] although the clinical significance of this measure has recently been questioned.[14]

Anal resting pressures Maximal resting anal pressure is defined as the difference between intrarectal pressure and the highest recorded anal sphincter pressure at rest,[4,18] and is generally recorded 1 to 2 cm cephalad to the anal verge, which corresponds to the condensation of smooth muscle fibers of the IAS; pressure at the level of the anal margin can alternatively be used as the zero baseline (**Fig. 1**).[16] Anal resting tone is subject to pressure oscillations caused by slow waves, of amplitude 5 to 25 mm Hg, occurring at a frequency of 6 to 20 min^{-1},[15,21] or high-amplitude ultraslow waves, 30 to 100 mm Hg in magnitude, occurring at 0.5 to 2 min^{-1} (although the latter are rarely observed in patients with low resting pressures).[22]

The primary component contributing to anal resting tone is IAS activity (55%–80%, of which most is nerve-induced, and the remainder is purely myogenic).[23] Symptoms of passive fecal incontinence correlate with low resting anal tone[24] and often a reversal of the anal pressure gradient;[25] this implies IAS weakness, typically caused by rupture of the smooth muscle ring, or secondary to IAS degeneration.[26] Patients with very low basal pressures may be fully continent, and conversely those with normal resting tone may be incontinent.[27] Consequently, measurement of resting tone, although of pathophysiologic significance in patients with incontinence, must be considered in combination with other functional findings.[14,27] Indeed, one large study showed that maximal anal resting tone had a sensitivity of only 32% for discriminating continent from incontinent patients;[28] this emphasizes the multifactorial nature of incontinence.[29,30]

Anal squeeze pressures The measure of a patient's ability to squeeze their striated anal musculature can be calculated as the maximal voluntary anal squeeze pressure (the difference between intrarectal pressure, or the pressure at the level of the anal margin, and the highest recorded pressure during anal squeeze),[4] or the maximal voluntary

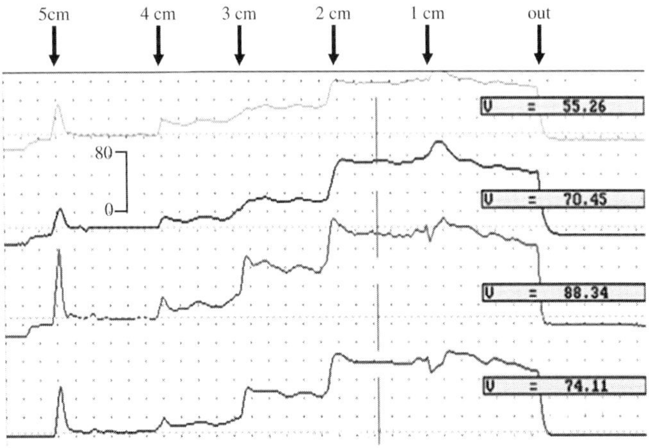

Fig. 1. Station-pull through manometry of the anal sphincter at rest. A perfused-tube catheter with four radially arranged channels (at 90 degrees) is pulled through the anal sphincter at 1-cm increments (*arrows*), using rectal pressure as baseline (*dashed lines*). Note radial pressure asymmetry (maximum resting pressure of 55 mm Hg in channel 1, and 88 mm Hg in channel 3).

anal squeeze increment (the difference between resting pressure at any given level of the anal canal, and the highest recorded pressure during anal squeeze);[4,16] the latter is probably a better determinant of anal squeeze function. The duration of the sustained squeeze can be defined as the time interval at which the subject can maintain squeeze pressure at greater than or equal to 50% of the maximum squeeze pressure.[4]

The squeeze increment is essentially contributed by the EAS, and also by contraction of the puborectalis sling. Low or poorly sustained squeeze pressures implies EAS weakness. Standard manometry cannot differentiate, however, between compromised muscle integrity or impaired innervation, or both (or indeed a poorly compliant patient[14]) as a cause of that weakness.

Symptoms of urge or stress fecal incontinence often correlate with low anal squeeze pressures,[24] with the major causative factor being obstetric injury.[29,31] In addition, squeeze duration is reduced[32] and fatigue rate is significantly shortened[33] in incontinent patients compared with controls. Of all standard measures of anorectal function, anal squeeze pressure has been shown to have the greatest sensitivity and specificity for discriminating patients with fecal incontinence from continent patients and controls;[27,28] nevertheless, the correlation between anal canal pressures and incontinence is not perfect,[34] given the wide range of normal values[16] and the contribution of those various other factors crucial to anorectal continence.[29]

An exciting recent technologic development is the advent of so-called "high-resolution manometry," which uses multiple closely spaced sensors simultaneously to measure circumferential pressures.[35] By interpolating between adjacent sensors, intraluminal pressure becomes a spatial continuum; recorded data are displayed as pressure topography plots, rather than overlapping line traces, with pressure magnitude indicated by color intensity.[36] As is happening in the field of esophageal function testing, it is feasible that high-resolution manometry may challenge conventional anorectal manometry, which has been in clinical use for 30 years, as the principal tool for the evaluation of anal sphincter function. Vector manometry, which was designed to assess the circumferential symmetry of anal canal pressures and permit the identification of localized pressure defects, has been superseded by endoanal ultrasound.[3]

Rectoanal Reflex Activity

Rapid distention of the rectum, mimicking the sudden arrival of a fecal bolus, induces a sequence of events:[21] (1) a transient increase in rectal pressure, probably caused by secondary rectal contractions, followed by; (2) a transient increase in anal pressure, associated with EAS contraction (the rectoanal contractile reflex), followed in turn by; (3) a more prolonged reduction in anal pressure, associated with relaxation of the IAS (the rectoanal inhibitory reflex). The rectoanal inhibitory reflex is thought to allow rectal contents to be sampled by the sensory area of the anal canal, allowing discrimination between flatus and fecal matter (ie, fine-tuning of the continence mechanism). By contrast, the rectoanal contractile reflex is a compensatory guarding mechanism that allows a positive anal-to-rectal pressure gradient to be maintained during transient increases in intra-abdominal or intrarectal pressure (eg, coughing), which is essential for preservation of continence.[19]

Technique

The rectoanal inhibitory reflex can be simply measured by concomitantly recording resting anal pressures during inflation of the rectal balloon with air,[14] using a rapid intermittent distention technique (incrementally in 10-mL or 50-mL aliquots). The threshold volume needed to elicit the reflex and the duration of the response at each distention volume should be recorded. The rectoanal contractile reflex can be measured simultaneously during the same procedure. Alternatively, this can be evaluated by instructing the patient to blow up a party balloon, blow against a fixed pressure level into a manometer, or cough strongly (the cough reflex).[14,16,28] The aim is to determine whether a positive anal-to-rectal pressure differential is maintained. This test is also useful for further evaluation of EAS function, especially in those patients with apparently attenuated voluntary anal squeeze pressures in whom poor compliance is suspected.[14]

Measurements and clinical use

The rectoanal inhibitory reflex is an intramural reflex mediated by the myenteric plexus, and modulated by the spinal cord.[21] The amplitude and duration of relaxation are correlated with the distending volume. Classically, the rectoanal inhibitory reflex is absent in patients with Hirschsprung's disease,[37] although the clinical use of this observation is negligible in an adult gastroenterologic practice, because undiagnosed Hirschsprung's disease in this population is exceptionally rare.[14] Differences in reflex parameters have been shown between incontinent patients and healthy subjects,[38] but the clinical significance of these findings is unclear.

The rectoanal contractile reflex is a polysynaptic sacral reflex,[39] which results in a contraction of the EAS. Under normal circumstances, intra-anal pressure should exceed intrarectal pressure, and the duration of the reflex anal contraction should be longer than the intra-abdominal pressure peak.[14] An abnormal reflex response, along with attenuated voluntary squeeze pressures, indicates neural damage of the sacral arc, either of the spinal sacral segments or the pudendal nerves;[14] such patients usually suffer from urge incontinence, and may have a lesion of the cauda equina or sacral plexus, a pudendal neuropathy, or more generalized peripheral neuropathy (eg, diabetes). The reflex is preserved in patients with a supraconal spinal cord lesion,[8] but in such individuals, voluntary squeeze pressures are impaired or absent.[28] There are no data on the specificity of this reflex. In clinical practice, it may be most useful to check a patient's compliance with instructions to squeeze, but in those without overt neurologic signs or evidence of spinal damage, an abnormal reflex may be interpreted as a subclinical neuropathy.[14]

Rectoanal Pressure Relationships During Defecatory Maneuvers

In patients with symptoms of disordered rectal evacuation, which are suspected to be caused by pelvic floor dysfunction, simple manometric assessment of rectoanal coordination during defecatory maneuvers, such as bearing down or straining, can be performed. Normally, these result in an increase in intrarectal pressure caused by the Valsalva maneuver, associated with a decrease in intra-anal pressure, caused by coordinated relaxation of the EAS. This process is under voluntary control, and is most likely a learned response. The cough reflex is likely inhibited concomitantly by descending inhibitory pathways.[14] These mechanisms facilitate the process of defecation. An inability to perform this coordinated movement has been proposed to represent the principal pathophysiologic mechanism in patients with a functional defecation disorder, variably termed "dyssynergic defecation," "anismus," "outlet dysfunction," "functional outlet obstruction," or "pelvic floor dyssynergia".[40–44]

Technique

Intra-anal and intrarectal pressures (from within the rectal balloon, which may or may not be distended[14]) should be recorded simultaneously while the patient is asked to strain as if to defecate. There is no agreed method for this technique.[14] It is important to limit movement of the pressure-sensing device within the anal canal.

Measurements and clinical use

Straining should induce a relaxation of the anal canal in asymptomatic subjects (**Fig. 2**A). Three dyssynergic patterns of defecation, however, may be evidenced (see **Fig. 2**B):[3,45] (1) type 1, a paradoxic increase in intra-anal pressure in the presence of adequate expulsive forces (increase in intrarectal pressure); (2) type 2, an inability to generate adequate expulsive forces (no increase in intrarectal pressure), together with a paradoxic increase in intra-anal pressure; and (3) type 3, generation of adequate expulsive forces (increase in intrarectal pressure), but absent or incomplete (<20%) reduction in intra-anal pressure.[41] These findings alone, however, are not diagnostic for a functional defecation disorder, which requires further supportive clinical evidence.[44] Nevertheless, the test may be useful in identifying patients who are amenable to biofeedback therapy.[46]

In constipated patients, a positive yield for dyssynergia using anorectal manometry has been shown to vary between 20% and 75%.[46] The test has been criticized, however, on a number of fronts: notably, manometry is conducted in the horizontal position, and expulsion efforts do not mimic normal defecation; patient cooperation is the key component, and some patients' embarrassment at the nature of this test may inhibit normal evacuation.[42] Taken together, these factors likely lead to an overdiagnosis of dyssynergia.

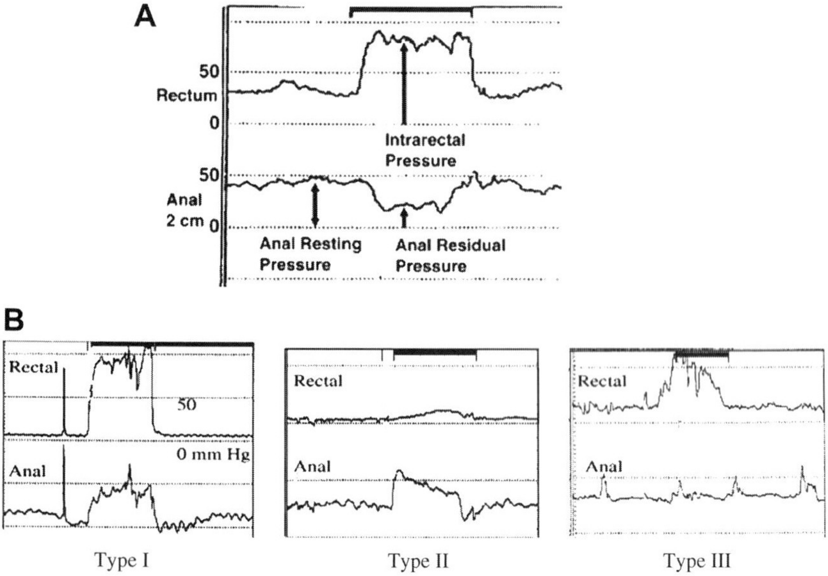

Fig. 2. Relationship between rectal and anal pressures during defecatory maneuvers in a normal subject (*A*), and three patients with different types of dyssynergia (*B*). (*Adapted from* Rao SS, Azpiroz F, Diamant N, et al. Minimum standards of anorectal manometry. Neurogastroenterol Motil 2002;14:553–9; and Rao SS, Mudipalli RS, Stessman M, et al. Investigation of the utility of colorectal function tests and Rome II criteria in dyssynergic defecation (anismus). Neurogastroenterol Motil 2004;16:589–96; with permission.)

hemorrhoids,[59,61] and mucosal prolapse.[61] Assessment of anal canal sensation, however, is not of established clinical value.[11]

Anal motor function

This is covered in the previous section on anal sphincter function and the later section on pudendal nerve terminal motor latencies (PNTML) and electromyography (EMG).

Evaluation of Rectal Sensorimotor Function

Evaluation of rectal sensitivity involves the presentation of a stimulus and the measurement of the perceived response to the stimulus. The available techniques are shown in **Table 3**. For the assessment of rectal (efferent) motor function (**Table 4**), manometry and balloon expulsion are discussed previously; consequently, this section concentrates on the evaluation of rectal biomechanic properties.

Equipment

Latex balloon distention For simplicity and economy, rectal sensorimotor function can be assessed using a latex balloon secured to a catheter that is distended (manually or pump-assisted) with air or water,[11,65]. Incorporating water-perfused catheters or microtransducers within the rectal balloon allows the simultaneous acquisition of intra-balloon (rectal) pressures and distending volumes, and thus calculation of rectal compliance (see later).

Barostat assembly The barostat is a computer-driven device that consists of a pressure transducer coupled through an electronic relay servomechanism and an electric motor to a pneumatic pump. The assembly required to study rectal sensorimotor function consists of an oversized polyethylene bag (infinitely compliant within the range of distention) connected to the barostat by means of a closed-tip double-lumen polyvinyl tube rectal catheter. One lumen is used for inflation, whereas the other is connected to the pressure transducer port of the barostat and is used to monitor pressure directly within the barostat bag. The use of this equipment has certain advantages over the use of latex balloon that is manually distended: (1) the bag is secured at both ends to the catheter, which ensures distention in the circumferential axis by eliminating axial migration into the sigmoid colon; (2) simultaneous acquisition of volume and pressure

Table 3
Techniques used in the measurement of rectal sensory function

Stimulation	Response
Mechanical Distention	**Subjective Assessment of Conscious Perception**
Latex balloon with hand-held syringe	Quantification of sensory thresholds
Polyethylene bag attached to a barostat	Verbal descriptive (Likert) scales
	Visual analog scales
Direct stimulation of rectal mucosa	**Quantification of reflex response**
Electrical	RIII reflex
Thermal	
Multimodal	**Objective central representation**
Mechanical, thermal, electrical, impedance planimetry	Cortical evoked potentials
	Functional MRI

Abbreviation: MRI, magnetic resonance imaging.

Table 4
Techniques used in the measurement of rectal motor function

Method	Measurement	Rationale
Static / ambulatory manometry	Intraluminal pressure changes	Reflects rectal contractile activity
Barostat / impedance planimetry	Rectal biomechanical properties (tone, compliance, strain, stress, and so forth)	Reflects, in part, neurogenic function of rectal smooth muscle
Evacuation proctography, balloon expulsion	Rectal evacuatory function	Summated end-product of motor function

data is possible, and it is not subject to the same limitations as volume-based (simple balloon) distention techniques;[66] and (3) the distention is computerized, which allows distention parameters known to affect visceral sensitivity (see later), such as rate and pattern of inflation, to be tightly controlled and standardized using the barostat computer software. In addition, the influence of response bias may be minimized.

Patient preparation To enable accurate evaluation, all variables that may influence measurements should be kept constant between studies. Certain guidelines have been detailed in the report of an international working group.[66] Whether subjects should receive bowel preparation remains a contentious issue; cleansing the studied segment of gut is preferable, but the use of bowel preparation may influence the sensorimotor properties of that segment. The subject should be positioned prone.[66]

Rectal Sensation

The importance of rectal sensory dysfunction is increasingly recognized in the development of functional bowel disorders.[7,52,67] Although the rectum is sensitive to electrical[68] and thermal stimulation,[69] mechanical distention is the most reliable and physiologic stimulus for the assessment of sensation.[70]

Technique

Simple balloon distention Rectal sensation is most effectively and conveniently quantified in everyday clinical practice by manually distending a latex balloon with air, using a hand-held syringe.[11] Two techniques are used for inflation: ramp (continual) or intermittent, which can be either phasic (volumes injected and then withdrawn)[71] or stepwise (volumes maintained between inflations).[72] Sensory responses are altered by (1) the type of inflation; (2) the distending medium (air or water); (3) speed of inflation;[71] (4) the distance of the balloon from the anal verge;[11] (5) the position of the patient;[11] and (6) the biomechanic and structural properties of the rectum.[7,73,74]

Barostat distention The computerized barostat is now the method of choice for the evaluation of various components of rectal sensorimotor function.[14,66] For assessment of rectal sensitivity, either phasic or stepwise isobaric distention paradigms may be used with good reproducibility for both being reported.[75] The "ascending method of limits," which involves the presentation of an increasing stimulus until perceived by the subject, is usually used to measure sensory thresholds during distention. The use of such a predictable protocol, however, may incur response bias. Various approaches have been adopted to reduce this. Recently, the Mayo group has assessed visceral sensitivity using stepwise distention from 0 to 60 mm Hg in 4–mm Hg steps every 1 minute (ascending method of limits) and four random-order phasic distentions of pressures set at 12, 24, 36, and 48 mm Hg above the basal operating pressure.[76,77] Measurement of rectal sensitivity (and compliance and tone) are only reproducible after a conditioning distention,[75] however, which usually involves distention from 0 to 36 mm Hg (or to maximum toleration) in 4–mm Hg increments at 30-second intervals.

Direct stimulation of the rectal mucosa (nonmechanical distention): thermal and electrostimulation The application of an electrical stimulus of 500-μs duration and 10-Hz frequency to the rectal mucosa has been successfully used to assess rectal sensory function.[68] Similarly, thermal (cold or warm) stimulation may be applied to the rectum using intraluminal water-filled bags[78] or thermal probes.[69] A specifically designed thermal probe, capable of achieving temperatures from 38°C to 51°C, has proved useful in the investigation of rectal sensory function.[69]

Measurements and clinical use

Simple balloon distention During distention, subjects are instructed to volunteer a range of sensations: first sensation; constant (flatus) sensation (optional); desire to defecate; and maximum toleration.[4,11,65] The distending volume (or pressure) at each of these sensory thresholds is then recorded. Despite large intersubject variation, several studies have reported a high degree of reproducibility with regard to recorded sensory thresholds,[69,71] notably for maximum tolerable volume.[21,79] In recent years, consensus statements and technical and performance reviews have acknowledged that evaluation of rectal sensory function using simple balloon distention is useful in the assessment of functional gastrointestinal disorders,[4,11,14,72] has an accepted place in the clinical management of patients with anorectal disorders,[4,11] and is of established value in terms of diagnostic potential.[2,80] It is important, however, to consider that this technique measures "rectal perception of distention" and not (necessarily) "afferent nerve function."

Barostat distention Conscious perception can be measured by recording the volumes or pressures required to trigger rectal sensations, as with simple balloon distention. Alternatively, perception can be recorded using a rating scales, such as verbal descriptive (Likert) scales and visual analog scales.[66] The Mayo group has evaluated rectal sensitivity by recording sensory pressure thresholds during an "ascending method of limits" stepwise distention and by recording symptom ratings for gas, urgency, discomfort, and pain during four random order phasic distentions.[76,77]

Direct stimulation of the rectal mucosa (nonmechanical distention): thermal and electrostimulation Electrical stimulation of the rectal mucosa results in the perception of a discomfort, tingling or burning.[68] Previously, it has been shown that it is safe and reproducible, and that the results correlate well with the findings of simple balloon distention.[69] It has been criticized, however, because results may be influenced by loss of contact with the rectal mucosa, and the presence of feces in the rectum.[81] Thermal stimulation is most commonly described by subjects as a prickling or sharp feeling, or an aching or throbbing sensation.[69] A recent study has confirmed that a sensory response is perceived by all subjects at temperatures above 43°C, and that heat stimulation is a reproducible, simple technique that agrees well with simple balloon distention in the assessment of rectal sensitivity in healthy volunteers.[69] At the current time, the value of both these techniques is yet to be established and they remain confined to the research setting.[11]

Overall, irrespective of stimulation technique used, once normal ranges have been determined in healthy control subjects, abnormalities of rectal sensitivity may be defined. Heightened sensory awareness (rectal hypersensitivity) is suggested by sensory threshold volumes (or pressures) reduced below the normal range or verbal descriptive or visual analog scale scores elevated above the normal range. By contrast, impaired or blunted rectal sensitivity (rectal hyposensitivity) is suggested by the presence of elevated sensory threshold volumes (or pressures) or reduced verbal descriptive or visual analog scale scores compared with the normal range.[14] Both rectal hypersensitivity and hyposensitivity have been reported in functional bowel disorders.[7,28,49,50,67,82]

Limitations and implications for the assessment of rectal sensitivity in clinical practice

Traditionally, it has been considered that alteration of perception of rectal distention automatically indicates afferent nerve dysfunction, such as that which may occur following nerve or spinal injury.[83] Abnormal sensory threshold volumes during simple balloon distention may not accurately reflect the function of visceral afferents under certain circumstances, however, because such volumes may be influenced by structural or biomechanic properties of the rectum.[73] For example, in the presence of increased rectal diameter or compliance, greater volumes are required to distend and stimulate the rectum,[74,84] and elevated sensory threshold volumes may conceivably reflect increased rectal size and inadequate stimulation, rather than dysfunction of the rectal afferent pathway itself.[7]

Some advocate the measurement of sensory threshold pressures rather than volumes. Changes in pressure are not the direct stimulus for rectal perception, however, because rectal mechanoreceptors are stimulated by forces (strains) and deformations (stresses) acting in the rectal wall.[85,86] Isobaric distention is not guaranteed to control adequately for differing biomechanic properties. Furthermore, the measurement of threshold pressures in the evaluation of rectal sensitivity is less practical in the clinical setting.

Techniques that involve direct stimulation of the rectal mucosa have the advantage of not being influenced by abnormal rectal wall properties, because they rely solely on direct contact with the mucosa, and they offer more accurate evaluation of the rectal afferent nerve pathway.[68,69] Their impact on clinical management, however, remains less certain.[11] In patients with abnormal sensory threshold volumes to balloon distention, however, the use of such complementary techniques may be indicated.

Rectal Compliance

Rectal compliance refers to the ability of the rectum to distend, and is defined as the "volume response to an imposed pressure".[86] The rectum initially actively relaxes in response to distention,[87] and this "adaptive relaxation," facilitated by its viscoelastic properties, allows accommodation of significant increases in volume while maintaining low intraluminal pressures,[88] so that continence is not threatened. With continued distention, the rectal wall becomes more resistant to stretch as its elastic limit is approached, and there are regular contractions of the rectal wall,[89] causing intrarectal pressure to rise.

Technique

Although feasible using conventional latex balloon distention, rectal compliance can be most accurately assessed using the barostat, which minimizes both observer bias and error.[66] Measurement by means of latex (or equivalent) balloons requires correction to account for their intrinsic elasticity.[4,14] Oversized polyethylene bags are favored; provided that the range of volumes used for the study remains below 90% of the maximum volume of the bag, polyethylene can be regarded as infinitely compliant, in that its own properties have no influence on the internal pressure.[66] Using an intermittent balloon distention technique, intrabag (intrarectal) volumes and pressures are recorded concomitantly.[4] The pressure-volume relationship of the rectum during distention, necessary for the calculation of rectal compliance, can be evaluated using a variety of paradigms, although phasic distention is most commonly used, often with simultaneous assessment of sensitivity.[66] It is important that each distending level is maintained for some time (typically 30–60 seconds) to enable the rectum to adapt to a steady state and for accurate measurements to be obtained.[14] A typical recording of pressures and volumes during phasic isobaric distention using a barostat is shown in **Fig. 3**A.

Measurements and clinical use

Rectal compliance is calculated as change in volume divided by change in pressure ($\Delta V/\Delta P$).[11,14] For technical and physiologic reasons, however, the pressure-volume curve is nonlinear, and calculating a single value to describe the slope of that curve (ie, ascribing a linear measurement for compliance) is too simplistic and imprecise.[4,11,90] It is more accurate to express compliance values as a graphic plot of all volumes tested.[4,11] Such a plot reveals a characteristic triphasic sigmoid curve (**Fig. 3**B). A more accurate measure of compliance can be obtained by calculating the slope of the pressure-volume curve.[66,73] Alternatively, compliance can be approximated to an exponential function.[17]

Rectal compliance reduced below the normal range (indicative of a "stiff" rectum) occurs because of rectal fibrosis (eg, due to chronic inflammatory diseases), chronic ischemia, or pelvic irradiation.[14] In such cases, the slope of the pressure-volume curve is reduced (ie, it is closer to the horizontal position). Reduced rectal compliance has also been noted in patients with diarrhea-predominant irritable bowel syndrome[91] and certain patients with urge fecal incontinence.[52] By contrast, rectal compliance increased above the normal range is indicative of an excessively lax (floppy) rectum. The slope of the pressure-volume curve is displaced toward the vertical position. Increased rectal compliance has been reported in patients with gross dilatation of the rectum (megarectum)[92] and certain patients with chronic constipation.[74]

There is no clear consensus about the value of rectal compliance measurement and its impact on clinical management.[90] Given the potential influence of abnormal rectal biomechanic properties on sensitivity,[14] however, many specialist centers are now assessing rectal compliance on a routine or selective basis.[3]

Rectal Tone

Rectal tone reflects fixed physical properties of the tissues (passive resistance) and myogenic and neurogenic activity in the contractile apparatus of the rectal smooth muscle.[93] Changes in tone, both at rest and in response to physiologic (food) or pharmacologic stimuli, can be measured with the barostat by using a prolonged isobaric distention technique, with the pressure in the bag set at 2 mm Hg above the minimum distending pressure, defined as the pressure that prevents complete collapse of the bag. Because the barostat maintains a constant pressure by aspirating air from the bag during rectal contraction, and injecting air into it during relaxation, movement of the rectal wall may be closely followed. The volume of air aspirated or injected provides an indirect measure of the magnitude of the contraction or relaxation,[66] and hence tone. Currently, however, the value of measuring rectal tone remains uncertain and it is performed only in research laboratories.

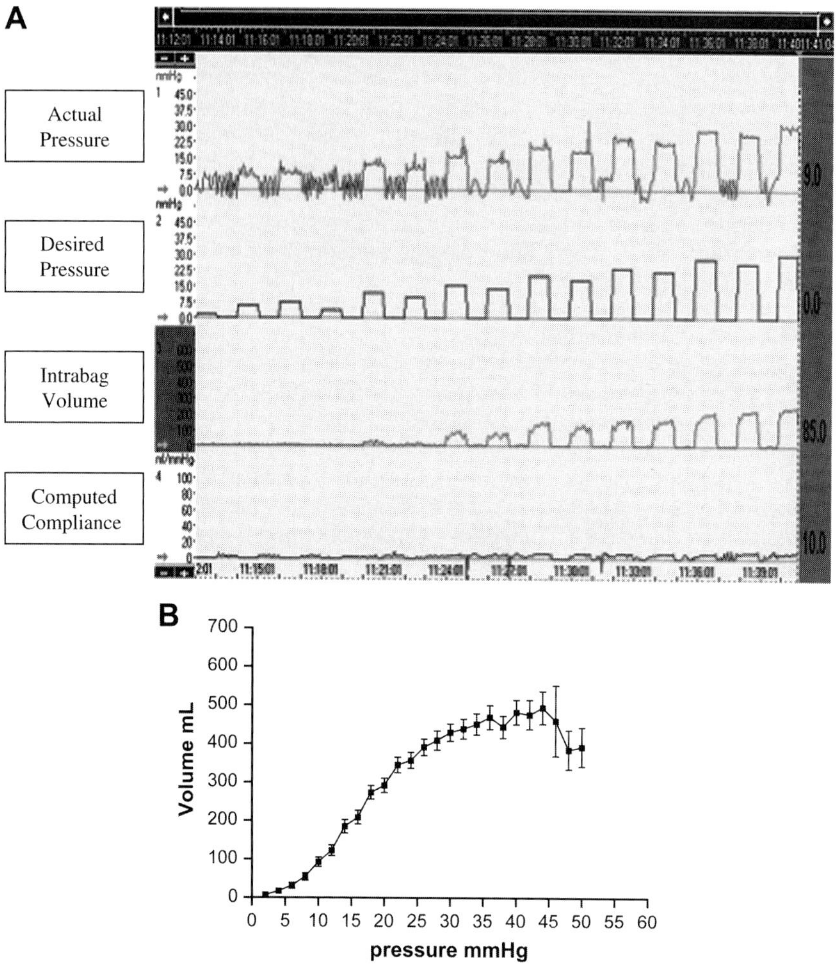

Fig. 3. (*A*) Typical barostat recording during random phasic isobaric distention. The computer display shows the actual and desired pressure during phasic distention. The actual intrabag pressures obtained accurately reflected the preprogrammed desired pressures. The intrabag volumes, required to obtain the desired pressure, are also shown. The computed compliance measurement is not used during the analysis. (*B*) Pressure-volume relationship during phasic isobaric distention. A plot of volume against pressure reveals the classic sigmoid-shaped curve that summarizes the pressure-volume relationship of the rectum. Mean rectal compliance is taken as the slope of the steep linear part of the curve.

Limitations and Implications for the Assessment of Rectal Compliance and Tone in Clinical Practice

Although the need to consider rectal wall biomechanic properties when evaluating rectal sensitivity is not in doubt,[14,73] the assessment of compliance and tone for this purpose has attracted considerable criticism.[86] Accordingly, the use of alternative methodologies for studying rectal biomechanics has been proposed by the Aalborg group. Impedance planimetry is a novel technology that combines rectal balloon inflation with measurement of intrabag (ie, intraluminal) impedance, and provides an accurate appreciation of capacity (cross-sectional area) and tension-strain relationships.[94,95] It offers a more informative evaluation of rectal biomechanics in comparison with studies using the barostat.[96]

NEUROPHYSIOLOGIC EVALUATION

It has long been recognized that anal sphincter dysfunction may be related to denervation injury,[97] and neurophysiologic assessment of the pelvic floor may be indicated in patients with fecal incontinence. Electrodiagnostic tests principally enable characterization of nerve, muscle, and neuromuscular junction integrity, help localize the nerve injury, and provide a measure of severity. In addition, EMG studies may help diagnose altered rectoanal co-ordination in patients with a functional outlet obstruction. Tests of both peripheral and central neural function are considered.

Pudendal Nerve Terminal Motor Latency

The pudendal nerve is a mixed nerve providing efferent and afferent pathways to the EAS, urethral sphincter, perineal musculature, mucosa of the anal canal, and perineal skin, but not the mid or distal rectum.[56] The branches of the pudendal nerve, which course over the pelvic floor, are vulnerable to stretch injury, which leads to denervation of the EAS, and may result in muscle weakness and incontinence.[97,98] Stimulation of the pudendal nerve generates a compound muscle action potential (CMAP) response of the EAS, which can be recorded by surface electrodes. Pudendal nerve terminal motor latency (PNTML) is a measurement of the conduction time from stimulation of the pudendal nerve at the level of the ischial spines, to the EAS contraction. Prolonged latencies are used as a surrogate marker of pudendal neuropathy, and to ascertain whether EAS weakness is secondary to pudendal nerve injury, a sphincter defect, or both.[11] Before the advent of endoanal ultrasound, most cases of idiopathic or neurogenic fecal incontinence were believed to be a result of pudendal nerve injury.[99] It is now recognized, however, that structural damage to the anal sphincters rather than pudendal neuropathy is the underlying pathogenic mechanism in most patients[100] and true isolated neuropathy may be rare.[101]

Technique

Evaluation of pudendal nerve function is achieved using a disposable bipolar electrode (St. Mark's pudendal electrode), developed 20 years ago,[102] consisting of flexible printed circuits and pairs of stimulating and recording electrodes, attached to a suitable EMG machine. This is mounted on the index finger of a gloved hand, which is then inserted into the anorectum so that the recording electrodes, located at the base of the finger, are sited within the anus at the level of the EAS.[16] The pudendal nerve courses around the pelvic brim, and can be stimulated by the stimulating electrodes located at the tip of the finger, by palpating the ischial spines on either side and applying intermittent electrical pulses; to ensure that all motor fibers within the nerve are stimulated, a supramaximal stimulus should be used. A number of CMAP responses should be elicited bilaterally to provide reproducibility of the response. The PNTML, in milliseconds, is measured as the time interval between the stimulus artifact and the onset of the CMAP response. An alternative method to per rectal stimulation in women is by a transvaginal technique, which may be less uncomfortable and is well described.[103]

Measurements and clinical use

The recorded latency primarily reflects integrity of myelin insulation of the nerve, but may also indicate damage to the largest and fastest conducting fibers. A prolonged latency indicates either demyelination[103] or irreparable damage of a number of fast firing fibers. Although amplitude of the CMAP response is a better measure of axonal injury than the latency, in clinical practice this is not routinely measured.[103,104] The upper limit of normal for PNTMLs has often been reported as 2.2 milliseconds;[16,103] however, latencies are known to increase with age, independent of continence status,[105–107] and in healthy subjects over 50 years of age, normal latency values of greater than 2.5 milliseconds have been reported.[52,105,107] The normal upper limit for latency, which is a continuous variable, not a dichotomous one, has been ill-defined for a robust diagnosis of pudendal neuropathy.

The principal clinical use for the measurement of pudendal nerve function has been in fecal incontinence.[6,8,103] Prolonged latencies have been demonstrated particularly in those incontinent patients who have suffered obstetric trauma,[108] but also in patients who have abnormal perineal descent[109] (perhaps because of excessive straining at stool[110]), rectal prolapse,[111] or a recognized neurologic disorder.[112] Indeed, grouped data show that incontinent patients with bilaterally prolonged PNTMLs have reduced anal squeeze pressures compared with controls, supporting the concept that a neuropathic process impairs EAS function.[113] In addition, prolonged latencies have been proposed as a prognostic indicator of the outcomes of interventional treatment, either conservative[114] or surgical.[8,115]

Limitations

The value, and indeed the validity, of pudendal nerve latency testing has come under increasing scrutiny,[3,8,11,14,104,133] given that most incontinent patients are now recognized as having identifiable muscle damage or degeneration.[26,100] Recording of latencies is less sensitive than needle EMG studies to disclose anal sphincter denervation.[116,117] There are also a number of concerns related to methodology and interpretation:

1. The sensitivity and specificity of this test is poor; many patients with delayed latencies have squeeze pressures within the normal range and vice versa[116,117]
2. The known increase in PNTMLs with age is rarely accounted for, and normative data are inadequate[3]
3. Normal latencies may be recorded in a damaged nerve, as long as some fast-conducting fibers remain[106]
4. The test is operator dependent[8,11] and may be technically difficult to perform in some patients, notably those with a high body mass index or a long anal canal
5. The close proximity of the stimulating and recording electrodes may lead to a motor artifact, which can be mistaken for the true CMAP[104]
6. Reproducibility of the test is unknown[3]
7. Reports suggesting that prolonged latencies can predict clinical outcomes after surgery are conflicting and inconsistent[11,119]
8. The significance of a unilateral neuropathy is unclear, although with recent evidence of laterality of pudendal nerve innervation of the EAS,[120] this perhaps merits further investigation[121]

On the evidence to date, the routine use of PNTML testing is no longer advocated[3,11,14,104] because it contributes little to the management of individual patients.

Electromyography

Recording of pelvic floor EMG (both the EAS and levator ani muscles) can be used in a variety of ways:[11,104,122] (1) to map the EAS to identify areas of injury or congenital abnormality; (2) to determine striated muscle function (ie, whether the muscle contracts or relaxes appropriately, based on recruitment of firing motor units); (3) to assess denervation-reinnervation potentials, indicative of neural injury; and (4) in conjunction with other tests of anorectal motor function (eg, manometry, proctography) to provide an integrated assessment.

Technique

Studies of EMG activity can be performed using a needle electrode (either a concentric needle, which samples approximately 30 motor units simultaneously, or a single-fiber electrode, which samples only one motor unit at a time), a skin electrode, or an anal plug electrode. The choice is dependent on the modality under study. Disposable needle electrodes are usually favored and are inserted transcutaneously with or without topical anesthesia into the four quadrants of the EAS and also through the EAS into the deeper puborectalis, by a midline approach between the anus and tip of the coccyx; in experienced hands, this is not accompanied by severe discomfort.[3] Concentric needle electrodes enable various parameters to be measured: insertional and spontaneous activities; and motor unit action potential (MUAP) morphology (duration, amplitude, percentage polyphasia) and recruitment during voluntary or reflex (eg, to cough) muscle contraction.[17,104,122] With single-fiber electrodes, fiber density can be calculated, which is an index of motor unit grouping, a consequence of denervation, and subsequent reinnervation.[98,122] For either method, 20 motor unit potentials are traditionally recorded at each site.[98] Conventionally, only striated muscular activity is assessed, although EMG studies of the IAS have been performed using fine-wire electrodes.[123]

Measurements and clinical use

Using a concentric needle electrode, the EAS, under normal conditions, shows tonic activity during the resting state (**Fig. 4**A); in a muscle replaced by scar tissue (eg, with obstetric injury), there is no insertional activity.[103] Denervation injury is indicated by abnormal spontaneous activity, such as fibrillation potentials and high-frequency discharges,[103,104] and increased temporal recruitment of MUAPs. Maximal activity during voluntary muscle contraction is reduced, and there may be reinnervation (signs of collateral sprouting) where MUAP morphology is disturbed (eg, prolonged duration, altered amplitude, and increased polyphasia [**Fig. 4**B]).[103,104,122] Adjacent normal muscle shows normal patterns of innervation on insertion, at rest, and during voluntary activity. Automated computer analysis enables quantification of MUAP parameters.[104]

Fiber density, as recorded by single-fiber EMG, is defined as the mean number of muscle fibers belonging to an individual motor unit per detection site.[104] Normal fiber density in the EAS is greater than 2; an increase is a sensitive indicator of collateral reinnervation. This test has been shown to be highly repeatable.[124]

In the striated anal musculature of patients with fecal incontinence, MUAP activity, fiber density, and jitter (the stability of consecutive muscle fiber discharges, reflecting the stability of terminal motor axons and neuromuscular transmission[104]) have been shown to be altered in comparison with controls.[98,116–118,122,125] However, such neurogenic changes may be caused by injury at any level along the motor neurone, from sacral spinal cord to muscle fascicles entering the sphincter, and a firm diagnosis of pudendal neuropathy can only be determined if these changes are seen both in the anal sphincter and ischiocavernosus muscle.[3] The routine use of EMG studies for the assessment of patients with fecal incontinence is diminishing in clinical practice,[11] given the widespread availability of endoanal ultrasonography, which has superseded EMG for identifying muscle defects, and the fact that technique and interpretation may require specialized training and expertise. Nevertheless, EMG assessment of the pelvic floor may be considered in patients with clinically suspected neurogenic

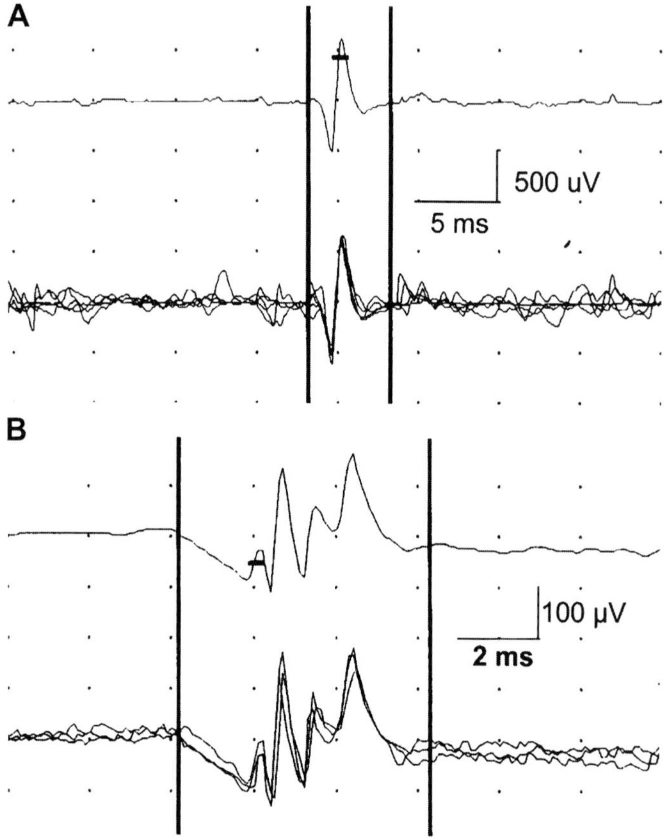

Fig. 4. Typical examples of a normal motor unit (*A*) and an abnormal motor unit (*B*), as recorded by concentric needle EMG. (*From* Bharucha AE. Update of tests of colon and rectal structure and function. J Clin Gastroenterol 2006;40:96–103; with permission.)

weakness, particularly if there are signs of proximal (spinal cord, sacral roots) involvement.[3] Furthermore, EMG signals, using an anal plug electrode, are commonly used as a tool to facilitate biofeedback for pelvic floor retraining, either in patients with fecal incontinence or a functional outlet obstruction.[14]

Somatosensory (Cortical) Evoked Potentials

Somatosensory evoked potentials allow evaluation of afferent pathways and are measured by applying a peripheral stimulus and recording evoked potentials from the central nervous system. The transmission and processing of sensory information from the anus or rectum to the brain may be assessed using cortical evoked potentials, which are measurements of the electrical potentials generated by cortical neurons in response to a series of repeated sensory stimuli.[126] The technique involves the brief presentation of a sensory stimulus, which is time and phase locked to the recording of the electroencephalogram by surface electrodes placed on the scalp. The stimulus-specific cortical evoked potentials occur at a fixed time after each stimulus, whereas other brain activity does not, and it can be extracted from the background electrical activity of the brain.[126] Both mechanic[127,128] and electrical stimulation[129] have been used, with the latter being more reliable for recording cortical evoked potentials.[129]

The rectal cortical evoked potential response provides an objective correlate of perceived sensation, with the response increasing in amplitude while decreasing in latency, as the stimulation intensity increases.[130] Nevertheless, despite resurgence in the interest of cortical evoked potentials within the last few years, and the identification of prolonged latencies in certain groups of patients,[127] at the current time the technique remains confined to the research setting.

SUMMARY

Although rigorous laboratory assessment is not required for all patients, a number of tests do exist for the manometric and neurophysiologic evaluation of motor and sensory functions of the anorectum and pelvic floor. Judicious use of these tests is recommended, but in those patients in whom investigation is warranted, a comprehensive and structured assessment should be performed, given the multiple mechanisms involved in the physiologic processes of continence preservation and defecation, and the often multifactorial pathoetiology of anorectal dysfunction.[131] Several studies have looked at the clinical impact of such investigations in patients with fecal incontinence or constipation, and demonstrated that the information provided markedly improved diagnostic yield[80,132,133] and directly influenced or altered the management plan in a significant proportion of cases.[2,132,134–136] Although these investigations do not replace a careful and directed clinical assessment, they provide complementary information that may allow a decision regarding choice of suitable, rather than empiric therapy to be made on an individual basis. The major caveat is that there is no uniform standardization of tests, and results between centers are often difficult to compare. In addition, robust normative data for all measures of function remain inadequate, particularly with regard to age and gender stratification. Furthermore, the tests are not widely available, and there is a lack of specialized training.[137] To address these issues satisfactorily, particularly through education, must remain a principal focus for those actively involved in this field. A better critical examination of the diagnostic yield and accuracy of current investigations is also needed, and this is only feasible through large, well-designed, prospective studies.[46] Such an approach would enable the refinement of existing techniques, both in terms of test performance, indications for use, and data interpretation, which together with evolving newer modalities will further enhance the diagnostic capabilities available to the physician, and it is hoped contribute to the development of novel therapeutic options.

REFERENCES

1. Camilleri M, Talley NJ. Pathophysiology as a basis for understanding symptom complexes and therapeutic targets. Neurogastroenterol Motil 2004;16(2):135–42.
2. Rao SS, Patel RS. How useful are manometric tests of anorectal function in the management of defecation disorders? Am J Gastroenterol 1997;92:469–75.
3. Bharucha AE. Update of tests of colon and rectal structure and function. J Clin Gastroenterol 2006;40(2):96–103.
4. Rao SS, Azpiroz F, Diamant N, et al. Minimum standards of anorectal manometry. Neurogastroenterol Motil 2002;14(5):553–9.
5. Scott SM, Lunniss PJ. Investigations of anorectal function. In: Sultan AH, Thakar R, Fenner DE, editors. Perineal and anal sphincter trauma. London: Springer-Verlag; 2007. p. 102–22.

6. Madoff RD, Parker SC, Varma MG, et al. Faecal incontinence in adults. Lancet 2004;364(9434):621–32.
7. Gladman MA, Lunniss PJ, Scott SM, et al. Rectal hyposensitivity. Am J Gastroenterol 2006;101(5):1140–51.
8. Rao SS. Diagnosis and management of fecal incontinence. Am J Gastroenterol 2004;99(8):1585–604.
9. Simpson RR, Kennedy ML, Nguyen MH, et al. Anal manometry: a comparison of techniques. Dis Colon Rectum 2006;49(7):1033–8.
10. Chaliha C, Sultan AH, Emmanuel AV. Normal ranges for anorectal manometry and sensation in women of reproductive age. Colorectal Dis 2007;9(9):839–44.
11. Diamant NE, Kamm MA, Wald A, et al. American Gastroenterological Association medical position statement on anorectal testing techniques. Gastroenterology 1999;116(3):732–60.
12. Keighley MR, Henry MM, Bartolo DC, et al. Anorectal physiology measurement: report of a working party. Br J Surg 1989;76(4):356–7.
13. Corrazziari E. Anorectal manometry: a round table discussion. Gastroenterol Int 1989;2:115–7.
14. Azpiroz F, Enck P, Whitehead WE. Anorectal functional testing: review of collective experience. Am J Gastroenterol 2002;97(2):232–40.
15. Sun WM, Rao SS. Manometric assessment of anorectal function. Gastroenterol Clin North Am 2001;30(1):15–32.
16. Rao SSC, Hatfield R, Soffer E, et al. Manometric tests of anorectal function in healthy adults. Am J Gastroenterol 1999;94(3):773–83.
17. Bharucha AE. Outcome measures for fecal incontinence: anorectal structure and function. Gastroenterology 2004;126(1 Suppl 1):S90–8.
18. McHugh SM, Diamant NE. Anal canal pressure profile: a reappraisal as determined by rapid pullthrough technique. Gut 1987;28(10):1234–41.
19. Jorge JM, Wexner SD. Anorectal manometry: techniques and clinical applications. South Med J 1993;86(8):924–31.
20. Nivatvongs S, Stern HS, Fryd DS. The length of the anal canal. Dis Colon Rectum 1981;24(8):600–1.
21. OØ Rasmussen. Anorectal function. Dis Colon Rectum 1994;37(4):386–403.
22. Read NW, Sun WM. Anorectal manometry. In: Henry MM, Swash M, editors. Coloproctology and the pelvic floor. Second edition. Oxford (UK): Butterworth-Heinemann Ltd; 1992. p. 119–45.
23. Lestar B, Penninckx F, Kerrimans R. The composition of the anal basal pressure: an in vivo and in vitro study in man. Int J Colorectal Dis 1989;4(2):118–22.
24. Engel AF, Kamm MA, Bartram CI, et al. Relationship of symptoms in faecal incontinence to specific sphincter abnormalities. Int J Colorectal Dis 1995; 10(3):152–5.
25. Lindsey I, Jones OM, Smilgin-Humphreys MM, et al. Patterns of fecal incontinence after anal surgery. Dis Colon Rectum 2004;47(10):1643–9.
26. Vaizey CJ, Kamm MA, Bartram CI. Primary degeneration of the internal anal sphincter as a cause of passive faecal incontinence. Lancet 1997;349(9052): 612–5.
27. Felt-Bersma RJ, Klinkenberg-Knol EC, Meuwissen SG. Anorectal function investigations in incontinent and continent patients: differences and discriminatory value. Dis Colon Rectum 1990;33(6):479–85.
28. Sun WM, Donnelly TC, Read NW. Utility of a combined test of anorectal manometry, electromyography, and sensation in determining the mechanism of idiopathic faecal incontinence. Gut 1992;33(6):807–13.

29. Lunniss PJ, Scott SM. Pathophysiology of anal incontinence. In: Sultan AH, Thakar R, Fenner DE, editors. Perineal and anal sphincter trauma. London: Springer-Verlag; 2007. p. 89–101.
30. Bharucha AE, Fletcher JG, Harper CM, et al. Relationship between symptoms and disordered continence mechanisms in women with idiopathic faecal incontinence. Gut 2005;54(4):546–55.
31. Lunniss PJ, Gladman MA, Hetzer FH, et al. Risk factors in acquired faecal incontinence. J R Soc Med 2004;97(3):111–6.
32. Chiarioni G, Scattolini C, Bonfante F, et al. Liquid stool incontinence with severe urgency: anorectal function and effective biofeedback treatment. Gut 1993; 34(11):1576–80.
33. Telford KJ, Ali AS, Lymer K, et al. Fatigability of the external anal sphincter in anal incontinence. Dis Colon Rectum 2004;47(5):746–52.
34. Siproudhis L, Bellissant E, Pagenault M, et al. Fecal incontinence with normal anal canal pressures: where is the pitfall? Am J Gastroenterol 1999;94(6):1556–63.
35. Bharucha AE, Fletcher JG. Recent advances in assessing anorectal structure and functions. Gastroenterology 2007;133(4):1069–74.
36. Kahrilas PJ, Ghosh SK, Pandolfino JE. Challenging the limits of esophageal manometry. Gastroenterology 2008;134(1):16–8.
37. Aaronson I, Nixon HH. A clinical evaluation of anorectal pressure studies in the diagnosis of Hirschsprung's disease. Gut 1972;13(2):138–46.
38. Sangwan YP, Coller JA, Schoetz DJ, et al. Spectrum of abnormal rectoanal reflex patterns in patients with fecal incontinence. Dis Colon Rectum 1996;39(1):59–65.
39. Chan CL, Ponsford S, Swash M. The anal reflex elicited by cough and sniff: validation of a neglected clinical sign. J Neurol Neurosurg Psychiatr 2004; 75(10):1449–51.
40. Rao SS, Welcher KD, Leistikow JS. Obstructive defecation: a failure of rectoanal coordination. Am J Gastroenterol 1998;93(7):1042–50.
41. Rao SS. Constipation: evaluation and treatment. Gastroenterol Clin North Am 2003;32(2):659–83.
42. Duthie GS, Bartolo DC. Anismus: the cause of constipation? Results of investigation and treatment. World J Surg 1992;16(5):831–5.
43. Minguez M, Herreros B, Sanchiz V, et al. Predictive value of the balloon expulsion test for excluding the diagnosis of pelvic floor dyssynergia in constipation. Gastroenterology 2004;126(1):57–62.
44. Bharucha AE, Wald A, Enck P, et al. Functional anorectal disorders. Gastroenterology 2006;130(5):1510–8.
45. Rao SS, Mudipalli RS, Stessman M, et al. Investigation of the utility of colorectal function tests and Rome II criteria in dyssynergic defecation (anismus). Neurogastroenterol Motil 2004;16(5):589–96.
46. Rao SS, Ozturk R, Laine L. Clinical utility of diagnostic tests for constipation in adults: a systematic review. Am J Gastroenterol 2005;100(7):1605–15.
47. Chan CL, Scott SM, Knowles CH, et al. Exaggerated rectal adaptation: another cause of outlet obstruction. Colorectal Dis 2001;3(2):141–2.
48. Read NW, Timms JM, Barfield LJ, et al. Impairment of defecation in young women with severe constipation. Gastroenterology 1986;90(1):53–60.
49. Rao SS, Ozturk R, Stessman M. Investigation of the pathophysiology of fecal seepage. Am J Gastroenterol 2004;99(11):2204–9.
50. Gladman MA, Scott SM, Chan CL, et al. Rectal hyposensitivity: prevalence and clinical impact in patients with intractable constipation and fecal incontinence. Dis Colon Rectum 2003;46(2):238–46.

51. Scott SM. Manometric techniques for the evaluation of colonic motor activity: current status. Neurogastroenterol Motil 2003;15(5):483–513.
52. Chan CL, Lunniss PJ, Wang D, et al. Rectal sensorimotor dysfunction in patients with urge fecal incontinence: evidence from prolonged manometric studies. Gut 2005;54(9):1263–72.
53. Thorson AG. Anorectal physiology. Surg Clin North Am 2002;82(6):1115–23.
54. Delvaux M. Role of visceral sensitivity in the pathophysiology of irritable bowel syndrome. Gut 2002;51(Suppl 1):i67–71.
55. Hobday DI, Aziz Q, Thacker N, et al. A study of the cortical processing of anorectal sensation using functional MRI. Brain 2001;124(Pt 2):361–8.
56. Chan CL, Ponsford S, Scott SM, et al. Contribution of the pudendal nerve to sensation of the distal rectum. Br J Surg 2005;92(7):859–65.
57. Duthie HL, Gairns FW. Sensory nerve endings and sensation in the anal region of man. Br J Surg 1960;47:585–95.
58. Miller R. The measurement of anorectal sensation. In: Kumar D, Waldron DR, Williams NS, editors. Clinical measurement in coloproctology. London: Springer-Verlag; 1991. p. 60–6.
59. Roe AM, Bartolo DC, Mortensen NJ. New method for assessment of anal sensation in various anorectal disorders. Br J Surg 1986;73(4):310–2.
60. Miller R, Bartolo DC, Cervero F, et al. Anorectal temperature sensation: a comparison of normal and incontinent patients. Br J Surg 1987;74(6):511–5.
61. Felt-Bersma RJ, Poen AC, Cuesta MA, et al. Anal sensitivity test: what does it measure and do we need it? Cause or derivative of anorectal complaints. Dis Colon Rectum 1997;40(7):811–6.
62. Miller R, Bartolo DC, Cervero F, et al. Differences in anal sensation in continent and incontinent patients with perineal descent. Int J Colorectal Dis 1989;4(1):45–9.
63. Speakman CT, Kamm MA. Abnormal visceral autonomic innervation in neurogenic faecal incontinence. Gut 1993;34(2):215–21.
64. Vasudevan SP, Scott SM, Gladman MA, et al. Rectal hyposensitivity: evaluation of anal sensation in female patients with refractory constipation with and without faecal incontinence. Neurogastroenterol Motil 2007;19(8):660–7.
65. Farthing MJ, Lennard-Jones JE. Sensibility of the rectum to distension and the anorectal distension reflex in ulcerative colitis. Gut 1978;19(1):64–9.
66. Whitehead WE, Delvaux M. Standardization of barostat procedures for testing smooth muscle tone and sensory thresholds in the gastrointestinal tract. Dig Dis Sci 1997;42(2):223–41.
67. Mertz H, Naliboff B, Munakata J, et al. Altered rectal perception is a biological marker of patients with irritable bowel syndrome. Gastroenterology. 1995;109(1):40–52.
68. Kamm MA, Lennard-Jones JE. Rectal mucosal electrosensory testing-evidence for a rectal sensory neuropathy in idiopathic constipation. Dis Colon Rectum 1990;33(5):419–23.
69. Chan CL, Scott SM, Birch MJ, et al. Rectal heat thresholds: a novel test of the sensory afferent pathway. Dis Colon Rectum 2003;46(5):590–5.
70. Gebhart GF. Visceral pain-peripheral sensitisation. Gut 2000;47(Suppl 4):iv54–5.
71. Sun WM, Read NW, Prior A, et al. Sensory and motor responses to rectal distention vary according to rate and pattern of balloon inflation. Gastroenterology 1990;99(4):1008–15.
72. Whitehead WE, Schuster MM. Anorectal physiology and pathophysiology. Am J Gastroenterol 1987;82(6):487–97.

73. Camilleri M. Testing the sensitivity hypothesis in practice: tools and methods, assumptions and pitfalls. Gut 2002;51(Suppl 1):i34–40.
74. Gladman MA, Dvorkin LS, Lunniss PJ, et al. Rectal hyposensitivity: a disorder of the rectal wall or the afferent pathway? An assessment using the barostat. Am J Gastroenterol 2005;100(1):106–14.
75. Hammer HF, Phillips SF, Camilleri M, et al. Rectal tone, distensibility, and perception: reproducibility and response to different distensions. Am J Physiol 1998; 274(3 Pt 1):G584–90.
76. Bharucha AE, Camilleri M, Zinsmeister AR, et al. Adrenergic modulation of human colonic motor and sensory function. Am J Physiol 1997;273(5 Pt 1): G997–1006.
77. Cremonini F, Houghton LA, Camilleri M, et al. Barostat testing of rectal sensation and compliance in humans: comparison of results across two centres and overall reproducibility. Neurogastroenterol Motil 2005;17(6):810–20.
78. Villanova N, Azpiroz F, Malagelada JR. Perception and gut reflexes induced by stimulation of gastrointestinal thermoreceptors in humans. J Physiol 1997; 502(Pt 1):215–22.
79. Sorensen M, Rasmussen OO, Tetzschner T, et al. Physiological variation in rectal compliance. Br J Surg 1992;79(10):1106–8.
80. Wexner SD, Jorge JM. Colorectal physiological tests: use or abuse of technology? Eur J Surg 1994;160(3):167–74.
81. Meagher AP, Kennedy ML, Lubowski DZ. Rectal mucosal electrosensitivity: what is being tested? Int J Colorectal Dis 1996;11(1):29–33.
82. Lea R, Houghton LA, Calvert EL, et al. Gut-focused hypnotherapy normalizes disordered rectal sensitivity in patients with irritable bowel syndrome. Aliment Pharmacol Ther 2003;17(5):635–42.
83. Devroede G, Lamarche J. Functional importance of extrinsic parasympathetic innervation to the distal colon and rectum in man. Gastroenterology 1974; 66(2):273–80.
84. Gladman MA, Dvorkin LS, Scott SM, et al. A novel technique to identify patients with megarectum. Dis Colon Rectum 2007;50(5):621–9.
85. Lynn PA, Olsson C, Zagorodnyuk V, et al. Rectal intraganglionic laminar endings are transduction sites of extrinsic mechanoreceptors in the guinea pig rectum. Gastroenterology 2003;125(3):786–94.
86. Gregersen H, Kassab G. Biomechanics of the gastrointestinal tract. Neurogastroenterol Motil 1996;8(4):277–97.
87. Musial F, Crowell MD. Rectal adaptation to distention: implications for the determination of perception thresholds. Physiol Behav 1995;58(6):1145–8.
88. Arhan P, Faverdin C, Persoz B, et al. Relationship between viscoelastic properties of the rectum and anal pressure in man. J Appl Physiol 1976;41(5 Pt 1): 677–82.
89. Broens P, Vanbeckevoort D, Bellon E, et al. Combined radiologic and manometric study of rectal filling sensation. Dis Colon Rectum 2002;45(8):1016–22.
90. van der Schaar PJ, Lamers CB, Masclee AA. The role of the barostat in human research and clinical practice. Scand J Gastroenterol 1999;34(Suppl 230): 52–63.
91. Zar S, Benson MJ, Kumar D. Rectal afferent hypersensitivity and compliance in irritable bowel syndrome: differences between diarrhoea-predominant and constipation-predominant subgroups. Eur J Gastroenterol Hepatol 2006;18(2): 151–8.

92. Gladman MA, Knowles CH. Novel concepts in the diagnosis, pathophysiology and management of idiopathic megabowel. Colorectal Dis 2008; [Epub ahead of print].
93. Gregersen H, Christensen J. Gastrointestinal tone. Neurogastroenterol Motil 2000;12(6):501–8.
94. Dall FH, Jørgensen CS, Houe D, et al. Biomechanical wall properties of the human rectum: a study with impedance planimetry. Gut 1993;34(11):1581–6.
95. Andersen IS, Gregersen H, Buntzen S, et al. New probe for the measurement of dynamic changes in the rectum. Neurogastroenterol Motil 2004;16(1):99–105.
96. Krogh K, Ryhammer AM, Lundby L, et al. Comparison of methods used for measurement of rectal compliance. Dis Colon Rectum 2001;44(2):199–206.
97. Parks AG, Swash M, Urich H. Sphincter denervation in anorectal incontinence and rectal prolapse. Gut 1977;18(8):656–65.
98. Neill ME, Swash M. Increased motor unit fibre density in the external anal sphincter muscle in ano-rectal incontinence: a single fibre EMG study. J Neurol Neurosurg Psychiatr 1980;43(4):343–7.
99. Kiff ES, Swash M. Slowed conduction in the pudendal nerves in idiopathic (neurogenic) faecal incontinence. Br J Surg 1984;71(8):614–6.
100. Kamm MA. Faecal incontinence. BMJ 1998;316(7130):528–32.
101. Vaizey CJ, Kamm MA, Nicholls RJ. Recent advances in the surgical treatment of faecal incontinence. Br J Surg 1998;85(5):596–603.
102. Rogers J, Henry MM, Misiewicz JJ. Disposable pudendal nerve stimulator: evaluation of the standard instrument and new device. Gut 1988;29(8):1131–3.
103. Olsen AL, Rao SS. Clinical neurophysiology and electrodiagnostic testing of the pelvic floor. Gastroenterol Clin North Am 2001;30(1):33–54.
104. Lefaucheur JP. Neurophysiological testing in anorectal disorders. Muscle Nerve 2006;33(3):324–33.
105. Jameson JS, Chia YW, Kamm MA, et al. Effect of age, sex and parity on anorectal function. Br J Surg 1994;81(11):1689–92.
106. Cheong DM, Vaccaro CA, Salanga VD, et al. Electrodiagnostic evaluation of fecal incontinence. Muscle Nerve 1995;18(6):612–9.
107. Lefaucheur J, Yiou R, Thomas C. Pudendal nerve terminal motor latency: age effects and technical considerations. Clin Neurophysiol 2001;112(3):472–6.
108. Sultan AH, Kamm MA, Hudson CN. Pudendal nerve damage during labour: prospective study before and after childbirth. Br J Obstet Gynaecol 1994;101(1): 22–8.
109. Jones PN, Lubowski DZ, Swash M, et al. Relation between perineal descent and pudendal nerve damage in idiopathic faecal incontinence. Int J Colorectal Dis 1987;2(2):93–5.
110. Snooks SJ, Barnes PR, Swash M, et al. Damage to the innervation of the pelvic floor musculature in chronic constipation. Gastroenterology 1985;89(5): 977–81.
111. Pfeifer J, Salanga VD, Agachan F, et al. Variation in pudendal nerve terminal motor latency according to disease. Dis Colon Rectum 1997;40(1):79–83.
112. Pinna Pintor M, Zara GP, Falletto E, et al. Pudendal neuropathy in diabetic patients with faecal incontinence. Int J Colorectal Dis 1994;9(2):105–9.
113. Hill J, Hosker G, Kiff ES. Pudendal nerve terminal motor latency measurements: what they do and do not tell us. Br J Surg 2002;89(10):1268–9.
114. Leroi AM, Dorival MP, Lecouturier MF, et al. Pudendal neuropathy and severity of incontinence but not presence of an anal sphincter defect may determine the

response to biofeedback therapy in fecal incontinence. Dis Colon Rectum 1999; 42(6):762–9.
115. Gilliland R, Altomare DF, Moreira H Jr, et al. Pudendal neuropathy is predictive of failure following anterior overlapping sphincteroplasty. Dis Colon Rectum 1998; 41(12):1516–22.
116. Thomas C, Lefaucheur JP, Galula G, et al. Respective value of pudendal nerve terminal motor latency and anal sphincter electromyography in neurogenic fecal incontinence. Neurophysiol Clin 2002;32(1):85–90.
117. Gregory WT, Lou JS, Stuyvesant A, et al. Quantitative electromyography of the anal sphincter after uncomplicated vaginal delivery. Obstet Gynecol 2004; 104(2):327–35.
118. Wexner SD, Marchetti F, Salanga VD, et al. Neurophysiologic assessment of the anal sphincters. Dis Colon Rectum 1991;34(7):606–12.
119. Malouf AJ, Norton CS, Engel AF, et al. Long-term results of overlapping anterior anal-sphincter repair for obstetric trauma. Lancet 2000;355(9200):260–5.
120. Enck P, Hinninghofen H, Merletti R, et al. The external anal sphincter and the role of surface electromyography. Neurogastroenterol Motil 2005;17(Suppl 1):60–7.
121. Gooneratne ML, Scott SM, Lunniss PJ. Unilateral pudendal neuropathy is common in patients with fecal incontinence. Dis Colon Rectum 2007;50(4):449–58.
122. Swash M. Electromyography in pelvic floor disorders. In: Henry MM, Swash M, editors. Coloproctology and the pelvic floor. Second edition. Oxford (UK): Butterworth-Heinemann Ltd; 1992. p. 184–95.
123. Farouk R, Duthie GS, MacGregor AB, et al. Evidence of electromechanical dissociation of the internal anal sphincter in idiopathic fecal incontinence. Dis Colon Rectum 1994;37(6):595–601.
124. Rogers J, Laurberg S, Misiewicz JJ, et al. Anorectal physiology validated: a repeatability study of the motor and sensory tests of anorectal function. Br J Surg 1989;76(6):607–9.
125. Gee AS, Durdey P. Preoperative increase in neuromuscular jitter and outcome following surgery for faecal incontinence. Br J Surg 1997;84(9):1265–8.
126. Hobday DI, Hobson AR, Sarkar S, et al. Cortical processing of human gut sensation: an evoked potential study. Am J Physiol Gastrointest Liver Physiol 2002; 283(2):G335–9.
127. Loening-Baucke V, Yamada T. Cerebral potentials evoked by rectal distention in humans. Electroencephalogr Clin Neurophysiol 1993;88(6):447–52.
128. Loening-Baucke V, Anderson RH, Yamada T, et al. Study of the afferent pathways from the rectum with a new distention control device. Neurology 1995; 45(8):1510–6.
129. Hobday DI, Hobson A, Furlong PL, et al. Comparison of cortical potentials evoked by mechanical and electrical stimulation of the rectum. Neurogastroenterol Motil 2000;12(6):547–54.
130. Hobson AR, Aziz Q. Brain imaging and functional gastrointestinal disorders: has it helped our understanding? Gut 2004;53(8):1198–206.
131. Gladman MA, Scott SM, Williams NS. Assessing the patient with fecal incontinence. An overview. In: Zbar AP, Pescatori M, Wexner SD, editors. Complex anorectal disorders: investigation and management. London: Springer-Verlag; 2005. p. 547–94.
132. Keating JP, Stewart PJ, Eyers AA, et al. Are special investigations of value in the management of patients with faecal incontinence. Dis Colon Rectum 1997; 40(8):896–901.

133. Vaizey CJ, Kamm MA. Prospective assessment of the clinical value of anorectal investigations. Digestion 2000;61(3):207–14.
134. Halverson AL, Orkin BA. Which physiologic tests are useful in patients with constipation? Dis Colon Rectum 1998;41(6):735–9.
135. Felt-Bersma RJ, Poen AC, Cuesta MA, et al. Referral for anorectal function evaluation: therapeutic implications and reassurance. Eur J Gastroenterol Hepatol 1999;11(3):289–94.
136. Liberman H, Faria J, Ternent CA, et al. A prospective evaluation of the value of anorectal physiology in the management of fecal incontinence. Dis Colon Rectum 2001;44(11):1567–74.
137. Rao SS. A balancing view: fecal incontinence: test or treat empirically—which strategy is best? Am J Gastroenterol 2006;101(12):2683–4.

Urodynamic Evaluation of the Bladder and Pelvic Floor

Catherine S. Bradley, MD, MSCE[a,b,*], Karen E. Smith, MD[c], Karl J. Kreder, MD, MBA[c]

KEYWORDS

- Urodynamic testing • Cystometry • Uroflowmetry
- Lower urinary tract disorders • Voiding dysfunction

The female pelvic floor is remarkable for the close functional relationships between its gastrointestinal, genital, and urologic structures. Because of anatomic factors, shared pelvic organ vascular supply and nervous system control, and overlapping environmental and biologic risk factors, pelvic floor disorders often overlap in individual patients. For instance, epidemiologic studies have confirmed a link between fecal and urinary incontinence in women.[1–3] Obstructive defecation and vaginal prolapse are associated,[4,5] although it is unclear whether defecatory dysfunction is more often a cause or result of vaginal prolapse. Similarly, rectal prolapse and uterine and vaginal prolapse result from defects in pelvic floor support, and may coexist or share similar risk factors.[6,7] Given the high frequency of overlapping pelvic floor conditions and symptoms, the evaluation and treatment of women with anorectal dysfunction and other pelvic floor disorders often require a multidisciplinary approach.

Pelvic floor disorders that result in urinary symptoms are frequently evaluated using a set of tests collectively called "urodynamic testing." Urodynamic tests evaluate lower urinary tract and pelvic floor function and dysfunction, and provide objective information about manometric, sensorimotor, and neurophysiologic parameters related to the bladder and pelvic floor. This article describes urodynamic tests and their

The opinions or assertions contained herein are the private views of the authors and are not to be construed as reflecting the views of the Department of the Army or the Department of Defense.

[a] Department of Obstetrics and Gynecology, University of Iowa Carver College of Medicine, University of Iowa Hospitals and Clinics, 200 Hawkins Drive, Iowa City, IA 52242, USA
[b] Department of Epidemiology, University of Iowa College of Public Health, 200 Hawkins Drive, Iowa City, IA 52242–1089, USA
[c] Department of Urology, University of Iowa Carver College of Medicine, University of Iowa Hospitals and Clinics, 200 Hawkins Drive, Iowa City, IA 52242–1089, USA
* Corresponding author. Department of Obstetrics and Gynecology, University of Iowa Carver College of Medicine, University of Iowa Hospitals and Clinics, 200 Hawkins Drive, Iowa City, IA 52242.
E-mail address: catherine-bradley@uiowa.edu (C.S. Bradley).

Gastroenterol Clin N Am 37 (2008) 539–552
doi:10.1016/j.gtc.2008.06.006 gastro.theclinics.com
0889-8553/08/$ – see front matter

parameters and discusses the role that urodynamic testing plays in the evaluation of common pelvic floor disorders.

ANATOMY AND INNERVATION OF THE BLADDER AND PELVIC FLOOR

Before discussing the urodynamic tests and their parameters, it is important to have a basic understanding of the anatomy and physiology of the bladder and pelvic floor. The lower urinary tract, including the bladder and urethra, must carry out both urine storage (bladder filling) and evacuation (micturition or bladder emptying) functions. The smooth muscle of the bladder walls (detrusor muscle) must relax during the filling phase and contract during micturition; and conversely, the smooth and striated portions of the urethra must contract during filling and relax during emptying. The bladder and urethra are intimately related to structures of the pelvic floor; consequently, optimal bladder function depends not only on an intact lower urinary neuromuscular system, but also on a well-functioning pelvic floor that provides adequate anatomic support.[8]

The supportive functions of the pelvic floor are performed by both muscular and connective tissue components. The pelvic floor muscles are the levator ani (including the puborectalis, pubococcygeus, and iliococcygeus) and coccygeus muscles. These muscles are attached laterally along the pelvic sidewalls, creating a hammock-like sling between the pubis and coccyx. The levator ani muscle is tonically contracted, providing a firm posterior shelf to support the pelvic contents and aid with urinary continence.[8] The connective tissue of the pelvic floor, sometimes called "endopelvic fascia," is a loose network of connective tissue, small vessels, lymphatics, and nerves, which surrounds and supports the pelvic organs and the vagina through its connections to the pelvic floor muscles.

Bladder filling and voiding functions are controlled by closely coordinated autonomic and somatic neurologic pathways.[9] The autonomic controls of the bladder include sympathetic and parasympathetic functions. The sympathetic (thoracolumbar) nerves promote urine storage by relaxing the detrusor muscle and contracting smooth muscle in the bladder neck and urethra. These nerves are inhibited during voiding. In contrast, parasympathetic (sacral) nerves cause the detrusor muscle to contract and are stimulated during micturition. The somatic nervous system controls the striated external urethral sphincter and levator ani muscle through the pudendal nerve and the sacral nerve roots (S2–S4). Inhibition of these nerves causes relaxation of the bladder outlet and pelvic floor, which must occur during voiding. The central nervous system provides voluntary control and modification of micturition reflexes.

COMPONENTS OF URODYNAMICS

Lower urinary tract dysfunction is often categorized into disorders of bladder storage and disorders of bladder emptying. Various urodynamic tests may aid in the evaluation of one or both functions. Individual urodynamic tests include cystometry, uroflowmetry, pressure flow studies, electromyography (EMG), and videourodynamics. In practice, several or all of these components are often combined and performed together as "urodynamic testing."

Cystometry

Cystometry refers to the measurement of intravesical bladder pressure during bladder filling, and most consider it the cornerstone of urodynamic testing.[10] Several standard parameters are evaluated during a cystometrogram including bladder storage pressure, capacity, sensation, bladder stability, and compliance.

In preparation for this phase of urodynamics, both urethral and rectal (or vaginal) catheters are placed. The bladder is then filled with contrast, saline, or water through the urethral catheter, and several parameters are continuously measured. The direct measurement of bladder pressure during cystometry, or intra vesical pressure (Pves), reflects the total pressure within the bladder. This is defined as the sum of the pressure within the bladder caused by "bladder wall events," or detrusor pressure (Pdet), and the pressure exerted on the bladder by external sources, or intra-abdominal pressure (Pabd). Pabd is measured by the rectal catheter. The actual pressure within the bladder caused by "bladder wall events," or Pdet, is not a directly measurable entity, and is calculated by subtracting Pabd from Pves.[10] A typical videourodynamic setup illustrating these parameters is shown in **Fig. 1**.

Bladder sensation during filling is studied by questioning the patient during the test. Sensation during cystometry is subjective, and can be influenced by the rate of filling; temperature of the fluid medium; position of the patient (supine versus upright); and the patient's level of concentration. Determining the volumes at which different degrees of fullness occur, and the report of pain during filling, and evidence of decreased sensation during filling may all be subtle predictors of disease processes. The greatest value of the cystometrogram with respect to sensation occurs when a symptom arises, and sensation is correlated to actual Pves changes.[11]

Bladder capacity that is measured during urodynamics, or the maximum cystometric capacity, reflects the volume at which a subject with normal bladder sensation can no longer delay voiding.[12] This measurement is different from the functional bladder capacity, which is usually determined by the voiding diary, and the maximum anesthetic capacity, which is obtained under anesthesia.

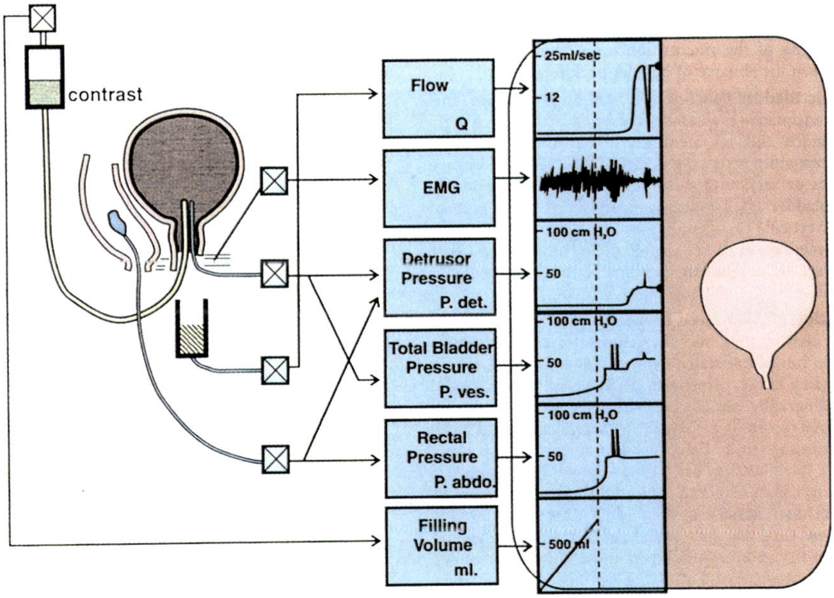

Fig. 1. Schematic of video-urodynamic setup, illustrating commonly monitored variables. (*From* Peterson AC, Webster GD. Urodynamic and videourodynamic evaluation of voiding dysfunction. In: Wein AJ, Kavoussi LR, Novick AC, et al, editors. Campbell-Walsh urology. Philadelphia: WB Saunders; 2007. p. 1990; with permission.)

A "stable" bladder refers to the accommodation of increasing bladder volumes without evidence of an involuntary detrusor contraction, or detrusor overactivity. According to the most recent definition from the International Continence Society (ICS), detrusor overactivity is an observation of involuntary detrusor contractions during urodynamics, which may be either spontaneous or provoked.[12] Detrusor overactivity is demonstrated on a cystometrogram tracing in **Fig. 2**.

Bladder compliance is another important parameter that can be measured during cystometry. Compliance (C) has been described simply as the "inverse of stiffness," and is formally defined as the change in bladder pressure for a given change in volume.[13] Compliance is calculated by dividing the volume change (V) by the Pdet (C = V/Pdet) and is expressed as milliliter per centimeter of H_2O.[10] A normal bladder displays low pressures during filling because of its spherical shape and viscoelastic

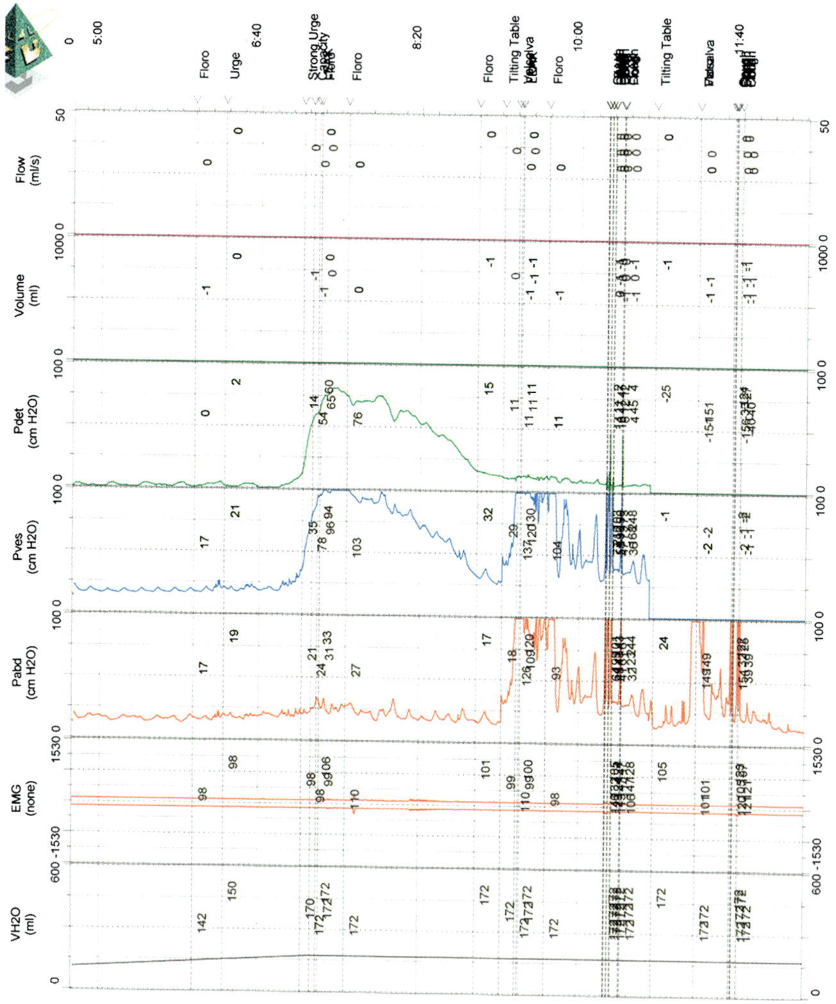

Fig. 2. The cystometrogram of a 72-year-old woman who presented with urinary incontinence symptoms. Detrusor overactivity (an involuntary bladder contraction) is seen and is illustrated by an abrupt rise in Pdet and Pves, without rise in Pabd.

properties. Loss of elasticity results from replacement of the muscle with collagen, and can be caused by a number of disease processes including neurologic conditions, prolonged catheter drainage, radiation therapy, prior pelvic or urethral surgery, interstitial cystitis, and obstructive uropathy.[13] A poorly compliant bladder displays an abnormal, often linear increase in Pdet during filling (**Fig. 3**). This can result in dangerously high detrusor storage pressures. High storage pressures can distort the normal detrusor anatomy resulting in the development of vesicoureteral reflux, and can be transmitted to the upper tracts, causing the development of hydronephrosis and renal failure. Early studies by McGuire and associates[14] have shown that sustained Pdet greater than 40 cm H_2O is specifically linked to renal or upper tract damage.

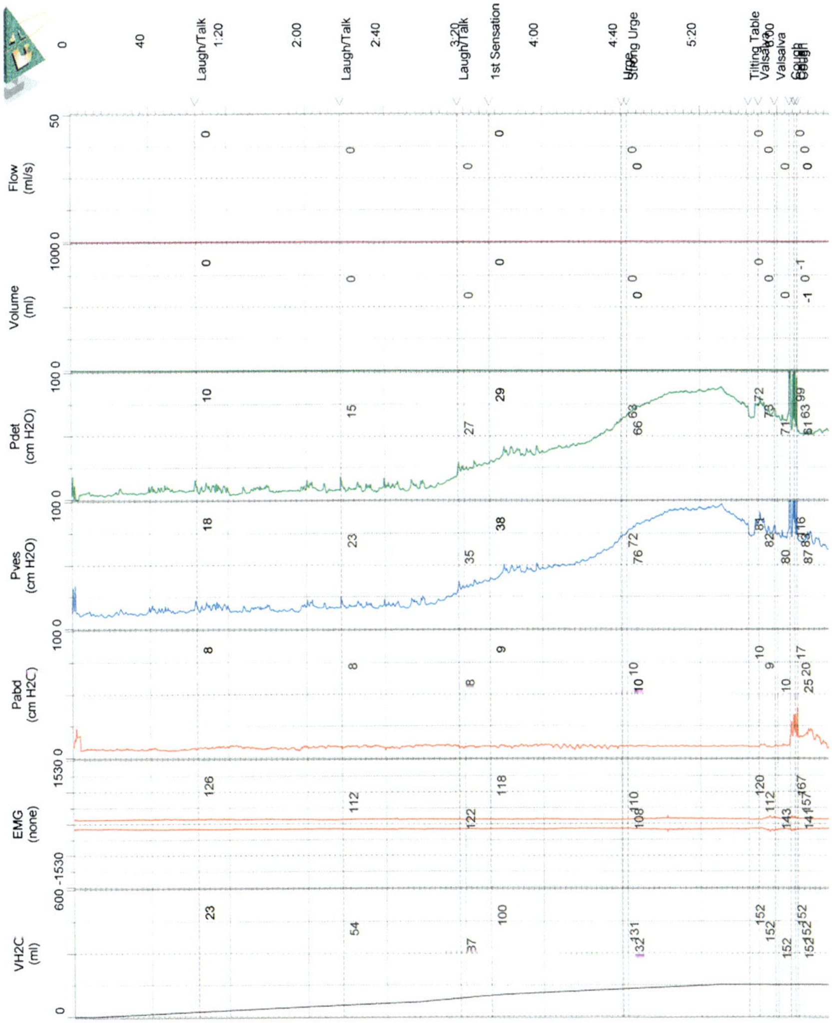

Fig. 3. The cystometrogram of a 63-year-old woman with history of abdominoperineal resection and adjuvant chemotherapy and radiation therapy for rectal cancer, who presented with elevated creatinine and severe bilateral hydronephrosis. The tracing demonstrates a poorly compliant bladder, with high detrusor storage pressures (seen in Pdet and Pves).

Lastly, bladder compliance can be calculated using two standard points: the Pdet at the start of filling with the corresponding bladder volume; and the Pdet and volume at cystometric capacity, or before the start of any detrusor contraction that causes any significant leakage.[12] Many clinicians, however, rely less on the actual calculated value of compliance and more on the actual bladder pressure during filling, because compliance can vary depending on the volume over which it is calculated.[11]

Uroflowmetry

Uroflowmetry is one of the most commonly used forms of urodynamic testing. It is a noninvasive test that measures the rate of urine flow over time. Uroflowmetry involves a well-hydrated patient voiding into a uroflowmeter, which in turn generates a "flow curve." The flow curve is plotted with the urine flow on the y-axis and time on the x-axis. **Fig. 4** demonstrates a typical uroflowmetry curve. Uroflowmetry is extremely useful as a screening test, especially to determine which patients may need further testing with more formal urodynamics, although it cannot determine the exact cause of a patient's voiding dysfunction.[15]

There are several important variables to consider when interpreting the results of a uroflow test. First, the voided volume influences the validity of the test, because peak flow rates vary with the volume voided.[10] For example, a voided volume less than 150 mL may indicate an invalid test, because flow patterns and parameters are inaccurate below this volume. Also, the voiding of a very large volume may lead to an abnormal flow test result in a patient with no significant pathology. This results from overstretching of the detrusor muscle, which can cause an inefficient contraction.

Next, maximum flow, or Qmax, is the maximum measured rate of flow, and can be determined by evaluating the flow curve during uroflowmetry (see **Fig. 4**).[10] Qmax can be influenced by a number of factors, including age, gender, and volume voided. One must interpret this value in the setting of additional clinical information. For example, flow rates in men decrease with age. Also, women generate higher flow rates on average than men because of the presence of a shorter urethra, which offers less resistance.[10] Finally, there can be variability among uroflow tests in the same patient, depending on several factors, including time of day, hydration status, and even "learning" by repetition. It is important to repeat an abnormal test on a patient who is being considered for surgery or invasive therapy.

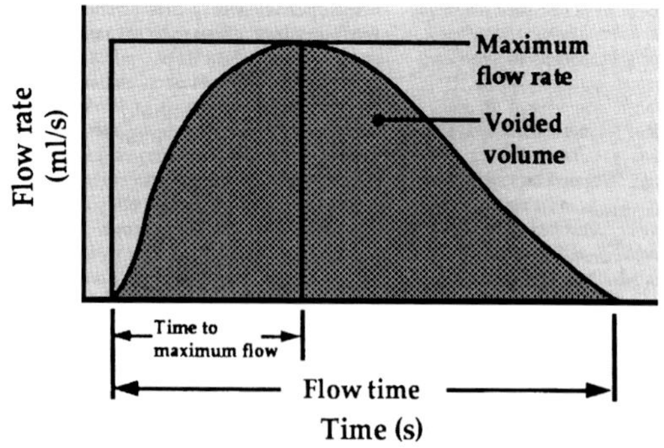

Fig. 4. Schematic of a normal uroflowmetry curve, with flow rates measured over time. Note Qmax (maximum flow rate) at peak of curve and normal "bell-shaped" flow pattern. (*From* Peterson AC, Webster GD. Urodynamic and videourodynamic evaluation of voiding dysfunction. In: Wein AJ, Kavoussi LR, Novick AC, et al, editors. Campbell-Walsh urology. Philadelphia: WB Saunders; 2007. p. 2001; with permission.)

Finally, the pattern of flow is also important to consider when evaluating uroflow data, although this may be subject to the interpretation of the individual clinician because there is no standard against which to compare these patterns. Flow patterns can be described in various ways, such as "intermittent," which may indicate obstruction. Abnormal uroflowmetry results are often further evaluated using a more invasive test, typically a pressure flow study.

Pressure Flow Studies

Although uroflow studies are good screening tests for identifying patients with low flow rates or abnormal voiding patterns, they cannot identify whether this is caused by outlet obstruction or poor detrusor contractility. Pressure flow studies are useful in determining a patient's voiding mechanism and the cause that underlies abnormal voiding. Pressure flow studies combine uroflowmetry with simultaneous measurement of Pdet, and require placement of a rectal (or vaginal) catheter for Pabd measurement, and a urethral catheter, which measures Pves and allows the calculation of Pdet during voiding. The bladder is filled until the patient feels sufficiently full, and then the patient is asked to void. By measuring the Pdet during voiding, specifically at maximum flow, one can determine whether poor flow is caused by obstruction (high pressures) or whether it is caused by detrusor failure (low or absent Pdet). Similar to noninvasive uroflowmetry, flow rates (including Qmax) and the pattern of flow are also evaluated during pressure flow studies.

Whereas outlet obstruction may be seen frequently in men because of an enlarged prostate, in women it is most likely caused by pelvic organ prolapse, as a complication after surgery for stress incontinence, or from pelvic floor or external sphincter pathology, such as detrusor sphincter dyssynergia. **Fig. 5** is a pressure flow study from a female patient demonstrating bladder outlet obstruction occurring after a pubovaginal sling procedure performed for stress incontinence.

Electromyography

EMG is an additional part of standard urodynamic testing that can be performed during cystometry and during the pressure flow study to evaluate the striated urethral sphincter and pelvic floor. EMG monitoring is most commonly done with either perineal surface-patch electrodes or needle electrodes. Needle electrodes (the gold standard) are able to isolate electrical activity from specific muscle fibers within a 0.5-mm radius of the tip.[16,17] They are, however, invasive, uncomfortable, and can be easily dislodged with movement. Use of patch electrodes has the benefit of being essentially noninvasive, with a patch being placed on the perineum, but some argue that the signal source may be inferior.[16]

Although the striated urethral sphincter and levator ani are located in close proximity, they are anatomically and neurologically discontinuous.[18] Perineal surface measurements may not accurately reflect striated sphincter activity, but a compounding of motor unit signals from all muscles of the pelvic floor. A recent study evaluated patch versus needle electrodes during pressure flow studies, and found that needle electrode EMG was more often interpretable, and showed motor unit quiescence of the external sphincter more often, suggesting that the signal obtained from the pelvic floor musculature in the region may mask the actual signal obtained from the external sphincter.[17] Needle electrodes have been found to be more reliable in evaluating the urethral sphincter.

As with other aspects of urodynamics, it is important to recognize normal findings on EMG to interpret abnormal findings. A normal EMG study essentially rules out a neurologic cause in a patient's voiding dysfunction; however, an abnormal EMG

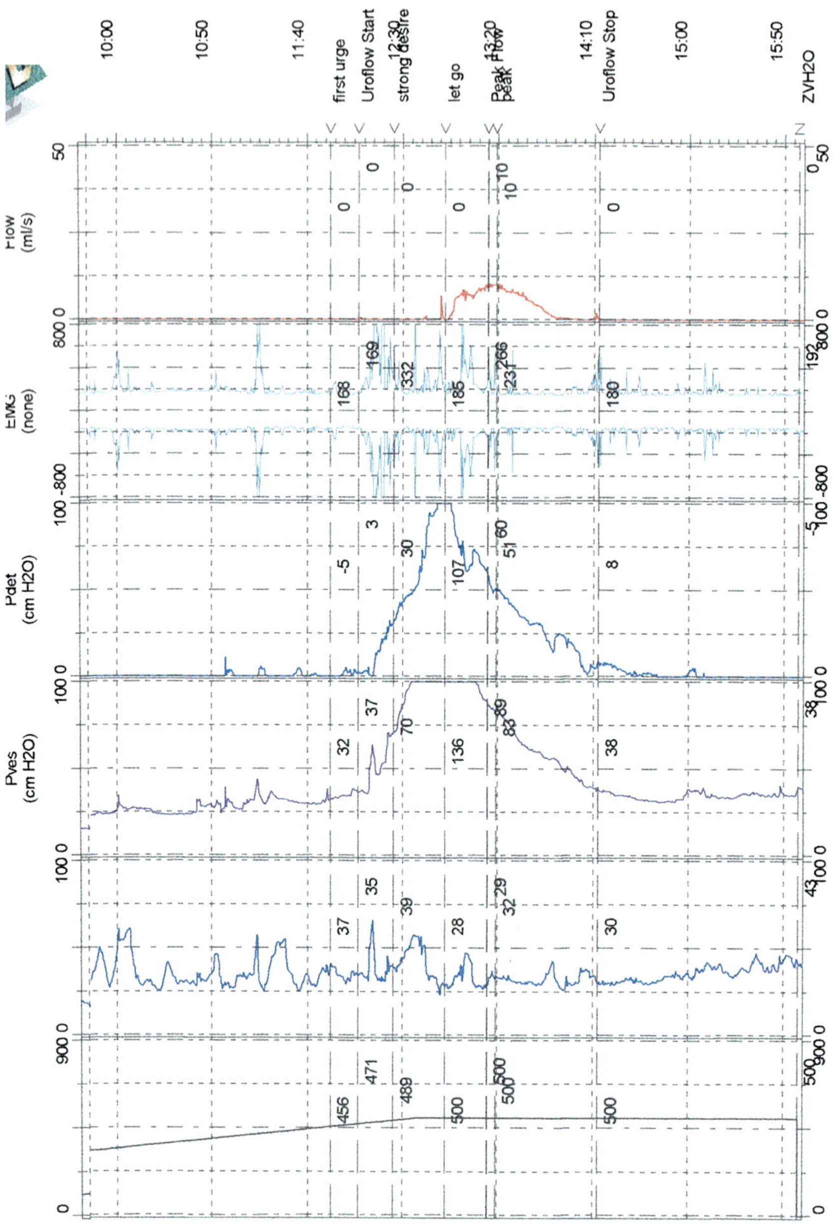

Fig. 5. A 54-year-old woman presented with new voiding complaints after pubovaginal sling surgery. Pressure flow study demonstrated high detrusor pressure, low flow, and incomplete bladder emptying (Pdet = 60 cm H_2O, Qmax = 10 mL/s, and postvoid residual = 100 mL).

study may signify that further work-up is warranted. For example, low-level firing of EMG is seen in normal subjects at rest, and it increases in amplitude and frequency with increases in Pabd, such as with coughing and laughing, and with bladder filling.[16] Patients may also exhibit an increased EMG activity during an involuntary detrusor contraction if they voluntarily try to contract their pelvic muscles to prevent leakage. Silence of the EMG signals is believed to be the first recognizable sign of the onset of micturition and should remain that way throughout flow.

Evaluation of the pelvic floor and external sphincter musculature by EMG is an integral component of the work-up of patients with obstructive voiding complaints to rule out sphincter or pelvic floor muscle dysfunction. Dysfunctional voiding is characterized by an intermittent flow rate caused by involuntary intermittent contractions of the periurethral striated muscle or pelvic floor during voiding in neurologically normal individuals.[12] In those patients with suspected bladder outlet obstruction caused by an anatomic source (eg, pelvic organ prolapse), evaluation with EMG during voiding is important to rule out sphincteric dysfunction. Patients with an underlying and undiagnosed neurologic disorder may also display urethral sphincter dysfunction, and may present with either irritative or obstructive voiding complaints. In the setting of neurologic disease, this abnormal EMG finding is termed "detrusor sphincter dyssynergia," and is defined as a detrusor contraction concurrent with an involuntary contraction of the urethral or periurethral striated muscle, which may prevent flow of urine.[12] Urodynamically, detrusor sphincter dyssynergia is seen as a confluence of large amplitude EMG spikes during flow, and can occur in patients with neurologic disorders, such as multiple sclerosis and suprasacral spinal cord injury.[9] In a patient without a known neurologic diagnosis, suspected detrusor sphincter dyssynergia should signal the physician that further work-up is warranted to exclude a neurologic etiology.

Video Urodynamics

Videourodynamic evaluation, which combines the use of fluoroscopy with the measurement of bladder and urethral pressures during cystometry or the pressure flow study, is desirable when simultaneous evaluation of structure and function is necessary to make a precise diagnosis.[19] Videourodynamics may be especially helpful in the work-up of urinary incontinence associated with pelvic organ prolapse (discussed later). It is also useful in the evaluation of voiding dysfunction, specifically to identify the presence of vesicoureteral reflux caused by poor bladder compliance. If reflux occurs at low volumes, it may act as a "pop-off mechanism," which may prevent elevation of a patient's Pdet on the urodynamic tracing. This phenomenon may go unnoticed without use of fluoroscopy. Bladder diverticula caused by chronic bladder outlet obstruction may also result in an artificially low Pdet during voiding and may not be recognized during urodynamics without fluoroscopy.

URODYNAMICS IN THE EVALUATION OF PELVIC FLOOR DISORDERS

Indications

Urodynamic tests may provide a better understanding of the underlying pathophysiologic mechanisms of urinary disorders. Although often considered an essential part of the evaluation and management of patients with lower urinary tract symptoms, the clinical use of urodynamics has not yet been clearly demonstrated.[20] Experts agree that the validity of urodynamics is linked to the patient's symptoms and the ability to reproduce those symptoms during the testing session. Urodynamic test results should also be interpreted alongside information obtained from the entire clinical evaluation, which includes symptom observation, medical history, physical examination, voiding diary, and other selected tests. When evaluating a patient with voiding dysfunction, it is important to have a specific set of questions in mind before performing urodynamics. As with any test, one should know what information one wants to obtain from the test before its execution, and the limitations of the test.

Urodynamic tests are not necessary in the evaluation of every patient with lower urinary tract symptoms. For instance, urodynamic tests are not recommended in the initial evaluation of uncomplicated female urinary incontinence when conservative treatments are planned.[20,21] Urodynamic tests should be performed in cases with complex features, when diagnosis is difficult, and before more invasive therapy is considered.[20]

Indications for urodynamic testing in women with urinary incontinence include the following:

- Urinary complaints with complex features
  - Incomplete bladder emptying
  - Prior anti-incontinence surgery
  - Symptomatic pelvic organ prolapse
  - Associated neurologic condition
- Before initiating invasive therapy
- Symptoms do not correlate with objective findings
- Failure to improve after initial treatment.

Stress Urinary Incontinence and Pelvic Organ Prolapse

Provocative cystometry is the key urodynamic test for the evaluation of stress urinary incontinence symptoms. According to the ICS terminology report,[12] urodynamic stress incontinence (previously "genuine stress incontinence") is the observation of urethral leakage during increased abdominal pressure, in the absence of a detrusor contraction. Studies suggest that cystometry has varying sensitivity and specificity for the symptom of stress incontinence, depending on whether other symptoms (often mixed urinary incontinence) are present. One review reported that the symptom of stress incontinence had a 56% positive predictive value for pure urodynamic stress incontinence and 79% for urodynamic stress incontinence with other abnormalities.[22]

In addition to the observation of urodynamic stress incontinence, urethral parameters measured during cystometry may be used to aid in determining prognosis and in patient counseling. A urethral pressure profile may be measured at rest with a urethral catheter by slowly withdrawing the catheter while measuring pressures. The maximum urethral closure pressure, identified during a urethral pressure profile, represents the highest pressure along the functional length of the urethra. The maximum urethral closure pressure has been reported to correlate with stress incontinence severity and with surgical outcomes in some studies, but not in others, and the reproducibility of urethral pressure profile parameters is poor.[20] If leakage is present, abdominal or Valsalva leak point pressures can be measured, representing the Pves at which urine leakage occurs because of increased abdominal pressure in the absence of a detrusor contraction.[12,23] Leak point pressures have been used to assign broad categories of stress incontinence, which may be used to guide treatment. Because leak point pressures are performed during stress maneuvers and maximum urethral closure pressure measured at rest, the leak point pressures may more accurately reflect the pathophysiologic processes associated with stress incontinence.[20] Research using leak point pressures is limited, however, by a lack of standardized definitions and techniques, and because data on reproducibility are sparse.[20]

The use of urodynamics plus fluoroscopy, or videourodynamics, is often useful in the evaluation of both urinary incontinence and prolapse. Under fluoroscopy, the urethra and bladder base are observed during the filling phase, looking specifically for whether or not the bladder neck is closed at rest, and for the position of the bladder in relation to the pubic symphysis. If significant prolapse exists, it may be necessary either to obtain fluoroscopic images with the patient in the oblique position to determine whether urethral hypermobility is present, or to repeat the images with either pessary or vaginal pack reduction of the prolapse. During stress maneuvers (straining and coughing), the bladder neck and urethra are evaluated for opening and leakage. The presence and degree of prolapse may also be assessed. **Fig. 6** demonstrates the use of fluoroscopy during cystometry in a woman with a cystocele (anterior vaginal wall prolapse).

Women with severe prolapse may not have stress incontinence symptoms, but may develop them when the prolapse is reduced. Many recommend that urodynamic testing be performed in women with moderate to severe pelvic organ prolapse to evaluate for "occult" stress incontinence before surgery and to identify which patients should have a concurrent incontinence surgery at time of their prolapse repair. In such patients, cystometry may be performed with the prolapse reduced using a pessary, vaginal pack, or speculum. "Occult" stress incontinence is demonstrated when the patient does not leak on urodynamics without reduction of the prolapse, but demonstrates urodynamic stress incontinence when the prolapse is reduced (see **Fig. 6**). Although most studies report high rates of occult stress incontinence among women with severe prolapse, it is unclear whether treatment outcomes are altered when these urodynamic techniques are performed. One study found that urodynamic testing before prolapse surgery was not cost-effective.[24] A review of the literature by the Third International Consultation on Incontinence found that there is no reliable test that can demonstrate which patients with prolapse are at risk for postoperative incontinence.[20]

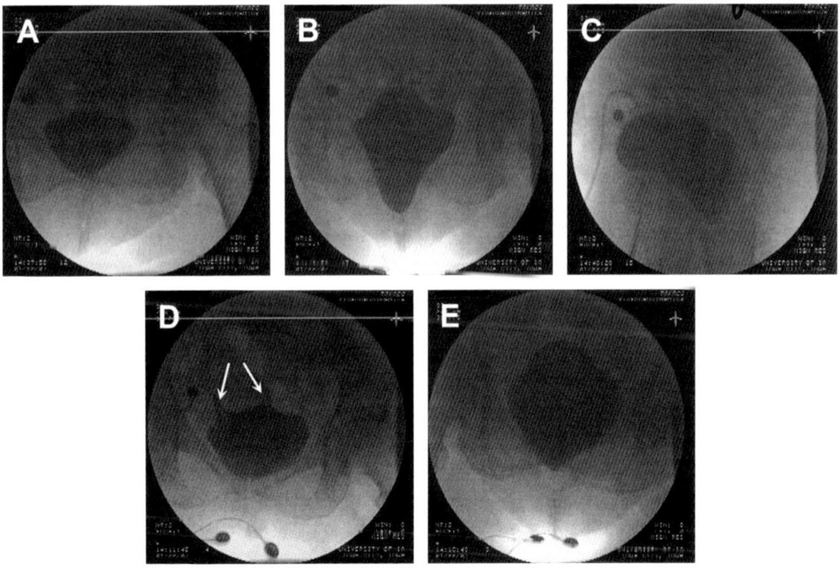

Fig. 6. A 71-year-old female patient presented with urge urinary incontinence and vaginal bulge symptoms. Fluoroscopic images taken during cystometry are shown, including rest (*A*), Valsalva (*B*), and oblique (*C*) perspectives. During cystometry, no urodynamic stress incontinence was initially demonstrated, but when the prolapse was reduced with a pessary (*D; arrows*), leakage was seen during Valsalva (*E*), consistent with "occult" stress incontinence.

Overactive Bladder

In 2002, the ICS defined overactive bladder as a symptom-based condition characterized by "urgency, with or without urge incontinence, usually with frequency and nocturia," in the absence of other etiologies.[12] This definition focuses on urgency, rather than urge incontinence, because it is increasingly recognized that approximately two thirds of patients with overactive bladder do not have urge incontinence.[25]

Overactive bladder symptoms are, however, poor predictors of urodynamic detrusor overactivity. Some studies suggest that sensitivity of clinical diagnosis is better than that obtained with urodynamic testing, because greater than 50% of patients with a subjective history of urge urinary incontinence have normal urodynamic studies[26] and, conversely, detrusor overactivity may be observed on cystometry in about 10% of asymptomatic women.[20] Given this, the Third International Consultation on Incontinence recommends that invasive urodynamic testing is not needed before instituting conservative therapies in patients with uncomplicated overactive bladder and urge incontinence (no symptoms of voiding difficulties).[20] Similar to the evaluation of stress urinary incontinence symptoms, urodynamics are recommended in complex cases.

If symptoms are not improved with typical conservative therapies, urodynamics should be pursued to rule out other causes of incontinence, including poor compliance and occult stress incontinence. Furthermore, evaluation of the pelvic floor by EMG may identify dysfunctional voiding, an entity that may respond well to biofeedback.

Neurologic Lesions

Normal storage and evacuation of urine requires a complex interplay among neural centers in the spinal cord, supraspinal, and peripheral nerve centers. Interruption or insult at any level can cause voiding dysfunction, and the complex symptoms resulting from neurologic lesions and disorders generally deserve full characterization using urodynamic tests.[20] Characteristic urodynamic findings may be seen, depending on the type of neurologic lesion (eg, suprapontine, suprasacral, or sacral) involved.

SUMMARY

Urodynamic testing plays an important role in the evaluation of women with pelvic floor disorders, including stress urinary incontinence, pelvic organ prolapse, and overactive bladder, especially in patients in whom conservative treatment efforts have failed. Urodynamic tests, which may include cystometry, uroflowmetry, pressure flow studies, EMG, or videourodynamics, can be used to provide objective measurements of lower urinary tract and pelvic floor function and to suggest underlying etiologies for bothersome lower urinary tract symptoms.

REFERENCES

1. Varma M, Brown J, Creasman J, et al. Fecal incontinence in females older than age 40 years: who is at risk? Dis Colon Rectum 2006;49:841–51.
2. Roberts RO, Jacobsen SJ, Reilly WT, et al. Prevalence of combined fecal and urinary incontinence: a community-based study. J Am Geriatr Soc 1999;47:837–41.
3. Markland AD, Kraus SR, Richter HE, et al. Prevalence and risk factors of fecal incontinence in women undergoing stress incontinence surgery. Am J Obstet Gynecol 2007;197:662.e1–662.e7.

4. Arya LA, Novi JM, Shaunik A, et al. Pelvic organ prolapse, constipation, and dietary fiber intake in women: a case-control study. Am J Obstet Gynecol 2005; 192:1687–91.
5. Morgan DM, DeLancey JO, Guire KE, et al. Symptoms of anal incontinence and difficult defecation among women with prolapse and a matched control cohort. Am J Obstet Gynecol 2007;197:509.e1–509.e6.
6. Peters WA III, Smith MR, Drescher CW. Rectal prolapse in women with other defects of pelvic floor support. Am J Obstet Gynecol 2001;184:1488–95.
7. Altman D, Zetterstrom J, Schultz I, et al. Pelvic organ prolapse and urinary incontinence in women with surgically managed rectal prolapse: a population-based case-control study. Dis Colon Rectum 2006;49:28–35.
8. DeLancey JO. Anatomy of the female bladder and urethra. In: Bent AE, Ostergard DR, Cundiff GW, editors. Ostergard's urogynecology and pelvic floor dysfunction. 5th edition. Philadelphia: Lippincott Williams & Wilkins; 2003. p. 3–18.
9. Benson JT, Walters MD. Neurophysiology and pharmacology of the lower urinary tract. In: Walters MD, Karram MM, editors. Urogynecology and reconstructive surgery. Philadelphia: Mosby Elsevier; 2007. p. 31–43.
10. Webster GD, Kreder KJ. The neurourologic evaluation. In: Walsh PC, Retik AB, Vaughan ED, editors. Campbell's urology. 7th edition. Philadelphia: Saunders; 1998. p. 927–52.
11. Nitti VW. Cystometry and abdominal pressure monitoring. In: Nitti VW, editor. Practical urodynamics. Philadelphia: Saunders; 1998. p. 38–51.
12. Abrams P, Cardozo L, Fall M, et al. The standardization of terminology of lower urinary tract function: report from the Standardization Sub-committee of the International Continence Society. Am J Obstet Gynecol 2002;187:116–26.
13. Ghoniem G. Disorders of bladder compliance. In: Kursh ED, McGuire EJ, editors. Female urology. Philadelphia: Lippincott; 1994. p. 83–92.
14. McGuire EJ, Woodside JR, Borden TA, et al. Prognostic value of urodynamic testing in myelodysplastic patients. J Urol 1981;126:205–9.
15. Boone TB, Kim YH. Uroflowmetry. In: Nitti VW, editor. Practical urodynamics. Philadelphia: Saunders; 1998. p. 28–37.
16. O'Donnell PD. Electromyography. In: Nitti VW, editor. Practical urodynamics. Philadelphia: Saunders; 1998. p. 65–71.
17. Mahajan ST, Fitzgerald MP, Kenton K, et al. Concentric needle electrodes are superior to perineal surface-patch electrodes for electromyographic documentation of urethral sphincter relaxation during voiding. BJU Int 2006;97:117–20.
18. Brostrom S, Jennum P, Lose G. Motor evoked potentials from the striated urethral sphincter and puborectal muscle: normative values. Neurourol Urodyn 2003;22: 306–13.
19. McGuire EJ, Cespedes RD, Cross CA, et al. Videourodynamic studies. Urol Clin North Am 1996;23:309–21.
20. Griffiths D, Kondo A, Bauer S, et al. Dynamic testing. In: Abrams P, Cardozo L, Khoury S, editors. Incontinence (3rd International Consultation on Incontinence). Paris: Health Publications, Ltd; 2005. p. 585–674.
21. Fantl JA, Newman DK, Colling J, et al. Urinary incontinence in adults: acute and chronic management. Clinical Practice Guideline No. 2. Rockville (MD): Agency for Health Care Policy and Research; 1996. AHCPR publication no. 96-0682.
22. Harvey MA, Versi E. Predictive value of clinical evaluation of stress urinary incontinence: a summary of the published literature. Int Urogynecol J Pelvic Floor Dysfunct 2001;12:31–7.

23. Cespedes RD, McGuire EJ. Leak point pressures. In: Nitti VW, editor. Practical urodynamics. Philadelphia: Saunders; 1998. p. 94–107.
24. Weber AM, Walters MD. The cost-effectiveness of urodynamic testing before surgery for women with pelvic organ prolapse and stress urinary incontinence. Am J Obstet Gynecol 2000;183:1338–47.
25. Milsom I, Abrams P, Cardozo L, et al. How widespread are the symptoms of an overactive bladder and how are they managed? A population-based prevalence study. BJU Int 2001;87:760–6.
26. Colli E, Artibani W, Goka J, et al. Are urodynamic tests useful tools for the initial conservative management of non-neurogenic urinary incontinence? A review of the literature. Eur Urol 2003;43:63–9.

Radiologic Evaluation of Pelvic Floor Disorders

Celine Savoye-Collet, MD, PhD[a,b,*], Edith Koning, MD[a,b], Jean-Nicolas Dacher, MD, PhD[a,b]

KEYWORDS

- Pelvic floor disorders • Defecography • Anal endosonography
- MR-defecography

Pelvic floor disorders refer to a group of clinical conditions that include pelvic organ prolapse, urinary and fecal incontinence, chronic constipation, and pelvic pain. Various imaging modalities are available, including ultrasound (US), MRI, and defecography. Over the last decade there have been considerable advances in several imaging techniques. High-resolution US and MRI not only provide superior depiction of the pelvic anatomy but also help to understand pathology and functional changes. MRI can also be used for a multicompartmental dynamic assessment of the pelvic floor (dynamic MRI defecography) and for the analysis of the sphincters (static MRI). Because MRI has enormous potential, it underscores the need for an integrated evaluation of pelvic floor disorders that involves the radiologist and a multidisciplinary team.

This article focuses on defecography, anal US, and dynamic MRI by discussing normal and abnormal patterns and clinical use. Particular emphasis has been placed on the gastroenterologist's point of view.

DEFECOGRAPHY

Defecography (evacuation proctography) is a dynamic fluoroscopic examination (**Box 1**). It began in 1964 with Burhenne's[1] dynamic barium studies of the defecation process. Defecography examines the dynamic changes of the perineum and the evacuation of the anorectum. This test is indicated in patients with constipation to identify an outlet obstruction caused by either anatomic or functional disorder.[2–4] The procedure requires rectal opacification. Additionally, small bowel opacification, or in women

[a] Radiology Department, Rouen University Hospital Charles Nicolle, 1 Rue de Germont, F-76031 Rouen, France

[b] LITIS EA 4108, University of Rouen, Avenue de l'Universite, Technopole du Madrillet, F-76801 Saint Etienne du Rouvray, Rouen, France

* Corresponding author. Radiology Department, Rouen University Hospital Charles Nicolle, 1 Rue de Germont, F-76031 Rouen, France.

E-mail address: savoyecel@hotmail.com (C. Savoye-Collet).

Gastroenterol Clin N Am 37 (2008) 553–567
doi:10.1016/j.gtc.2008.06.004 gastro.theclinics.com

Box 1
Defecography in clinical practice

Defecography is contraindicated in young women during menstruation and pregnancy.

The exact procedure should be clearly explained to obtain full cooperation from the patient. A quiet radiology suite is important, and the patient should be hidden from the view of the technologist to provide privacy during the act of defecation.

When an enterocele is suspected, a barium meal is administered 1.5 hours before the examination. In women, vaginal opacification with barium is recommended before rectal opacification. The latter is performed with a mixture of 150 to 200 mL of barium and a starchy component.

First, a lateral view is taken in the upright position to localize the bony landmarks and to check the quality of the various opacifications (small bowel, vagina, and rectum). Next, the patient is seated on a special commode for filming the dynamic process of defecation. Dynamic images are performed at rest, during squeeze, and during straining.

The pubococcygeal line is drawn on the lateral view. Then, the distance between this line and the anorectal junction is measured. The exact measurement of the anorectal angle is somewhat controversial.

vaginal opacification, may be performed. If bladder dysfunction is suspected, a cystography can be performed along with defecography in a one-session examination (cystodefecography).[5,6]

Normal Findings

Normal patterns have been described.[7,8] At rest, the anorectal junction is located above the ischium. During squeezing, the anorectal junction is elevated and located less than 3.5 cm below the pubococcygeal line. During the defecation process, the puborectalis muscle opens widely without anal or rectal prolapse and the anorectal junction descends below the pubococcygeal line. A rectocele, less than 2.5 cm in size, is inconsequential provided it empties completely at the end of defecation.

Pathology and Clinical Use

Defecography can reveal several structural abnormalities. The most frequent abnormal findings are perineal descent at rest or during squeezing; rectocele (significant if >3.5 cm in depth and with residual barium at the end of defecation); rectal prolapse; paradoxical contraction of the puborectalis muscle (dyssynergia); enterocele; and sigmoidocele (**Figs. 1** and **2**).[9,10] Interobserver agreement was shown to be good for the diagnosis of rectocele and enterocele but inadequate for perineal descent.[2–4,11] Functional findings are also important. For example, an incomplete and prolonged contrast evacuation seems more specific of dyssynergia than an inappropriate puborectal contraction.

Defecography is indicated when some of the aforementioned abnormalities are clinically suspected, but not proved at clinical examination or in patients with an unexplained anorectal disorder. Defecography can be useful in cases of dyschezia (incomplete or difficult rectal emptying) when the patient did not respond to the first-line treatment (**Fig. 3**). It can also be discussed in patients incontinent for solid stools before surgery if a pelvic static disorder (eg, a rectal prolapse) is suspected. Finally, it can be performed in patients with pelvic pain to rule out an enterocele. Rectocele and severe rectal prolapse could lead to surgery. This test is especially important when surgical treatment is being considered for a problem, such as rectal prolapse.[12] The association of an enterocele can modify the surgical option. The relevance of

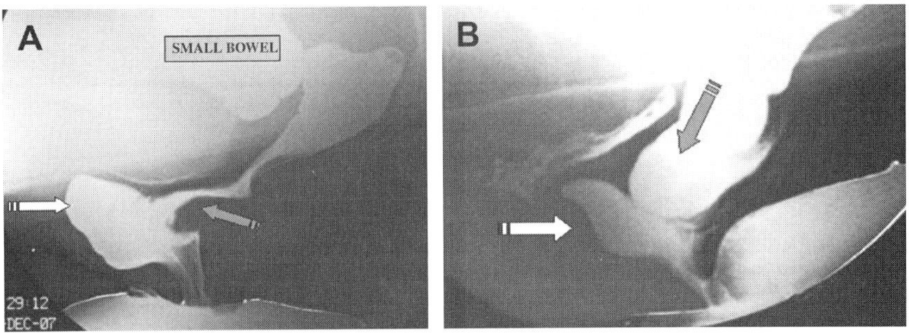

Fig. 1. Defecography: dynamic image drawn from the evacuation film (*A*). Anterior rectocele with residual barium storage (*white arrow*) associated with a paradoxical contraction of the puborectal muscle (*gray arrow*) (*B*). Anterior rectocele (*white arrow*) associated with an enterocele (*gray arrow*).

defecography findings, however, remains controversial.[2,13–16] In many instances, normal individuals show abnormal findings and hence the link between a clinical symptom and an abnormal defecography finding is difficult to establish.[3]

ULTRASONOGRAPHY

With the advent of the newest transducer technology, US imaging is gaining a key role in the understanding of pelvic floor disorders. The most commonly used technique is endoanal US but endovaginal and transperineal US techniques are being developed and represent potential new uses. Additionally, the use of three-dimensional software may provide an accurate diagnosis of complex diseases.

Anal Endosonography

Anal endosonography is a technique specially adapted for the examination of anal sphincters (**Box 2**). The main indication is the diagnosis of anal sphincter defect in

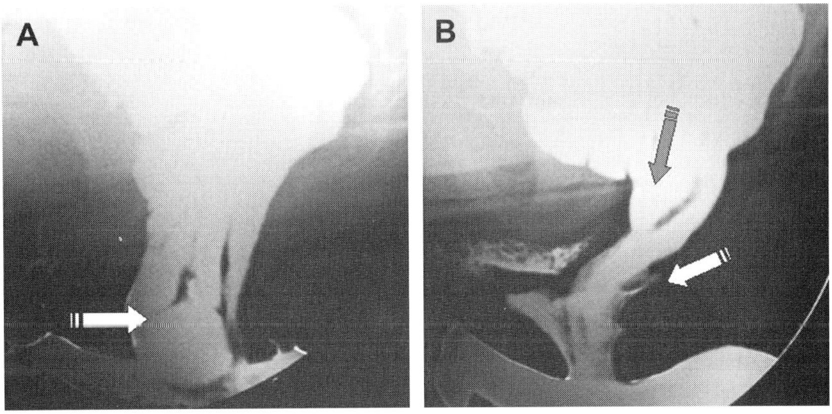

Fig. 2. Defecography: dynamic image drawn from the evacuation film. (*A*) Major enterocele (*arrow*) (*B*). Small enterocele (*gray arrow*) associated with moderate rectal procidence (*white arrow*).

Investigation	Indications	Expected Findings
DEFECOGRAPHY	**Difficult defecation/Dyschezia** unresponsive to initial treatment **Fecal incontinence (pre-op work up)** **Rectal prolapse** **Rectocele** **Unexplained pelvic pain** especially when enterocele is suspected	Internal rectal prolapse Rectocele, enterocele, sigmoidocele Pelvic floor descent Paradoxal puborectalis contraction Incomplete and prolonged contrast evacuation Poor Rectal Stripping
ANAL ENDOSONOGRAPHY	**Fecal incontinence** **After sphincteroplasty** if anal incontinence persists	External and/or internal anal sphincter defect Abnormality of external and/or internal anal sphincter thickness Postoperative status
MR DEFECOGRAPHY	**See defecography above** + **Evaluate global pelvic floor dysfunction**	See defecography above + Elytrocele Genito-urinary prolapse Abnormalities of the levator ani muscle
STATIC MR	**Fecal incontinence** **After sphincteroplasty** if anal incontinence persists	See anal endosonography above + Precise evaluation of external anal sphincter atrophy

Fig. 3. Summary table for the main imaging tests with their indications and expected findings.

the investigation of patients with fecal incontinence. Anal endosonography was first developed in the 1990s at Saint Mark's Hospital, London, UK.[17] It is also useful in the assessment of anal sepsis, anal cancer, and perineal pain.[18]

Normal Findings

A good knowledge of the anatomy of anal sphincters and pelvic floor is required. From the surface outward, several layers can be identified (**Fig. 4**). Mucosa and submucosa usually appear hyperechoic. The 2- to 3-mm thick internal anal sphincter (IAS) is in continuity with the circular muscular layer of the rectum. It is clearly delineated, homogeneously hypoechoic, and its thickness increases with age.[17,19–21] The hyperechoic longitudinal muscle layer of rectum is difficult to distinguish from the hyperechoic external anal sphincter (EAS).[20] At its upper part, the EAS is in continuity with the

Box 2
Anal endosonography in clinical practice

A rectal enema is recommended a few hours before the examination. An US machine equipped with an anorectal transducer (eg, Bruel and Kjaer) is required. The rigid cylindric transducer offers 360-degree high-resolution image with a frequency ranging from 6 to 16 MHz.

The patient is placed in the supine (or left lateral) position throughout the examination. The anal transducer is gently introduced and slowly withdrawn to obtain several images of the anal canal and surroundings: at the upper part of the anal canal the puborectalis muscle is identified, then both the external anal sphincter and internal anal sphincter are visible. Finally at the lower end, only the external anal sphincter is visible. The patient may be asked to contract voluntarily during the examination. Location and size of abnormalities are based on quadrants using a standard clock face, 12 o'clock being the anterior midline point. The external anal sphincter and internal anal sphincter thickness is also assessed.

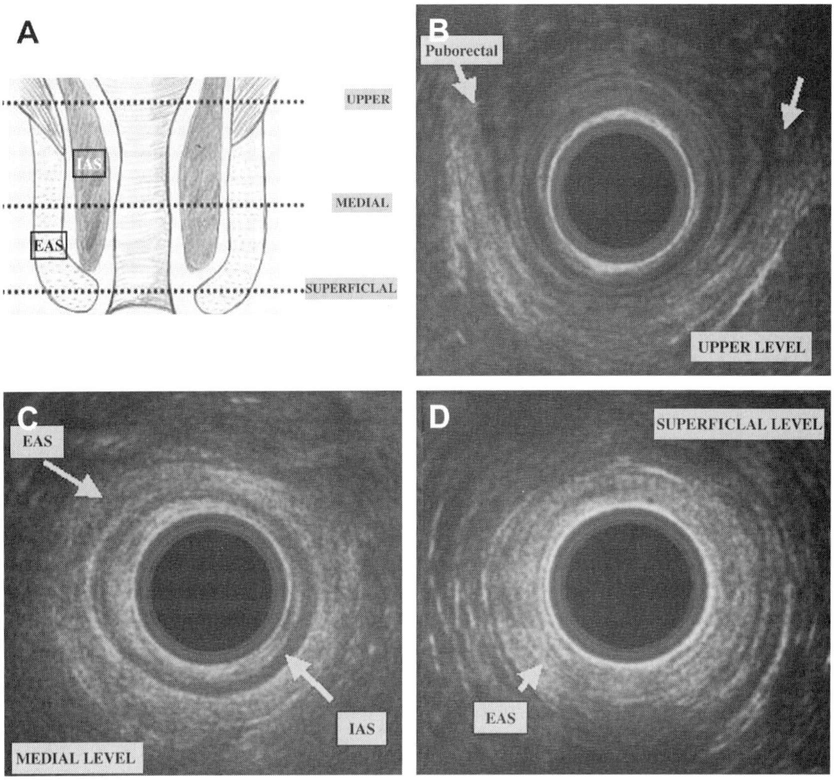

Fig. 4. Anal endosonography. (*A*) The anal canal in the coronal plane showing the internal (IAS) and external (EAS) anal sphincters. The three following different levels of anal endosonography (*B–D*) are shown (*dotted lines*). (*B*) Upper level showing the "U-shaped" puborectal muscle (*arrows*). (*C*) Medial level showing both the EAS (*superior arrow*) and IAS (*inferior arrow*). (*D*) Superficial level showing the EAS alone (*arrow*).

puborectalis muscle. It appears annular, thick, and symmetric in men and it is thinner and anteriorly opened in women.[19] Its subcutaneous part is highly hyperechoic. Its mean thickness is 6 to 8 mm.[22,23] Other elements can be identified: the "U-shaped" puborectalis muscle, the hypoechoic anococcygeal ligament, the ischioanal fatty spaces, the vagina, and the urethra.

Pathology and Clinical Use

Anal endosonography is commonly performed to identify an EAS or IAS defect that may cause fecal incontinence. An IAS defect is diagnosed based on a segmental loss of circumference and retraction of the torn ends (**Fig. 5**). An EAS defect is diagnosed based on a sharply delineated hypoechoic area that interrupts the normal echostructure (see **Fig. 5**). Both IAS and EAS defects can be present. The anterior part of the EAS in women needs to be analyzed carefully; it often appears thin and slightly heterogeneous because of its muscular insertion (tendinous arch of the pelvis). The anococcygeal ligament is responsible for a hypoechoic triangle, which should not be misdiagnosed as a pathologic defect.[24]

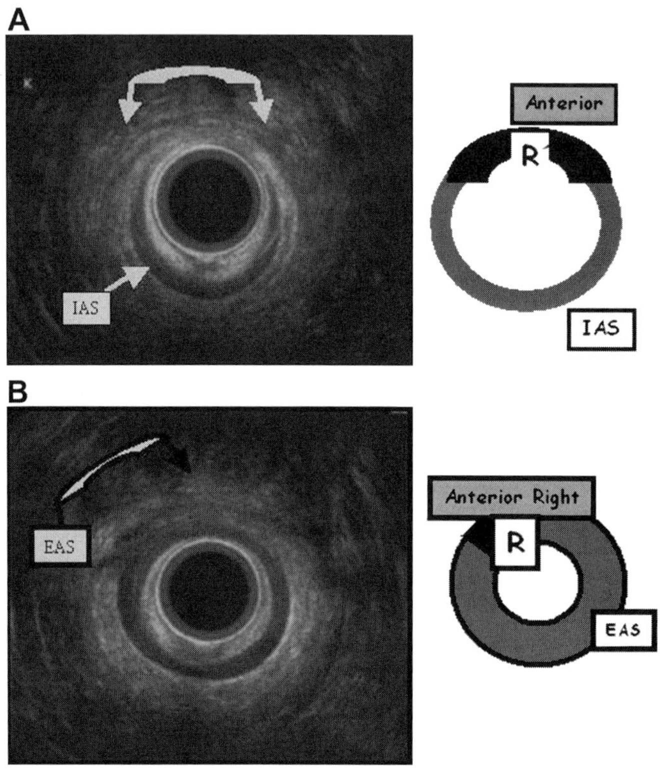

Fig. 5. Anal endosonography showing an anterior sphincter defect. (*A*) IAS defect with a posterior retraction of both ends. (*B*) EAS defect.

Anal endosonography can detect sphincter defects with great accuracy.[10,25] The sensitivity and specificity of anal endosonography for the diagnosis of anal sphincter defect is over 90%.[26,27] Obstetric trauma remains the main cause of sphincter disruption and represents a major health problem.[28] Anorectal trauma is a consequence of surgery for fistula in ano, hemorrhoids, or anal fissure. In these iatrogenic situations, the location of the defect correlates well with the surgical procedure.

Anal endosonography is clinically useful in patients with fecal incontinence when an anal sphincter disruption is suspected (see **Fig. 3**). Therapy can be directed based on US findings, such as the type (external or internal) and the size of the defect often expressed in degrees or percentage of the anal circumference. EAS defects that occupy less than 120 degrees of the anal circumference can be surgically corrected by overlapping sphincter repair.[29] Anal endosonography can also be performed after a sphincteroplasty to assess the morphology of the EAS and to correlate surgery with the functional results.[30,31] In patients with surgical repair of the EAS, the outcome was more favorable when there was evidence that the sphincter ends were overlapping.[30] Anal endosonography can accurately demonstrate abnormal IAS thickness because the borders of this smooth muscle are sharply limited.[32] In contrast, EAS atrophy is more difficult to identify by means of two-dimensional anal endosonography. Recently, three-dimensional anal endosonography has been described and seems promising.[32,33]

Endovaginal and Transperineal Ultrasonography

Pelvic floor dysfunction in women may occur secondary to morphologic and anatomic changes of the urogenital organs and these can be identified by perineal and transvaginal US.[34] US as part of the diagnostic work-up of stress urinary incontinence and urinary prolapse allows morphologic and dynamic assessment of the lower urinary tract. Anal sphincters can be analyzed by both approaches.[34,35]

Transperineal US, also called "translabial" or "introital" US, allows assessment of the bladder neck and urethral motility using a 5- to 7-MHz transducer.[36] For this test, the bladder should be full. The patient lies on her back and the probe is placed between the labia and gentle pressure is applied to the introitus and the external urethral orifice. The transducer axis corresponds to the body axis. The patient is asked to perform certain maneuvers (coughing and contraction of pelvic floor muscles) to evaluate the changes in position of the urethra and bladder.

Transvaginal US is a well-established procedure in gynecologic practice and can be useful. Here with the patient lying on her back, the transducer is gently applied to the dorsal vaginal wall. It provides very detailed information about the pelvic floor and in particular the area surrounding the urethral sphincter complex.

The aforementioned approaches are under clinical evaluation. There are no evidence-based data for their clinical use in patients with stress urinary incontinence or urinary prolapse.

DYNAMIC MRI DEFECOGRAPHY

In the assessment of pelvic floor disorders, MRI seems to be an innovative technique that does not expose the patient to ionizing radiation. Dynamic assessment of the pelvic floor is similar to defecography, but MRI overcomes some of the limitations of a radiograph examination. It can be performed either with a standard MRI machine or an open device that allows assessment of the subject in a seated position.[37–40] MRI defecography using a conventional MRI machine is a safe alternative for the diagnosis of clinically relevant abnormalities.[41] Real-time dynamic sequences are performed (dynamic MRI) for the analysis of the three compartments of the pelvis. A study of the rectal evacuation is also possible (MRI defecography) (**Box 3**).

MRI Normal Findings

All three compartments of the pelvis can be analyzed by dynamic MRI within one session. At rest, the anterior pelvic organs lie above that line. During straining, they are displaced posteriorly, but remain above the pubococcygeal line. The anorectal changes are similar to those observed with standard defecography. The muscles are directly visualized, however, especially the levator ani and its iliococcygeal and puborectalis portions (**Fig. 8**).

Pathology and Clinical Use

Several anomalies can be described by MRI (**Fig. 9**).[42] At the genitourinary level, various associations of prolapse can be identified. Two lines (pubococcygeal and pubohymenal) have to be drawn to differentiate between the normal and the prolapsed position of organs. Several classifications can be used similar to those used in practice. Regarding the posterior compartment, MRI findings can be grossly compared with those of standard defecography. MRI, however, provides additional information regarding the fatty spaces and muscles. Elytrocele or an abnormality of the levator ani muscle is easily identified by MRI. The analysis of the anorectal mucosa and the

Box 3
MRI defecography in clinical practice

First, one should check that there are no contraindications for the MRI test. An evacuating enema is recommended before the examination.

The cooperation and comfort of the subject is essential for a successful dynamic MRI examination. The patient receives instructions regarding the different maneuvers (rest, squeezing, straining). The bladder should not be emptied and may require further filling. A cloth is placed under the patient's buttocks to protect them on the MRI bed. In women, hydric sterile paste (eg, US jelly) is introduced into the vagina. The rectum is distended by 100 to 200 mL of hydric paste.

Two types of sequences are recorded by a pelvic coil. First, three-axis conventional T2-weighted sequences with a high spatial resolution are performed to assess morphologic changes. Second dynamic sagittal T2-weighted sequences are performed during maneuvers at rest, squeezing, and mild and maximum straining. Finally, a dynamic study of the rectal evacuation is performed using for example fast gradient-echo sequences with an image every 2 seconds. Images are reconstructed in real time and the patient is instructed and encouraged to expel the rectal contents (**Fig. 6**).

If necessary, the subject is asked to empty their bladder and rectum in a toilet and additional dynamic images are obtained during repeat straining maneuvers to enhance detection of other abnormalities. The total examination time is 20 to 25 minutes. Special marks are placed on images (eg, the inferior pubococcygeal and pubohymeneal lines) to enhance the understanding between the structural and functional changes of the pelvic floor (**Fig. 7**).

diagnosis of internal mucosal prolapse, however, remain a challenge. Caution is required when reporting, because an obvious prolapse can hide another one.

MRI can reveal the relative position of various pelvic organs during different maneuvers; the type and degree of anterior, medial, or posterior prolapse; and the morphology of the levator ani muscle. It also indicates the presence of an incidental lesion involving the uterus, ovaries, or digestive tract.[42] MRI is clinically relevant in patients who complain of dyschezia and do not respond to first-line treatment, or preoperatively when a pelvic static disorder is suspected (see **Fig. 3**). In patients suffering from fecal incontinence, MRI defecography has been shown to alter the surgical approach in 67% of cases.[40] Another indication of MRI is the global assessment of pelvic floor after urogenital surgery when new symptoms appear. MRI findings should be matched with the patient's symptoms and other clinical information to optimize treatment.

MRI of the pelvic floor is promising for several conditions, such as estimating the rectal mechanical properties, and these can be correlated with barostat findings and the anatomy of extrarectal structures.[43]

Static MRI

Another contribution of MRI in assessing pelvic floor disorders is the analysis of anal sphincters and their surrounding structures, especially in the clinical context of fecal incontinence.[44] Endoanal MRI technique permits multiplanar analysis and may provide high contrast, high spatial resolution imaging.[45] A disposable endoanal coil is well tolerated by most patients. After it is introduced, both axial T2-weighted fast spin echo and T1-weighted spin echo sequences are performed. An external phased-array coil, if used, prevents interference with physiology, but spatial resolution can deteriorate.[46] The IAS is visible on axial T2-weighted images as a sharply defined

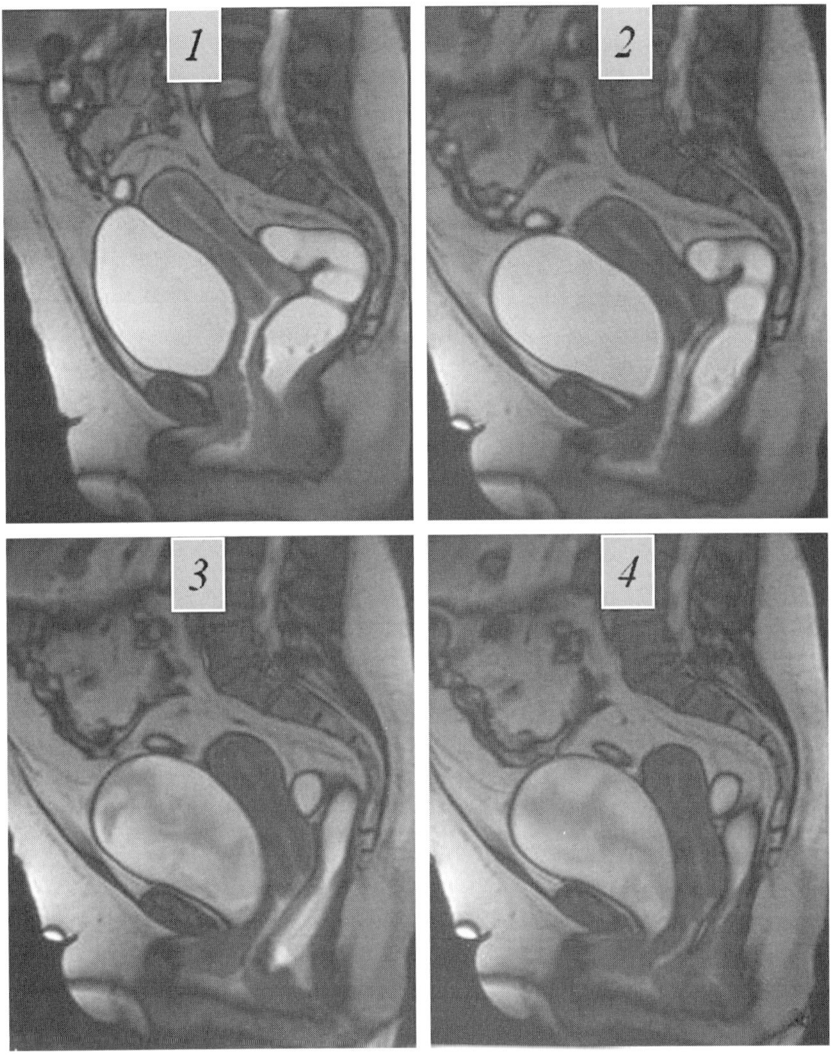

Fig. 6. Dynamic MRI defecography. Four dynamic consecutive images taken in the same woman during rectal evacuation: (*1*) squeeze, (*2*) anal sphincter opening, (*3* and *4*) rectal emptying.

hypersignal ring, whereas the EAS appears as a relatively hyposignal ring. Sphincter defects are defined by a disruption of the sphincter ring and scar tissue appears as a hyposignal deformation. EAS atrophy appears as global thinning or fatty replacement.[27]

There is lack of consensus as to whether endoanal MRI or US is superior for imaging the anal sphincter. In most studies, the yield of both techniques is comparable in detecting sphincter disruption. In others, MRI was less effective in showing IAS defects.[45] In contrast, endoanal MRI permits better identification of EAS atrophy.[27,47,48] Some authors believe that EAS atrophy could negatively affect continence after anterior anal sphincter repair.[27,45]

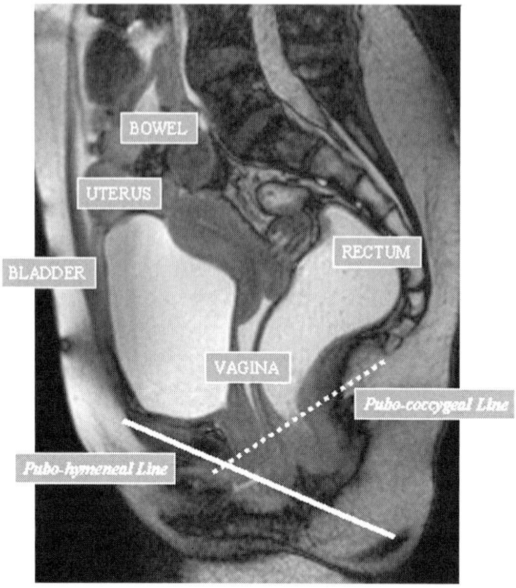

Fig. 7. Dynamic MRI defecography. Spontaneous visualization of bladder and small bowel. Vagina and rectum were opacified by hydric contrast. Sagittal view showing the pubococcygeal and pubohymeneal lines.

In women with chronic perineal pain, MRI can be used to identify pelvic venous dilatation. Such a diagnosis requires gadolinium-enhanced sequences. MRI can also be used for the detection of problems with sacral nerve roots by performing lumbosacral oriented sequences.

INTERVENTIONAL CT

CT is not commonly used for the diagnosis of pelvic floor disorders. This is related to the lack of contrast resolution of CT when compared with US or MRI. Moreover, CT examination exposes the patient to radiation. CT can provide useful information in

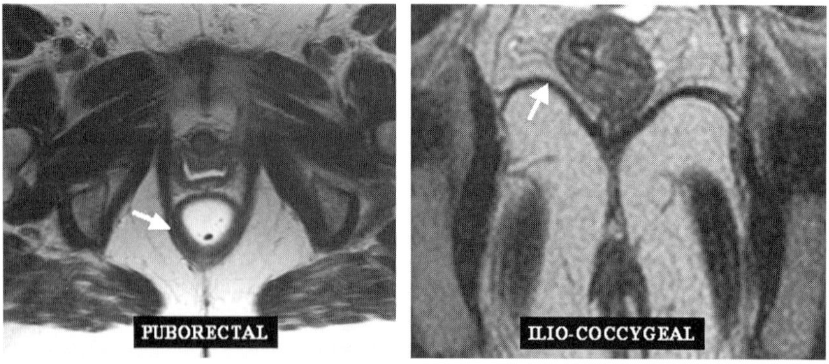

Fig. 8. Dynamic MRI defecography. Axial view showing the puborectal muscle (*arrow*) (*left*) and coronal view showing the iliococcygeal muscle (*arrow*) (*right*).

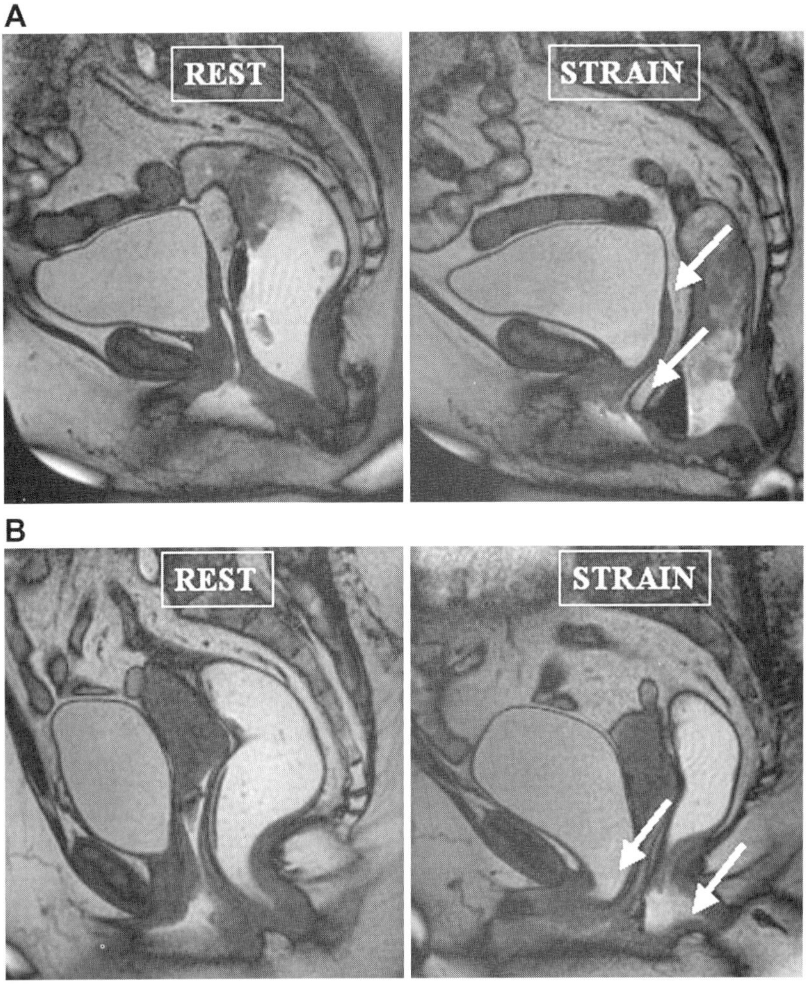

Fig. 9. Dynamic MRI defecography. (*A*) Sagittal view at the beginning (*left*) and at the end (*right*) of the evacuation showing the progressive appearance of an elytrocele (peritoneal pouch into the rectovaginal space) (*arrows*). (*B*) Sagittal view before (*left*) and after (*right*) the evacuation showing the association of urinary bladder and rectal prolapse (*arrows*).

certain situations, however, such as identifying the Alcock's canal to infiltrate the pudendal nerve (**Fig. 10**).[49] CT can also be used for sacral nerve stimulation in patients with refractory voiding disorders, such as urinary urge incontinence and fecal incontinence. For this procedure, an electrode is implanted in the third sacral vertebra and attached to an implantable pulse generator.[50] The exact position of the device can be checked by CT. The implantation of the sacral electrode can also be performed under CT guidance.[51]

SUMMARY

Several modalities are available for imaging the pelvic floor, and the choice between these techniques is determined by the availability of equipment and local expertise.

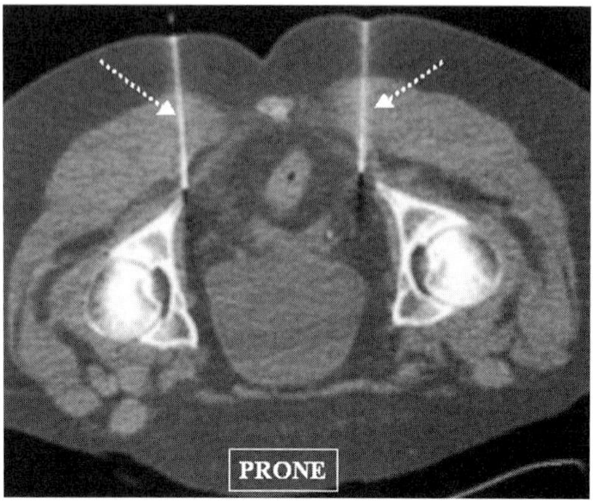

Fig. 10. Interventional CT. Visualization of the proper positioning of two needles before infiltration of the Alcock's canals.

Either endoanal US or MRI can be used for the detection of anal sphincter defects in patients with fecal incontinence. Endoanal US is an ideal screening test and is widely available. MRI offers additional advantages, such as the diagnosis of EAS atrophy. Although defecography provides valuable morphologic and functional information in constipated patients, MRI defecography permits a dynamic global approach for the assessment of pelvic floor structure and function. The lack of radiation exposure is an advantage. oreover, the pelvic floor muscles and the urogenital compartments can be clearly visualized in a single examination. It is now well recognized that pelvic floor disorders rarely occur in isolation and information regarding global pelvic floor structure and function is desirable.

Regarding US and MRI, technical improvements continue to provide high-resolution three-dimensional images. It is likely that radiologists will face an increasing demand for these examinations, because of the ageing population in western countries.[52] A more precise and global assessment of the morphology and function will improve decision making and outcome of patients with pelvic floor disorders.

REFERENCES

1. Burhenne HJ. Intestinal evacuation study: a new roentgenologic technique. Radiol Clin 1964;33:79–84.
2. Wiermsa TG, Mulder CJ, Rieders JW. Dynamic rectal examination: its significant clinical value. Endoscopy 1997;29:462–71.
3. Harvey JC, Halligan S, Bartram CI, et al. Evacuation proctography: a prospective study of diagnostic and therapeutic effects. Radiology 1999;211:223–7.
4. Choi JS, Wexner SD, Nam YS, et al. Intraobserver and interobserver measurements of the anorectal angle and perineal descent in defecography. Dis Colon Rectum 2000;43:1121–6.
5. Liu BH, Fang SW, Tong WD, et al. Role of pelvicography and colpocystodefecography in diagnosis of outlet obstructive constipation. Int J Colorectal Dis 2005; 20(4):317–20.
6. Bethoux A, Bory S. Les mécanismes statiques viscéraux pelviens chez la femme à la lumière de l'exploration fonctionnelle du dispositif en position debout. Ann Chir 1962;16:887–916.

7. Mahieu P, Pringot J, Bodart P. Defecography: I. Description of a new procedure and results in normal patients. Gastrointest Radiol 1984;9:247–51.
8. Shorvon PJ, Mc Hugh S, Diamant NE, et al. Defecography in normal volunteers: results and implications. Gut 1989;30:1737–49.
9. Agachan F, Pfeifer J, Wexner SD. Defecography and proctography: results of 744 patients. Dis Colon Rectum 1996;39:899–905.
10. Mellgren A, Bremmer S, Johansson C, et al. Defecography: results of investigations in 2816 patients. Dis Colon Rectum 1994;37:1133–41.
11. Muller-Lissner SA, Bartolo DC, Christiansen J, et al. Interobserver agreement in defecography: an international study. Z Gastroenterol 1998;36:273–9.
12. Jean F, Tanneau Y, Le Blanc-Louvry I, et al. Treatment of enterocele by abdominal colporectopexy: efficacy on pelvic pressure. Colorectal Dis 2002;4:321–5.
13. Felt-Bersma RJ, Luth WJ, Janssen JJ, et al. Defecography in patients with anorectal disorders: which findings are clinically relevant? Dis Colon Rectum 1990;33:277–84.
14. Hiltunen KM, Kolehmainen H, Matikainen M. Does defecography help in diagnosis and clinical decision-making in defecation disorders? Abdom Imaging 1994;19:355–8.
15. Bharucha AE, Fletcher JG, Harper CM, et al. Relationship between symptoms and disordered continence mechanisms in women with idiopathic faecal incontinence. Gut 2005;54:546–55.
16. Savoye-Collet C, Savoye G, Koning E, et al. Defecographic disorders in anal incontinent women: relation to symptoms and anal endosonographic patterns. Scand J Gastroenterol 2005;40:141–6.
17. Law PJ, Kamm MA, Bartram CI. Anal endosonography in the investigation of faecal incontinence. Br J Surg 1991;78:312–4.
18. Rottenberg GT, Williams AB. Endoanal ultrasound. Br J Radiol 2002;75:482–8.
19. Nielsen MB, Pedersen JF, Hauge C, et al. Endosonography of the anal sphincter: findings in healthy volunteers. AJR 1991;157:1199–202.
20. Sultan AH, Nicholls RJ, Kamm MA, et al. Anal endosonography and correlation with in vitro and in vivo anatomy. Br J Surg 1993;80:508–11.
21. Nielsen MB, Hauge C, Rasmussen O, et al. Anal sphincter size measured by endosonography in healthy volunteers: effect of age, sex, and parity. Acta Radiol 1992;33:453–6.
22. Sultan AH, Kamm MA, Hudson CN, et al. Endosonography of the anal sphincters: normal anatomy and comparison with manometry. Clin Radiol 1994;49:368–74.
23. Williams AB, Bartram CI, Halligan S, et al. Endosonographic anatomy of the normal anal canal compared with endocoil magnetic resonance imaging. Dis Colon Rectum 2002;45:176–83.
24. Deen KI, Kumar D, Williams JG, et al. The prevalence of anal sphincter defects in faecal incontinence: a prospective endosonic study. Gut 1993;34:685–8.
25. Karoui S, Savoye-Collet C, Koning E, et al. Prevalence of anal sphincter defects revealed by sonography in 335 incontinents patients and 115 continents patients. AJR 1999;173:389–92.
26. Deen KI, Kumar D, Williams JG, et al. Anal sphincter defects: correlation between endoanal ultrasound and surgery. Ann Surg 1993;218:201–5.
27. Dobben AC, Terra MP, Slors JF, et al. External anal sphincter defects in patients with fecal incontinence: comparison of endoanal MR imaging and endoanal US. Radiology 2007;242:463–71.
28. Sultan AH, Kamm MA, Hudson CN, et al. Anal sphincter disruption during vaginal delivery. N Engl J Med 1993;329:1905–11.

29. Nielsen MB, Hauge C, Pedersen JF, et al. Endosonographic evaluation of patients with anal incontinence: findings and influence on surgical management. AJR 1993;160:771–5.
30. Savoye-Collet C, Savoye G, Koning E, et al. Anal endosonography after sphincter anal repair: specific patterns related to clinical outcome. Abdom Imaging 1999; 24:569–73.
31. Savoye-Collet C, Savoye G, Koning E, et al. Endosonography in the evaluation of anal function after primary repair of a third degree obstetric tear. Scand J Gastroenterol 2003;38:1149–53.
32. Terra MP, Stoker J. The current role of imaging techniques in faecal incontinence. Eur Radiol 2006;16:1727–36.
33. Christensen AF, Nyhuus B, Nielsen MB, et al. Three-dimensional anal endosonography may improve diagnostic confidence of detecting damage to the anal sphincter complex. Br J Radiol 2005;78:308–11.
34. Lee JH, Pretorius DH, Weinstein M, et al. Transperineal three-dimensional ultrasound in evaluating anal sphincter muscles. Ultrasound Obstet Gynecol 2007; 30(2):201–9.
35. Timor-Tritsch IE, Monteagudo A, Smilen SW, et al. Simple ultrasound evaluation of the anal sphincter in female patients using a transvaginal transducer. Ultrasound Obstet Gynecol. 2005;25(2):177–83.
36. Tunn R, Petri E. Introital and transvaginal ultrasound as the main tool in the assessment of urogenital and pelvic floor dysfunction: an imaging panel and practical approach. Ultrasound Obstet Gynecol 2003;22(2):205–13.
37. Fielding JR, Griffiths DJ, Versi E, et al. MR imaging of pelvic floor continence mechanisms in the supine and sitting positions. AJR 1998;171:1607–10.
38. Pannu HK, Kaufman HS, Cundiff GW, et al. Dynamic MR imaging of pelvic organ prolapse: spectrum of abnormalities. Radiographics 2000;20:1567–82.
39. Roos JE, Weishaupt D, Wildermuth S, et al. Experience of 4 years with open MR defecography: pictorial review of anorectal anatomy and disease. Radiographics 2002;22:817–32.
40. Hetzer FH, Andreisek G, Tsagari C, et al. MR defecography in patients with fecal incontinence: imaging findings and their effect on surgical management. Radiology 2006;240(2):449–57.
41. Bertschinger KM, Hetzer FH, Roos JE, et al. Dynamic MR imaging of the pelvic floor performed with patient sitting in an open-magnet unit versus with patient supine in a closed-magnet unit. Radiology 2002;223:501–8.
42. Maubon A, Aubard Y, Berkane V, et al. MRI of the pelvic floor. Abdom Imaging 2003;28:217–25.
43. Bharucha AE, Fletcher JG. Recent advances in assessing anorectal structure and functions. Gastroenterology 2007;133(4):1069–74.
44. Fletcher JG, Busse RF, Riederer SJ, et al. Magnetic resonance imaging of anatomic and dynamic defects of pelvic floor in defecatory disorders. Am J Gastroenterol 2003;98:399–411.
45. Stoker J, Bartram CI, Halligan S. Imaging of the posterior pelvic floor. Eur Radiol 2002;12:779–88.
46. Schaefer O, Oeksuez MO, Lohrmann C, et al. Differentiation of anal sphincters with high-resolution magnetic resonance imaging using contrast-enhanced fast low-angle shot 3-dimensional sequences. J Comput Assist Tomogr 2004;28(2):174–9.
47. Bartram CI. Functional anorectal imaging. Abdom Imaging 2005;30(2):195–203.
48. Cazemier M, Terra MP, Stoker J, et al. Atrophy and defects detection of the external anal sphincter: comparison between three-dimensional anal

endosonography and endoanal magnetic resonance imaging. Dis Colon Rectum 2006;49(1):20–7.
49. Amarenco G, Savatovski I, Buet C, et al. Névralgies périnéales et syndrome du canal d'Alcock. Ann Urol 1989;23:488–92.
50. van Kerrebroeck PE, van Voskuilen AC, Heesakkers JP, et al. Results of sacral neuromodulation therapy for urinary voiding dysfunction: outcomes of a prospective, worldwide clinical study. J Urol 2007;178(5):2029–34.
51. Amoroso L, Pelliccioni G, Ghiselli R, et al. Sacral-neuromodulation CT-guided. Radiol Med 2005;109(4):421–9.
52. Savoye-Collet C, Koning E, Savoye G, et al. Defecography in symptomatic older women living at home. Age Ageing 2003;32:347–50.

Dyssynergic Defecation and Biofeedback Therapy

Satish S.C. Rao, MD, PhD, FRCP (LON)

KEYWORDS

- Dyssynergic defecation • Biofeedback therapy
- Constipation • Anorectal disorder

Neuromuscular dysfunction of the defecation unit can lead to disordered or difficult defecation. Likewise, neuromuscular dysfunction of the colon may lead to slow transit constipation. In many patients there is an overlap, because colonic transit is delayed in two thirds of patients with difficult defecation.[1,2] Preston and Lennard-Jones[3] first described the association of paradoxical anal contraction during attempted defecation in patients with constipation and coined the term "anismus." They believed that this condition was a spastic dysfunction of the anus, analogous to "vaginismus." The term "anismus" implies a psychogenic etiology, however, which is not true although psychologic dysfunction has been described in these patients. In the literature, a number of terms have been used to describe the constipation that is associated with anorectal dysfunction, which includes anismus,[3] pelvic floor dyssynergia,[4] obstructive defecation,[1,5] paradoxical puborectalis contraction,[6] pelvic outlet obstruction,[7,8] and spastic pelvic floor syndrome.[9] Pelvic floor is a complex muscular apparatus that serves three important functions: (1) defecation, (2) micturition, and (3) sexual function. All-encompassing terms, such as "pelvic floor dyssynergia" or "pelvic outlet obstruction," imply that this problem affects most of the pelvic floor, and possibly all of its functions. Although, some overlap has been described among patients with urinary obstruction and constipation,[10] most constipated patients do not report sexual or urinary symptoms.[11] Consequently, it misrepresents a functional disorder. Hence, these terms are not suitable. A consensus report from an international group of experts has recommended that the term "dyssynergic defecation" most aptly describes this form of constipation.[12]

EPIDEMIOLOGY

The prevalence of chronic constipation varies from 2% to 28%.[13] It is commonly encountered in primary care. Telephone interviews with 10,018 individuals, aged at least 18 years, produced an estimated prevalence of 14.7%.[14] In a questionnaire survey of

Division of Gastroenterology-Hepatology, University of Iowa Carver College of Medicine, University of Iowa Hospitals and Clinics, 4612 JCP, 200 Hawkins Drive, Iowa City, IA 52242, USA
E-mail address: satish-rao@uiowa.edu

Gastroenterol Clin N Am 37 (2008) 569–586
doi:10.1016/j.gtc.2008.06.011 gastro.theclinics.com
0889-8553/08/$ – see front matter

5430 households across the United States, functional constipation was reported by 3.6% of responders and difficult defecation by 13.8%.[15] Because most patients do not seek health care, its prevalence has been underestimated.[15]

Constipation is more common in women with an estimated female/male ratio of 2.2:1.[15,16] Its prevalence increases with advancing age, particularly after age 65, with the elderly reporting more problems with straining and hard stools than infrequency.[16] Its prevalence is twofold higher in African Americans;[16] in those of lower socioeconomic status (annual income ≤$20,000);[16] and in nursing home residents.[16] Pregnancy is also associated with higher prevalence of constipation, but no differences were seen between the first and the last trimester.[17]

Economic and Social Impact

Chronic constipation has a significant impact on the use of health care resources, including the cost of inpatient and outpatient care, laboratory tests, and diagnostic procedures.[18] In a recent study of 76,854 patients enrolled in Medical program, the total health care expenditure for patients with constipation over a 15-month period was $18,891,008, with an average cost of $246 per patient.[19] Approximately 0.6% of patients were hospitalized with an average cost of $2993 per admission.[19] In another study, expenditure for constipation was estimated at $235 million per year with 55% incurred from inpatient, 23% from emergency department, and 22% from outpatient care.[20]

Psychologic Distress, Abuse, and Impact on Quality of Life

Constipation is associated with increased psychologic distress. Several studies have shown higher prevalence for anxiety, depression, obsessive compulsiveness, psychoticism, and somatization.[21,22] Furthermore, paranoid ideation and hostility subscores were higher in patients with dyssynergia than slow transit constipation or healthy controls, providing evidence for significant psychologic distress, more so in dyssynergics than slow transit constipation patients.[22]

Sexual abuse was reported by 22% to 48% of subjects, mostly women, whereas physical abuse was reported by 31% to 74% of constipated subjects.[11,23] Another study found greater incidence of sexual abuse in women with pelvic floor dyssynergia.[23] Also, patients with abuse were more likely to seek health care and report feelings of incomplete evacuation or urge to defecate, but did not demonstrate rectal hypersensitivity.[24]

Patients with chronic constipation also showed significant impairment of health-related quality of life (**Fig. 1**).[22,25] Some domains were more affected in dyssynergics than slow transit constipation,[22] suggesting that dyssynergia is associated with greater impact on quality of life. Also, psychologic distress and lower quality of life were strongly correlated suggesting that these dysfunctions have synergistic effects on bowel function.[22]

ETIOLOGY AND PATHOPHYSIOLOGY

Origin

How, when, and why an individual develops dyssynergic defecation is unclear. The authors' prospective survey of 100 patients with dyssynergic suggested that the problem began during childhood in 31% of patients; after a particular event, such as pregnancy, trauma, or back injury in 29% of patients; and no identifiable precipitating cause in 40% of patients.[11] Two thirds acquire this condition during adulthood. In this group, 17% reported a history of sexual abuse, 43% the passage of hard stools

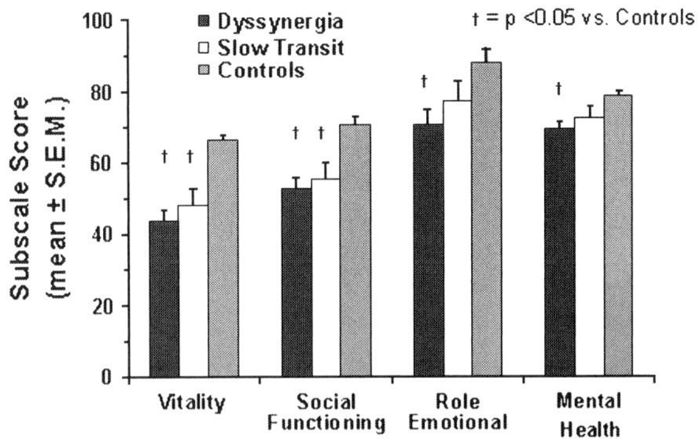

Fig. 1. Impact of chronic constipation on quality of life in patients with dyssynergic defecation, slow transit constipation, and healthy controls. (*From* Rao SS, Seaton K, Miller MJ, et al. Psychological profiles and quality of life differ between patients with dyssynergia and those with slow transit constipation. J Psychosom Res 2007;63:441–9; with permission.)

frequently, and 16% intermittently. Excessive straining to expel hard stools over time may also lead to dyssynergic defecation.

Pathophysiology

Earlier studies suggested that paradoxical anal contraction or involuntary anal spasm (anismus) during defecation may cause this problem.[3] Consequently, myectomy of the anal sphincter was performed,[8] but only 10% to 30% of patients improved.[26] Likewise, paralyzing the anal sphincter muscle with botulinum toxin injections produced minimal improvement.[27] Either spasm or inability to relax the external anal sphincter is unlikely to be the sole mechanism that leads to dyssynergic defecation.

A prospective study[1] showed that most patients with dyssynergic defecation demonstrate the inability to coordinate the abdominal, rectoanal, and pelvic floor muscles to facilitate defecation. This failure of rectoanal coordination consists of impaired rectal contraction (61%); paradoxical anal contraction (78%); or inadequate anal relaxation. Incoordination or dyssynergia of the muscles that are involved in defecation is primarily responsible for this condition. In addition, 50% to 60% of patients also demonstrate an impaired rectal sensation.[1]

CLINICAL FEATURES

Patients with dyssynergic defecation present with a variety of bowel symptoms. Often, patients do not volunteer or misrepresent their symptoms. For example, patients do not readily admit that they use digital maneuvers to disimpact stool or splint their vagina to facilitate defecation. By establishing a trustworthy relationship or through the help of symptom questionnaires or stool diaries, it may be possible to identify the precise nature of their bowel dysfunction. It is essential to determine this because only then can one approach this problem more rationally. In a prospective study, excessive straining was reported by 85%, a feeling of incomplete evacuation by 75%, the passage of hard stools by 65%, and a stool frequency of less than three bowel movements per week by 62% of patients.[11] In addition, 66% of patients used digital maneuvers to facilitate defecation. In another study of 134 patients, two or fewer stools per week, laxative dependence, and constipation since childhood was associated with slow transit constipation, whereas backache, heartburn, anorectal surgery, and a lower prevalence of normal stool frequency was reported by patients with pelvic floor dysfunction.[28] They concluded that symptoms are good predictors of transit time but poor predictors of pelvic floor dysfunction. A study of 190 constipated patients showed that stool frequency alone was of little value in constipation.[29] In contrast, a sense of obstruction or digital evacuation was specific but not sensitive for disordered dysfunction. They also concluded that symptoms alone cannot differentiate between the pathophysiologic subgroups that lead to constipation.[29]

Differential diagnosis includes many structural or functional abnormalities that may also lead to an evacuation disorder, such as rectocele, hypertensive anal sphincter, hemorrhoids, anal fissure, anorectal neoplasia, rectal prolapse, and proctitis. These conditions can be readily identified through appropriate testing. In contrast, functional evacuation disorders are less well recognized and poorly managed. These include dyssynergic defecation, excessive perineal descent, and mucosal intussusception. Also, paradoxical anal contraction has been described in patients after pouch reconstruction.[30] Many patients with the solitary rectal ulcer syndrome also exhibit dyssynergic defecation.[31]

Patients with defecation disorders have several psychologic abnormalities.[22] This includes such problems as obsessive-compulsive disorder, where the patient believes that having a bowel movement everyday or sometimes several times per day are the norm. A deviation from this process compels the individual to use laxatives, enemas, suppositories, or any other means to achieve an unphysiologic pattern of bowel movement. Others have phobia for stool impaction. This particularly affects children, who then learn quickly to exploit minor disturbance in defecation for seeking attention.[32] The problem may also be driven by psychosocial issues, such as interparental or parental-child conflicts or sibling rivalry. It has been shown that parental disattachment during childhood can lead to bowel dysfunction in adult life.[33] Finally, patients with bulimia or anorexia nervosa and others with a history of physical or sexual abuse may also develop profound defecation problems.[34]

DIAGNOSTIC PROCEDURES

General Issues

The first step in making a diagnosis of dyssynergic defecation is to exclude an underlying metabolic or pathologic disorder. Slow transit constipation may coexist with dyssynergic defecation,[1,35] and hence an assessment of colonic motor function and transit is useful. An evaluation of the distal colonic mucosa through flexible sigmoidoscopy may provide evidence for chronic laxative use and may reveal melanosis coli or other mucosal lesions, such as solitary ulcer syndrome, inflammation, or malignancy.

Digital Rectal Examination

A careful perianal and digital rectal examination is not only important but often the most revealing part of clinical evaluation. Anorectal inspection can detect skin excoriation, skin tags, anal fissures, or hemorrhoids. Assessment of perineal sensation and anocutaneous reflex by gently stroking the perianal skin with a cotton bud or blunt needle in all four quadrants elicits reflex contraction of the external anal sphincter. If this is absent, a neuropathy should be suspected. Digital rectal examination may reveal a stricture, spasm, tenderness, mass, blood, or stool. If stool is present, its consistency should be noted and the patient should be asked if they were aware of its presence. A lack of awareness of stool in the rectum may suggest rectal hyposensitivity. It is useful to assess the resting and squeeze tone of the anal sphincter and puborectalis muscle by asking the subject to squeeze. More importantly, the subject should be asked to push and bear down as if to defecate. During this maneuver, the examiner should perceive relaxation of the external anal sphincter or the puborectalis muscle, together with perineal descent. A hand placed on the abdomen can gauge the abdominal push effort. An absence of these normal findings should raise the index of suspicion for an evacuation disorder, such as dyssynergic defecation.[36] Digital rectal examination has a high sensitivity for identifying dyssynergia.[36] Even though digital rectal examination is a useful clinical tool, there is a lack of knowledge on how to perform a comprehensive evaluation. A survey of 256 final year medical students revealed that 17% had never performed a digital rectal examination and 48% were unsure of giving an opinion based on their findings.[37] A concerted effort is needed to improve the training of digital rectal examination.

Anorectal Manometry

This test provides a comprehensive assessment of pressure activity in the rectum and anal sphincter region together with an assessment of rectal sensation, rectoanal reflexes, and rectal compliance.[38,39,40] Anorectal manometry is essential for a diagnosis of dyssynergic defecation.[38,40] First, it excludes the possibility of Hirschsprung's disease. Normally, when a balloon is distended in the rectum there is reflex relaxation of the internal anal sphincter that is mediated by the myenteric plexus. This reflex response is absent in patients with Hirschsprung's disease. Second, it helps to detect abnormalities during attempted defecation. Normally, when a subject bears down or attempts to defecate, there is a rise in rectal pressure, which is synchronized with a relaxation of the external anal sphincter (**Fig. 2**). This maneuver is under voluntary control and is primarily a learned response. The inability to perform this coordinated movement represents the chief pathophysiologic abnormality in patients with dyssynergic defecation. This may either be caused by impaired rectal contraction, paradoxical anal contraction, impaired anal relaxation, or a combination of these mechanisms. Based on these features at least four types of dyssynergia can be recognized (see **Fig. 2**).

Type 1: Here, the patient can generate an adequate pushing force (rise in intra-abdominal pressure) along with a paradoxical increase in anal sphincter pressure.

Type 2: Here, the patient is unable to generate an adequate pushing force (no increase in intrarectal pressure) but can exhibit a paradoxical anal contraction.

Type 3: Here, the patient can generate an adequate pushing force (increase in intrarectal pressure) but either has absent or incomplete (<20%) sphincter relaxation (ie, no decrease in anal sphincter pressure).

Type 4: The patient is unable to generate an adequate pushing force and demonstrates an absent or incomplete anal sphincter relaxation.

In addition to the motor abnormalities described previously, sensory dysfunction may also be present. Both the first sensation and the threshold for a desire to defecate may be higher in about 60% of patients with dyssynergic defecation.[1,5] This may also be associated with increased rectal compliance. It must be noted that during attempted defecation some subjects may not produce a normal relaxation largely because of the laboratory conditions.[41,42] Hence, this pattern alone should not be considered diagnostic of dyssynergic defecation (see diagnostic criteria later).

By observing the attempts to defecate, it is possible to identify the recording that most closely resembles a normal pattern of defecation. This recording can then be

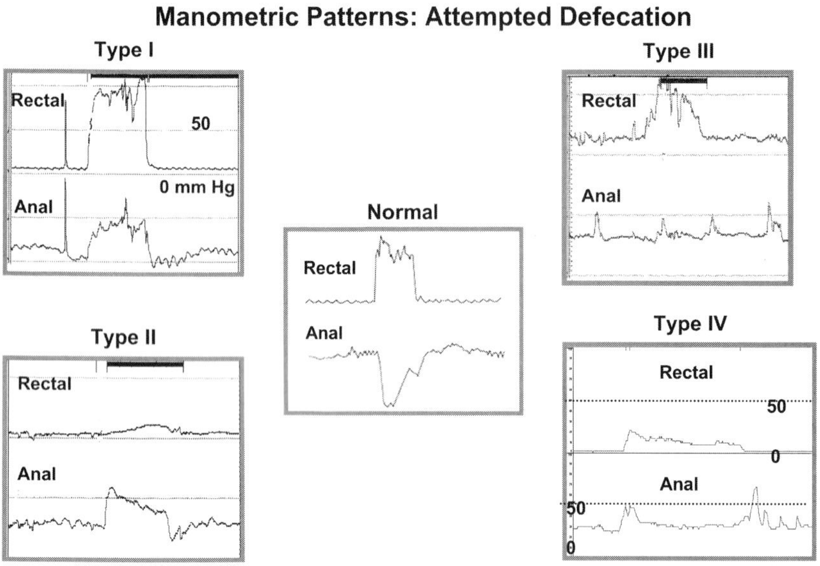

Fig. 2. This series reveals manometric patterns that are commonly seen during attempted defecation in a normal healthy individual (*central panel*) and in patients with dyssynergic defecation. They were obtained after placing a multisensor solid-state manometry catheter into the rectum: changes from a single sensor in the rectum and one from the anal canal are shown. In the center panel, it can be seen that the subject can generate a good pushing force (increase in intrarectal pressure) and simultaneously relax the anal sphincter. This is a normal pattern of defecation. In contrast, patients with dyssynergic defecation exhibit one of four abnormal patterns of defecation. In type I dyssynergia, the subject can generate an adequate propulsive force (rise in intrarectal pressure ≥40 mm Hg) along with paradoxical increase in anal sphincter pressure. In type II dyssynergia, the subject is unable to generate an adequate propulsive force; additionally there is paradoxical anal contraction. In type III dyssynergia, the subject can generate an adequate propulsive force but there is either absent relaxation (a flat line) or incomplete (≤20%) relaxation of anal sphincter. In type IV dyssynergia, the subject is unable to generate an adequate propulsive force together with an absent or incomplete relaxation of anal sphincter.

used to measure the intrarectal pressure, the anal residual pressure, and the percentage of anal relaxation. The residual anal pressure is defined as the difference between the baseline pressure and the lowest (residual) pressure within the anal canal when the subject is bearing down.[1,39] The percent of anal relaxation is calculated using the formula, percent anal relaxation = anal relaxation pressure/anal resting pressure × 100. From these measurements it is possible to derive an index of the forces required to perform defecation (the defecation index). The defecation index may serve as a simple and useful quantitative measure of the rectoanal coordination during defecation.[1,39]

Balloon Expulsion Test

In this test, either a silicone-filled stool-like device, such as the fecom,[43] or a 4-cm-long balloon filled with 50 mL of warm water is placed in the rectum.[39,43] A stop watch is started and the attendant leaves the room to provide privacy for the patient during balloon expulsion. The patient is then asked to expel the device and to stop the clock. Most normal subjects can expel a stool-like device within 1 minute, failing which

dyssynergic defecation should be suspected. Although quite specific for dyssynergia, its sensitivity is approximately 50%.

Defecography

Defecography is commonly performed by placing approximately 150 mL of barium paste into the patient's rectum. The patient is asked to sit on a special commode adjacent to a videofluoroscopic imaging system. The patient is instructed to squeeze or to evacuate the barium, and simultaneously the structural and functional changes of the anorectum are monitored by fluoroscopy and recorded on a videotape. This test provides useful information about anatomic and functional changes. In patients with dyssynergic defecation, the test may reveal poor activation of levator muscles, prolonged retention of contrast material or inability to expel the barium, or the absence of a stripping wave in the rectum.

Patients often, however, find this test embarrassing. Also, the type and consistency of barium paste varies considerably among different centers.[44] Because of these inherent deficiencies, this test should be regarded as an adjunct to clinical and manometric assessment of anorectal function and should not be relied on as a sole test for assessing an evacuation disorder.[44]

Diagnostic Criteria for Dyssynergic Defecation

Most published studies have used arbitrary or symptomatic diagnostic criteria. F
example, paradoxical anal contraction has been considered to be a sine qua
for dyssynergic defecation. One study reported during attempted defecation, h
ever, that five patients showed either no change in the anal resting pressure
insignificant (<20%) decrease;[1] all of these patients failed to expel a balloc
also had greater than 50% retention of barium material during defeco
Similarly, two other patients were able to expel the balloon but had par
anal contraction. Others have found that paradoxical anal contraction or in
(<20%) decrease in anal electromyographic (EMG) activity, colonic transit,
cographic abnormalities were not exclusively seen in patients with diffic
tion and none of the three tests showed significant differences in the
of anismus between patients with or without slow transit constipation
about two thirds of patients with constipation had objective evidenc
transit or pelvic floor dysfunction and no single test could reliably i
the pathophysiologic groups of constipation.[46] Because a given patie
some but not all of the aforementioned dysfunctions, it is important t
one yardstick to diagnose this condition. In a prospective study,
constipation symptoms together with dyssynergic pattern of defec
one additional abnormal test (eg, prolonged balloon expulsion
colonic transit, or excessive barium retention with defecography
nostic yield of identifying dyssynergic defecation.[47] To diagno
has been proposed that a patient must satisfy both the sympt
iologic criteria set forth in **Box 1**.[48]

TREATMENT

The treatment of a patient with dyssynergic defecation con
ment for constipation; (2) specific treatment (ie, neuromusc
therapy); and (3) other measures including, botulinum to
ileostomy.

Box 1
Criteria for dyssynergic defecation

A. Patients must satisfy the diagnostic criteria for functional chronic constipation (Rome III) and

B. Patients must demonstrate dyssynergia during repeated attempts to defecate

Dyssynergic or obstructive pattern of defecation (types 1–4) is defined as paradoxical increase in anal sphincter pressure (anal contraction) or less than 20% relaxation of the resting anal sphincter pressure or inadequate propulsive forces observed with manometry, imaging, or EMG recordings and

C. One or more of the following criteria during repeated attempts to defecate

1. Inability to expel an artificial stool (50 mL water-filled balloon) within 1 minute
2. A prolonged colonic transit time (ie, greater than five markers [>20% marker retention]) on a plain abdominal radiograph taken 120 hours after ingestion of one sitzmark capsule containing 24 radiopaque markers
3. Inability to evacuate or greater than or equal to 50% retention of barium during defecography

Modified from Rao SSC, Mudipalli RS, Stessman M, et al. Investigation of the utility of colorectal function tests and Rome II criteria in dyssynergic defecation (anismus). Neurogastroenterol Motil 2004;16:589–96; with permission.

Standard Treatment

This should consist of a detailed assessment and correction of coexisting issues, such as avoiding constipating medications, increasing fiber and fluid intake, and exercise activity. In a recent study, dietary instructions had little impact on fiber or nutrient intake in patients with dyssynergia, but about a third of patients were consuming a low-fiber diet, and in this group their fiber intake increased.[49] In addition, patients should receive instructions regarding timed toilet training and laxatives. Timed toilet training consists of educating the patient to attempt a bowel movement at least twice a day, usually 30 minutes after meals and to strain for no more than 5 minutes. During attempted defecation, they must be instructed to push at a level of 5 to 7, assuming evel 10 as their maximum effort of straining. They should be encouraged to capitalize n intrinsic physiologic mechanisms that stimulate the colon, such as after waking[50,51] nd after a meal.[51] It is important to emphasize that stool impaction should be pre-nted at all costs. Patients should be advised to refrain from manual maneuvers, ch as digital disimpaction of stools.

er supplements

anic polymers, such as bran or psyllium, have the ability to hold extra water and n resist digestion and absorption in the uppor gut. There is no evidence that stipated patients in general consume less fiber than nonconstipated patients, ever, and studies show similar levels of fiber intake.[49,52] Furthermore, constipated nts with slow transit or pelvic floor dysfunction respond poorly to dietary supple-ation with 30 g of fiber per day, whereas those without an underlying motility der improved.[53] A fiber intake of 20 to 30 g per day is optimal. Recently, both merican College of Gastroenterology task force[54] and a systematic review[55] ıded that psyllium, a natural fiber supplement, increases stool frequency and his compound a grade B recommendation, but there were insufficient data to

make a recommendation for the synthetic polysaccharide methylcellulose, or calcium polycarbophil or bran in patients with constipation.

Pharmacologic Approaches

In one report, $821 million was spent on over-the-counter laxatives in the United States.[56] Several types of laxatives are available.

Stool softeners

Sodium and calcium docusate compounds (Colace, Surfak) are anionic surfactants that lower the surface tension of stool and facilitate the mixing of aqueous and fatty substances and also stimulate intestinal fluid secretion. There are four randomized controlled trials that have compared stool softeners with either placebo or other laxatives. The sample sizes were small and the data were conflicting.[55] Consequently, these compounds were afforded a grade B recommendation.[54,55]

Stimulant laxatives

This group consists of anthraquinones (senna, casacara sagrada, danthron, and casanthronol); diphenylmethane derivatives (bisacodyl, sodium picosulphate); and ricinoleic acid (castor oil). Stimulant laxatives affect electrolyte transport across the intestinal mucosa and enhance colonic transport and motility, and usually work within several hours of administration.

Their long-term safety has not been established. Four randomized controlled trials were identified but none of them were placebo-controlled, the study design was of low quality, and hence a grade B recommendation was given.[55]

Osmotic laxatives

Osmotic laxatives include saline laxatives (salts of magnesium, phosphate, and sulfate); poorly absorbed synthetic disaccharides, such as lactulose; sugar alcohols, such as sorbitol or mannitol; and an inert polymer, polyethylene glycol (PEG-3350 [Miralax; Braintree Labs, Braintree, Massachusetts]). This group includes ions or molecules that are not well absorbed by the intestine and require retention of water by the intestinal lumen to maintain osmotic balance with plasma.

PEG-3350 is a large polymer that is poorly absorbed, is metabolically inert, and is not degraded by bacteria. It has been widely used as lavage solution in preparation for colonoscopy. There are at least eight placebo-controlled randomized control trials of PEG compounds and two randomized control trials comparing PEG with lactulose. PEG was superior to placebo in increasing stool frequency and stool consistency.[55] A recent study reported relief of constipation in 52% of patients on PEG-3350 versus 11% of patients on placebo.[57]

Chloride channel activators

Chloride channels are located in the apical and serosal membranes of the enterocyte and they facilitate chloride transport.[58] There are four subtypes.[59] Lubiprostone (Amitiza, Takeda Pharmaceuticals, Chicago, Illinois) is a gastrointestinal-targeted bicyclic fatty acid that selectively activates type 2 chloride channels. In a randomized controlled trial involving 237 patients, lubiprostone, 24 μg twice daily for 28 days, was more effective than placebo in increasing the number of spontaneous bowel movements, decreasing straining, improving stool consistency, and relieving symptoms of chronic constipation.[60] Long-term studies show that the compound is efficacious and safe.[61]

Miscellaneous and emerging therapies

Colchicine, a plant alkaloid used to treat gout and misoprostol, a prostaglandin analogue used to treat peptic disorders, induce diarrhea as a side effect. Consequently, they have been tried in patients with chronic constipation.[62,63] Another compound, linaclotide, a guanylate cyclase agonist, has been shown to accelerate gut transit in healthy subjects and in female patients with constipation-predominant irritable bowel syndrome.[64]

Specific Treatment

Biofeedback therapy

The goal of neuromuscular training using biofeedback techniques is to restore a normal pattern of defecation. Neuromuscular training or biofeedback therapy is an instrument-based learning process that is based on "operant conditioning" techniques. The governing principal is that when any behavior, be it a complex maneuver, such as eating, or a simple task, such as muscle contraction, is reinforced its likelihood of being repeated and perfected increases several fold. In patients with dyssynergic defecation, the goal of neuromuscular training is twofold:[2,65,66] to correct the dyssynergia in coordination of the abdominal, rectal, and anal sphincter muscles to achieve a normal and complete evacuation (**Fig. 3**); and to enhance rectal sensory perception in patients with impaired rectal sensation.

Improve or correct dyssynergia This training consists of improving the abdominal push effort (diaphragmatic muscle training) together with manometric-guided pelvic floor relaxation followed by simulated defecation training. An outline of the protocol used at Iowa for biofeedback training is shown in **Box 2**.

Rectoanal coordination The purpose of this training is to produce a coordinated defecatory movement that consists of an adequate abdominal push effort as reflected by a rise in intrarectal pressure on the manometric tracing that is synchronized with relaxation of the pelvic floor and anal canal as depicted by a decrease in anal sphincter pressure (see **Fig. 3**). To facilitate this training, ideally the subject should be seated

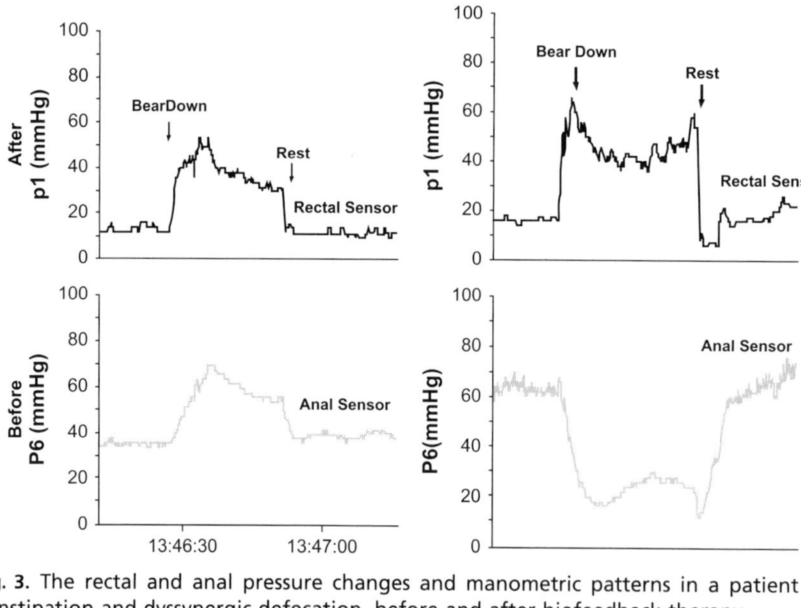

Fig. 3. The rectal and anal pressure changes and manometric patterns in a patient with constipation and dyssynergic defecation, before and after biofeedback therapy.

Box 2
Biofeedback therapy for constipation: Iowa protocol

- Phase I: evaluation and enrollment
  - Interview, stool diary
  - Tests of anorectal and colonic function
  - Symptom assessment (visual analog scale)
  - Diaphragmatic breathing exercises
  - Laxatives, timed-toilet training
- Phase II: active phase of biofeedback therapy
  - Visual, auditory, verbal feedback techniques (biweekly for six sessions)
  - Duration of each session: 60 minutes
  - Home devices
- Phase III: reinforcement
  - At 6 weeks, and 3, 6, and 12 months

on a commode with the manometry probe in situ. After correcting the patient's posture (eg, keeping the legs apart as opposed to keeping them together) and the sitting angle at which he or she will attempt the defecation maneuver (ie, leaning forward) the subject is asked to take a good diaphragmatic breath and to push and bear down as if to defecate.[2,65,66] The subject is encouraged to watch the monitor while performing this maneuver. The subject's posture and breathing techniques are continuously monitored and corrected. The visual display of the pressure changes in the rectum and anal canal on the monitor provides instant feedback to the subject regarding their performance and helps them to understand and learn quickly (see **Fig. 3**). At least 10 to 15 maneuvers are performed.

Next, the balloon in the rectum is distended with 60 mL of air to provide the subject with a sensation of rectal fullness or desire to defecate. As soon as the subject experiences this desire, he or she is then encouraged to push and attempt defecation while observing the pressure changes in the rectum and anal canal on the display monitor. Once again, the breathing and postural techniques are corrected. The maneuvers are repeated approximately 5 to 10 times. During the attempted defecation, the patient is instructed to titrate the degree of abdominal push and the anal relaxatory effort and in particular not to push excessively, because this is often counterproductive and leads to voluntary withholding. After each attempt, the balloon is deflated and reinflated before the next attempt. After completion of this maneuver, the balloon is fully deflated and the probe is removed. If using an EMG device, the goal is to teach the subject either to reduce the amplitude of electrical wave forms on the monitor or to decrease the intensity of sound signals.[67]

Simulated defecation training The goal of this training is to teach the subject to expel an artificial stool in the laboratory using the correct technique. This maneuver is performed by placing a 50-mL water-filled balloon in the rectum or by using an artificial stool such as Fecom.[65,68] After placement of balloon in the left lateral position, the subject is asked to sit on a commode and to attempt defecation. While the subject attempts to pass the balloon, assistance is provided, and the subject is taught to relax the pelvic floor muscles and to correct the posture and breathing techniques. If the subject is unable to expel the balloon, gentle traction is applied to the balloon to supplement the patient's efforts. Gradually, the subject learns how to coordinate the defecation maneuver and to expel the balloon.

Sensory training The goal of this training is to improve the thresholds for rectal sensory perception and to promote better awareness for stooling.[65,68] This is performed by intermittent inflation of the balloon in the rectum. The primary objective is to teach the subject to perceive a particular volume of balloon distention but with the same intensity as they had previously experienced with a larger volume of balloon distention. The first step here is progressively to inflate the balloon until the subject experiences an urge to defecate. This threshold volume is noted. After deflation, the balloon is reinflated to the same volume and the maneuver is repeated two or three times to educate the subject and to trigger appropriate rectal sensations. Thereafter, with each subsequent inflation the balloon volume is decreased in a stepwise manner by about 10%. During each distention, the subject is encouraged to observe the monitor and to note the pressure changes in the rectum and simultaneously pay close attention to the sensation they are experiencing in the rectum. They are encouraged to use the visual cues for volumes that are either not readily perceived or only faintly perceived. If the patient fails to perceive a particular volume or reports a significant change in the intensity of perception, the balloon inflation is repeated after a 5-second warning either by using the same volume or by using the previously perceived (higher) volume. By repeated inflations and deflations and through a process of trial and error, by the end of each session, newer thresholds for rectal perception are established.

Duration and frequency of training The number of neuromuscular training sessions and the length of each training session should be customized for each patient depending on their individual needs. Typically, each training session takes 1 hour. Patients are usually asked to visit the motility laboratory once in 2 weeks. On average, four to six training sessions are required.[65,68] At the outset, it is difficult to predict how many sessions a particular subject needs. After completion of neuromuscular training, periodic reinforcements at 6 weeks, 3 months, 6 months, and 12 months may provide additional benefit, and also improve the long-term outcome of these patients,[65] but its role has not been examined.

Devices and techniques for biofeedback Because neuromuscular training is an instrument-based learning technique, several devices and methods are available, and newer techniques continue to evolve. These include manometric-based biofeedback treatment with a solid-state manometry system, EMG biofeedback, balloon defecation training, and home training devices.[66] The solid-state manometry probe with microtransducers and a balloon is ideally suited for biofeedback therapy. Here, the transducers that are located in the rectum and anal canal provide a visual display of pressure activity throughout the anorectum. This display provides visual feedback to the subject. If required, surface EMG electrodes can be incorporated on the probe to provide both visual and auditory feedback. Sensory training can also be performed with the same probe. This system can serve as a comprehensive device for neuromuscular training.

Alternatively, an EMG biofeedback system that consists of a surface EMG electrode that is mounted on a probe or affixed to the surface of the external anal sphincter muscle can be used.[67,69] These electrodes pick up EMG signals from the surface of the anal sphincter muscle and these are in turn displayed on the monitor. This provides

Table 1
Summary of the randomized controlled trials of biofeedback therapy for dyssynergic defecation

	Chiarioni et al[71]	Rao et al[68]	Chiarioni et al[67]	Heymen et al[69]
Trial design	Biofeedback versus polyethylene glycol, 14.6 g	Biofeedback versus standard versus sham biofeedback	Biofeedback for slow transit versus dyssynergia	Biofeedback versus diazepam, 5 mg, versus placebo
Subjects and randomization	104 women 54 biofeedback 55 polyethylene glycol	77 (69 women) 1:1:1 distribution	52 (49 women) 34 dyssynergia 12 slow transit 6 mixed	84 (71 women) 30 biofeedback 30 diazepam 24 placebo
Duration and number of biofeedback sessions	3 months and 1 year, 5 weekly, 30-minute training sessions performed by physician investigator	3 months, biweekly, 1 hour, maximum of six sessions over 3 months, performed by biofeedback nurse therapist	Five weekly 30-minute training sessions, performed by physician investigator	Six biweekly, 1-hour sessions
Primary outcomes	Global improvement of symptoms Worse = 0 No improvement = 1 Mild = 2 Fair = 3 Major improvement = 4	1. Presence of dyssynergia 2. Balloon expulsion time 3. Number of complete spontaneous bowel movements 4. Global satisfaction	Symptom improvement None = 1 Mild = 2 Fair = 3 Major = 4	Global symptom relief
Dyssynergia corrected or symptoms improved	79.6% reported major improvement at 6 and 12 months 81.5% reported major improvement at 24 months	Dyssynergia corrected at 3 months in 79% with biofeedback versus 4% sham and 6% in standard group; CSBM = biofeedback group versus sham or standard, $P < .05$	71% with dyssynergia and 8% with slow transit alone reported fair improvement in symptoms	70% improved with biofeedback compared with 38% with placebo and 30% with diazepam
Conclusions	Biofeedback was superior to laxatives	Biofeedback was superior to sham feedback and standard therapy	Biofeedback benefits dyssynergia and not slow transit constipation	Biofeedback is superior to placebo and diazepam

instant visual feedback. The pitch of the auditory signals can be used to provide instant feedback regarding the changes in electrical activity of the anal sphincter. Such feedback responses can augment the learning process by helping the patient to titrate the defecation effort.

Home training devices largely use an EMG home trainer or silicon probe device attached to a hand-held monitor with an illuminated liquid crystal display. The pressure or electrical activity of the patient's sphincter responses can be displayed on a simple gauge, on a strip chart recorder, or on a color liquid crystal display and these are used to provide visual feedback for the subject.

Efficacy of biofeedback therapy The symptomatic improvement rate has varied between 44% and 100% in several uncontrolled clinical trials.[70] When interpreting the outcome of these studies, however, one should exercise caution because the end point for a successful treatment has been poorly defined and the duration of follow-up and the selection of patients has been quite variable. In the last few years, however, several randomized controlled trials of adults with dyssynergic defecation have been reported and are summarized in **Table 1**. There are significant methodologic differences between the studies and in the recruitment criteria and in the end points and outcomes. All of these studies have concluded, however, that biofeedback therapy is superior to controlled treatment approaches, such as diet, exercise, and laxatives,[68] or use of polyethylene glycol,[67] diazepam, or placebo,[69] balloon defecation therapy,[72] or sham feedback therapy.[68]

Biofeedback therapy is a labor-intensive and multidisciplinary approach but has no adverse effects; however, it is only offered in a few centers. To treat the vast number of constipated patients in the community, a home-based, self-training program is essential. A large statewide study that used home trainers demonstrated the feasibility of home training, but the efficacy of therapy was not compared and objective parameters of anorectal function were not assessed.[73] In another European study, significant improvement was reported in most subjects receiving home therapy,[7] but there was no control group.

Other measures for treating dyssynergic defecation

Injection of botulinum toxin into the anal sphincter has been tried with mixed results.[27] In both studies there was some improvement in less than one half of patients but troublesome incontinence occurred in one study.[74] The surgical aspects of managing dyssynergic defecation are discussed in the article by Scott and Gladman, elsewhere in this issue.

SUMMARY

Constipation caused by dyssynergic defecation is common and affects up to one half of patients with this disorder. This acquired behavioral problem is caused by the inability to coordinate the abdominal and pelvic floor muscles to evacuate stools. Today, it is possible to diagnose this problem through history, prospective stool diaries, and anorectal physiologic tests. Randomized controlled trails have now established that biofeedback therapy is not only efficacious but superior to other modalities and that the symptom improvement is caused by a change in underlying pathophysiology. Development of user-friendly approaches to biofeedback therapy and use of home biofeedback programs will significantly enhance the adoption of this treatment by gastroenterologists and colorectal surgeons. Improved reimbursement for this proved and relatively inexpensive treatment will carry a significant impact on the problem, and this could translate into significant improvement of symptoms for patients with this disorder.

REFERENCES

1. Rao SSC, Welcher K, Leistikow J. Obstructive defecation: a failure of rectoanal coordination. Am J Gastroenterol 1998;93:1042–50.
2. Rao SSC. Dyssynergic defecation. Gastroenterol Clin North Am 2001;30: 97–114.
3. Preston DM, Lennard-Jones J. Anismus in chronic constipation. Dig Dis Sci 1985; 30:413–8.
4. Whitehead WE, Wald A, Diamant N. Functional disorders of the anorectum. International Working Party Consensus Rome Criteria II. Gut 1999;45(Suppl 2):II55–9.
5. Papachrysostomou M, Smith A. Effects of biofeedback on obstructive defecation: reconditioning of the defecation reflex? Gut 1994;35(2):242–5.
6. Glia A, Gylin M, Gullberg K, et al. Biofeedback retraining in patients with functional constipation and paradoxical puborectalis contraction: comparison of anal manometry and sphincter electromyography for feedback. Dis Colon Rectum 1997;40:889–95.
7. Kawimbe BM, Pappachrysostomou M, Binnie NR, et al. Outlet obstruction constipation (anismus) managed by biofeedback. Gut 1991;32:1175–9.
8. Martelli H, Devroede G, Arhan P, et al. Mechanisms of idiopathic constipation: outlet obstruction. Gastroenterology 1978;75:623–31.
9. Bieijenberg G, Kuipers H. Treatment of spastic pelvic floor syndrome with biofeedback. Dis Colon Rectum 1987;30:101–11.
10. Thorpe AC, Williams NS, Badenoch DF, et al. Simultaneous dynamic electromyographic portography and cystometrography. Br J Surg 1993;80(1):115–20.
11. Rao SSC, Tuteja AK, Vellema T, et al. Dyssynergic defecation: demographics, symptoms, stool patterns and quality of life. J Clin Gastroenterol 2004;38: 680–5.
12. Bharucha AE, Wald A, Enck P, et al. Functional anorectal disorders. Gastroenterology 2006;130:1510–8.
13. Pare P, Ferrazzi S, Thompson D, et al. An epidemiological survey of constipation in Canada: definitions, rates, demographics, and predictors of health care seeking. Am J Gastroenterol 2001;96:3130–7.
14. Stewart WF, Liberman JN, Sandler RS, et al. Epidemiology of constipation (EPOC) study in the United States: relation of clinical subtypes to sociodemographic features. Am J Gastroenterol 1999;94(12):3530–40.
15. Drossman DA, Li Z, Andruzi E, et al. US householder survey of the functional gastrointestinal disorders: prevalence, sociodemography and health impact. Dig Dis Sci 1993;38:1569–80.
16. Higgins PD, Johanson JF. Epidemiology of constipation in North America: a systematic review. Am J Gastroenterol 2004;99:750–9.
17. Bradley CS, Kennedy CM, Turcea AM, et al. Constipation in pregnancy: prevalence, symptoms, and risk factors. Obstet Gynecol 2007;110(6):1351–7.
18. Dennison C, Prasad M, Lloyd A, et al. The health related quality of life and economic burden of constipation. Pharmacoeconomics 2005;23:461–76.
19. Singh G, Lingala V, Wang H, et al. Use of health care resources and cost of care for adults with constipation. Clin Gastroenterol Hepatol 2007;5(9):1053–8.
20. Martin BC, Barghout V, Cerulli A. Direct medical costs of constipation in the United States. Manag Care Interface 2006;19:43–9.
21. Nehra V, Bruce BK, Rath-Harvey DM, et al. Psychological disorders in patients with evacuation disorders and constipation in a tertiary practice. Am J Gastroenterol 2000;95:1755–8.

22. Rao SS, Seaton K, Miller MJ, et al. Psychological profiles and quality of life differ between patients with dyssynergia and those with slow transit constipation. J Psychosom Res 2007;63(4):441–9.
23. Leroi AM, Berkelmans I, Denis P, et al. Anismus as a marker of sexual abuse: consequences of abuse on anorectal motility. Dig Dis Sci 1995;40:1411–6.
24. Ringel Y, Whitehead WE, Tober BB. Sexual and physical are not associated with rectal hypersensitivity in patients with irritable bowel syndrome. Gut 2004;53: 838–42.
25. Irvine EJ, Ferrazzi S, Pare P, et al. Health-related quality of life in functional GI disorders: focus on constipation and resource utilization. Am J Gastroenterol 2002;97:1986–93.
26. Pinho M, Yoshioka K, Keighley MRB. Long term results of anorectal myectomy for chronic constipation. Br J Surg 1989;76:1163–4.
27. Joo JS, Agachan F, Wolff B, et al. Initial North American experience with botulinum toxin type A for treatment of anismus. Dis Colon Rectum 1996;39:1107–11.
28. Glia A, Lindberg F, Nilsson LH, et al. Clinical value of symptom assessment in patients with constipation. Dis Colon Rectum 1999;42(11):1401–8.
29. Koch A, Voderholzer WA, Klauser AG, et al. Symptoms in chronic constipation. Dis Colon Rectum 1998;40(8):902–6.
30. Hull TL, Fazio VW, Schroeder T. Paradoxical puborectalis contraction in patients after pelvic pouch construction. Dis Colon Rectum 1995;38(11):1144–6.
31. Rao SS, Ozturk R, De Ocampo S, et al. Pathophysiology and role of biofeedback therapy in solitary rectal ulcer syndrome. Am J Gastroenterol 2006;101(3):613–8.
32. Wald A, Chandra R, Chiponis D. Anorectal function and continence mechanisms in childhood encopresis. J Pediatr Gastroenterol Nutr 1986;5:346–51.
33. Hobbis ICA, Turpin G, Read NW. Examination of the role of psychosocial factors in the pathogenesis of functional bowel disorders. Gastroenterology 1995;108: A614.
34. Chiaioni G, Bassotti G, Monsignori A, et al. Anorectal dysfunction in constipated women with anorexia nervosa. Mayo Clin Proc 2000;75(10):1015–9.
35. Kacasick S, Ehrlich SM. Is constipation a disorder of defecation or impaired motility? AJR Am J Roentgenol 1996;166(1):63–6.
36. Rao P, Tantiphlachiva K, Attaluri A, et al. How useful is digital rectal examination in the diagnosis of dyssynergia? Am J Gastroenterol 2007;102:51.
37. Lawrentschuk N, Bolton DM. Experience and attitudes of final-year medical students to digital rectal examination. Med J Aust 2004;181:323–5.
38. Rao SSC, Patel RS. How useful are manometric tests of anorectal function in the management of defecation disorders. Am J Gastroenterol 1997;92:469–75.
39. Rao SSC, Hatfield R, Soffer E, et al. Manometric tests of anorectal function in healthy adults. Am J Gastroenterol 1999;94(3):773–83.
40. Rao SSC, Azpiroz F, Diamant N. Minimum standards of anorectal manometry. Neurogastroenterol Motil 2002;14:553–9.
41. Duthie GS, Bartolo DCC. Anismus: the cause of constipation? Results of investigation and treatment. World J Surg 1992;16:831–5.
42. Rao SSC, Kavlock R, Rao S. Influence of body position and stool characteristics on defecation in humans. Am J Gastroenterol 2006;101:2790–6.
43. Pelsang RE, Rao SSC, Welcher K. FECOM: a new artificial stool for assessing defecation. Am J Gastroenterol 1999;94:183–6.
44. Diamant NE, Kamm MA, Wald A, et al. AGA technical review on anorectal testing techniques. Gastroenterology 1999;116(3):735–60.

45. Schounten WR, Briel JW, Auwerda JJ, et al. Anismus: fact or fiction? Dis Colon Rectum 1997;40(9):1033–41.
46. Glia A, Lindberg G, Nilsson LH, et al. Constipation assessed on the basis of colorectal physiology. Scand J Gastroenterol 1998;33(12):1273–9.
47. Rao SSC, Mudipalli RS, Stessman M, et al. Investigation of the utility of colorectal function tests and Rome II criteria in dyssynergic defecation (anismus). Neurogastroenterol Motil 2004;16:589–96.
48. Longstreth GF, Thompson WG, Chey WD, et al. Functional bowel disorders. Gastroenterology 2006;130:1480–91.
49. Stumbo PJ, Hemmingway D, Paulson J, et al. How useful is dietary management in the treatment of chronic constipation?. Supplement to. Gastroenterology 2008; 134(4):A469.
50. Bassoti G, Gavurri M. Manometeric investigation of high amplitude propagated contractile activity of the human colon. Am J Physiol 1988;255:G660–4.
51. Rao SSC, Sadeghi P, Beaty J, et al. Ambulatory 24-hour colonic manometry in slow-transit constipation. Am J Gastroenterol 2004;99:2405–16.
52. Muller-Lissner SA, Kamm MA, Scarpignato C, et al. Myths and misconceptions about chronic constipation. Am J Gastroenterol 2005;100:232–42.
53. Voderholzer WA, Schatke W, Muhldorfer BE, et al. Clinical response to dietary fiber treatment of chronic constipation. Am J Gastroenterol 1997;92:95–8.
54. Brandt LJ, Prather CM, Quigley EM, et al. Systematic review on the management of chronic constipation in North America. Am J Gastroenterol 2005;100(Suppl 1): S5–21.
55. Ramkumar D, Rao SSC. Efficacy and safety of traditional medical therapies for chronic constipation: systematic review. Am J Gastroenterol 2005;100:936–71.
56. Kline C. Non prescription drugs USA 2000.
57. Dipalma JA, DeRidder PH, Orlando RC, et al. A randomized, placebo-controlled, multicenter study of the safety and efficacy of a new polyethylene glycol laxative. Am J Gastroenterol 2000;95(2):341–2.
58. Cuppoletti J, Malinowska DH, Tewari KP, et al. SPI-0211 activates T84 cell chloride transport and recombinant human ClC-2 chloride currents. Am J Physiol Cell Physiol 2004;287:C1173–83.
59. Lipecka J, Bali M, Thomas A, et al. Distribution of ClC-2 chloride channel in rat and human epithelial tissues. Am J Physiol Cell Physiol 2002;282:C805–16.
60. Johanson JF, Morton D, Geenen J, Multicenter. 4-week, double-blind, randomized, placebo-controlled trail of lubiprostone, a locally-acting type-2 chloride channel activator, in patients with chronic constipation. Am J Gastroenterol 2008;103(1):170–7.
61. Johanson JF, Panas R, Holland PC, et al. Long-term efficacy of lubiprostone for the treatment of chronic constipation. Gastroenterology 2006;130:M117.
62. Verne GN, Eaker EY, David RD. Colchicine is an effective treatment for patients with severe idiopathic constipation. Gastroenterology 1995;108:A70.
63. Roarty TP, Weber F, Soykan I, et al. Misoprostol in the treatment of chronic refractory constipation: results of a long-term open label trial. Aliment Pharmacol Ther 1997;11:1059–66.
64. Andersen V, Camilleri M, Busciglio IA, et al. Effects of 5 days linaclotide on transit and bowel function in females with constipation-predominant irritable bowel syndrome. Gastroenterol 2007;133(3):761–8.
65. Rao SSC, Welcher K, Pelsang RE. Effects of biofeedback therapy on anorectal function in obstructive defecation. Dig Dis Sci 1997;42:2197–205.

66. Rao SSC. The Technical aspects of biofeedback therapy for defecation disorders. Gastroenterologist 1998;6:96–103.
67. Chiarioni G, Salandini L, Whitehead WE. Biofeedback benefits only patients with outlet dysfunction, not patients with isolated slow transit constipation. Gastroenterology 2005;129:86–97.
68. Rao SS, Seaton K, Miller M, et al. Randomized controlled trial of biofeedback, sham feedback, and standard therapy for dyssynergic defecation. Clin Gastroenterol Hepatol 2007;5:331–8.
69. Heymen S, Scarlett Y, Jones K, et al. Randomized, controlled trail shows biofeedback to be superior to alternative treatments for patients with pelvic floor dyssynergia-type constipation. Dis Colon Rectum. 2007;50(4):428–41.
70. Heymen S, Jones KR, Scarlett, et al. Biofeedback treatment of constipation: a critical review. Dis Colon Rectum 2003;46(9):1208–17.
71. Chiarioni G, Whitehead WE, Pezza V, et al. Biofeedback is superior to laxatives for normal transit constipation due to pelvic floor dyssynergia. Gastroenterology 2006;130:657–64.
72. Koutsomanis D, Lennard-Jones J, Kamm MA. Prospective study of biofeedback treatment for patients with slow and normal transit constipation. Eur J Gastroenterol Hepatol 1994;6:131–7.
73. Patankar SK, Ferrara A, Levy JR, et al. Biofeedback in colorectal practice: a multicenter, statewide, three-year experience. Dis Colon Rectum 1997;40:827–31.
74. Hallan RI, Williams NS, Melling J, et al. Treatment of anismus in intractable constipation with botulinum A toxin. Lancet 1988;2:714–7.

Fecal Incontinence and Biofeedback Therapy

Christine Norton, PhD, MA, RN[a,b,*]

KEYWORDS

- Fecal incontinence • Biofeedback • Pelvic floor muscle training
- Conservative management

Fecal incontinence (FI) may be defined as involuntary loss of stool that is a social or hygienic problem.[1] It affects between 1% and 15% of adults to at least some extent,[2–5] depending on the definition used, and is probably a significant limitation on quality of life for 0.5% to 1% of adults.[2] Although FI increases in prevalence with advancing age and disability, it also affects large numbers of healthy adults in middle age. Somewhat surprisingly, in most large community studies the prevalence in men and women is similar, although women tend to have more severe and frequent symptoms, and certainly present more often for clinical care.

FI has an understandably profound impact on a patient's quality of life, leading to major social and psychologic impact in many cases.[6,7] As a stigmatized condition, it leads to embarrassment and shame, often combined with reluctance to admit the problem and present for help from health care professionals. Some people lack a vocabulary with which to explain their symptoms, or assume that FI is an inevitable consequence of childbirth, diarrheal disease, or anal surgery. The impact seems to be very individual, and some cope well, but others live in fear of being caught out in public and map all activities around the likely availability of easy access to toilet facilities.[8] Increasing recognition of the importance of the patient perspective and impact on quality of life has led to recent efforts to develop standardized and validated tools to add this dimension to outcome measures for FI,[9–11] in addition to the somewhat simplistic "scores" that presume that number of episodes equate to "severity".[12,13] Those patients with the most severe symptoms and impact on quality of life are the most likely to seek help.[4]

FI is a symptom arising from diverse etiologies, which often coexist in the same individual. Typically, patients complain of urgency and urge incontinence, often

[a] King's College London, Florence Nightingale School of Nursing and Midwifery, James Clark Maxwell Building, 57 Waterloo Road, London SE1 8WA, UK
[b] Burdett Institute of Gastrointestinal Nursing, St. Mark's Hospital, Watford Road, Harrow HA1 3UJ, UK
* Corresponding author. Burdett Institute of Gastrointestinal Nursing, St Mark's Hospital, Watford Road, Harrow HA1 3UJ, UK.
E-mail address: christine.s.norton@kcl.ac.uk

Gastroenterol Clin N Am 37 (2008) 587–604
doi:10.1016/j.gtc.2008.06.008 gastro.theclinics.com

indicating external sphincter weakness or damage,[14] or passive soiling secondary to internal anal sphincter disruption or atrophy.[15] Both symptoms can be present in the same individual. Stool consistency, bowel motility, sensation, completeness of evacuation, and physical or mental abilities for self-care may each have an impact. The most common causes and contributing factors are summarized in **Table 1**.

It is this multiple pathology that often enables FI symptoms to be reversed by conservative means. Even in patients with sphincter trauma, there may well be an element of residual function that can be improved, or other factors, such as stool consistency, toilet habit, complete evacuation, psychologic coping, and toilet access, can be optimized. In practice, although sphincter damage is commonly found when these patients are imaged, careful history often reveals that the patient has not been symptomatic continuously following the trauma incident. Other factors have contributed to symptom development, and these can be modified.

PATIENT ASSESSMENT

Because FI is a symptom of multiple etiologies, it is highly unlikely that the same treatment suits all patients. For this reason, careful assessment of history, symptoms, and contributing factors is mandatory (**Box 1**), as is a basic physical assessment including anal, abdominal, and rectal examination.[16–18] Various investigations are commonly used, including manometry, electrophysiologic tests to assess reflexes and sensory function, and imaging of the sphincters using anal ultrasound or MRI. There is almost

Table 1
Causes of fecal incontinence

External sphincter disruption or internal sphincter disruption	Obstetric injury; congenital anomaly; iatrogenic following colorectal surgery (eg, hemorrhoidectomy or sphincterotomy); impalement injuries; idiopathic degeneration
Diarrhea or loose stool	Inflammatory bowel disease; irritable bowel syndrome; gastrointestinal infections; dietary sensitivities (eg, lactose or fructose intolerance, caffeine sensitivity, excess alcohol, artificial sugars); medications (eg, orlistat, antibiotics); celiac disease; anxiety; radiation enteropathy
Loss of sensation	Neurologic disease or injury (eg, spinal cord injury, spina bifida, multiple sclerosis, diabetic neuropathy)
Constipation or incomplete evacuation	Frailty, immobility, stool impaction, rectocele or pelvic floor dysfunction, neurologic disease or injury, medications
Anorectal pathology	Rectal prolapse, third-degree hemorrhoids, anal fistula
Physical disabilities with toileting difficulties	Neurologic disease or injury, frail elderly people, poor toileting facilities, lack of caregiver availability
Mental capacity to comply with social norms for toilet behavior	Severe learning difficulties, confusion, advanced dementia
Idiopathic	Cause unknown

Box 1
Checklist for FI assessment

Onset of symptoms

Usual bowel habit

Changes in bowel habit

Stool consistency

Amount and frequency of FI

Urgency or urge FI

Passive soiling

Difficulty wiping clean after toilet

Nocturnal bowel symptoms

Abdominal pain and bloating

Evacuation difficulty

- Straining
- Incomplete evacuation
- Pain
- Digitation

Control of flatus

Rectal bleeding or mucus

Products used to manage FI

Diet: pattern and constituents

Fluid intake and types

Obstetric and surgical history

Comorbidities and physical abilities

Medications

Mental status

Abdominal, anal, perineal, and rectal examination

no evidence that the results of these tests change management or influence patient outcomes, however, and expert opinion suggests that evaluation of FI does not necessarily include manometry and imaging in the first instance for all patients.[16] In the United Kingdom, national guidelines[19] now encourage a step-wise approach to patients (in the absence of alarm symptoms, such as rectal bleeding or unexplained change in bowel habit, which warrant investigation in their own right), except those with acute sphincter rupture or complete rectal prolapse who should normally obtain imaging and a surgical opinion as first-line management. Other patients should normally have a targeted history and physical examination[17,20] and then consideration of a range of conservative options, which can be combined according to individual need.

ELEMENTS OF CONSERVATIVE CARE

In the United Kingdom a step-wise approach has been recommended by the National Health Service (**Fig. 1**).[21] This includes identifying and addressing such factors as toilet

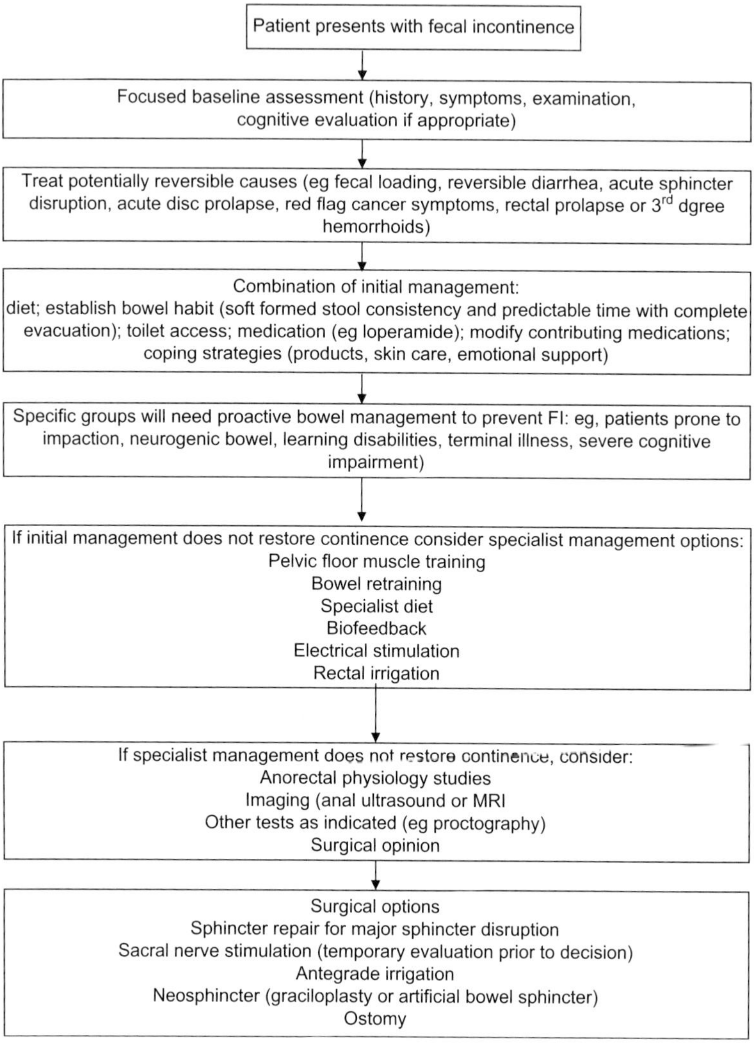

Fig. 1. Step-wise algorithm for management of fecal incontinence.

access, diet, mobility, and cognitive factors. Medical management without any exercises or biofeedback has been found to improve symptoms in one third to one half of patients.[22,23]

Patient Education and Understanding

Few patients understand how the gastrointestinal tract works and many have misconceptions, leading to counterproductive coping strategies.[24] Patients often benefit from verbal and written information to enhance understanding of normal gut function and why their symptoms have arisen.[25]

Bowel Habit

For most patients there should be an attempt to address bowel habit to enable the patient to achieve a complete evacuation of a formed stool at a predictable time each day.[16,17] Even if FI persists, this makes the symptom much more tolerable and less limiting of activities. This might mean addressing constipation or evacuation difficulties for some patients (see the article by Rao, elsewhere in this issue), or reducing frequency and firming the stool for those with urgency and loose stool.

Diet Modification

There is an obvious relationship between dietary intake and defecation. Changing the amount, content, and timing of food and drink can make a major difference to bowel habit and stool consistency for some people, maybe particularly when there is an element of irritable bowel syndrome (IBS) also present. Patients with FI secondary to loose stool have been found to respond to addition of soluble fiber to their diet. In one randomized controlled trial (RCT) of 39 patients, placebo was compared with two types of fiber supplement, both of which produced less FI than placebo,[26] although another RCT has suggested that response to fiber is individual with some patients reporting benefit from either high- or low-fiber diets.[27]

Other diet modification approaches should be individualized. Diarrhea-predominant IBS patients may benefit from fiber reduction, especially if intake is high to excessive.[28] Lactose intolerance, undiagnosed celiac disease, and excess caffeine or alcohol intake may each contribute and be easily overlooked. Fructose intolerance affects up to one third of IBS patients and a diet with restricted fruit intake may improve symptoms.[29]

Other Lifestyle Modifications

There are several other known risk factors for FI that have yet to be subjected to trials treating the symptom. Obesity,[5,30] particularly morbid obesity,[31] has been found to increase risk of FI,[32,33] with rates over 60% reported, and such medications as Olestra to treat obesity have been reported to increase FI (probably by causing loose stool).[34] It is not known if weight loss reverses symptoms once present. Depression is also found to coexist,[5] but again treatment studies are lacking. Group therapy may be of benefit to some.[35] Smoking can stimulate colonic motility[36] and might in theory exacerbate urgency.

Urge Resistance Training

It is not difficult to imagine how patients with the socially devastating symptom of FI might become hypersensitive to any rectal or anal sensation and respond by an immediate search for toilet facilities. This seems to initiate a vicious circle of increasing urgency and anxiety for some patients, with urge FI resulting when the panic is overwhelming or no facilities can be located. Patients seem to lose all confidence in the ability to defer defecation and all rectal sensation is interpreted as an impending incontinence episode. This vicious circle can be broken in some patients by careful explanation and coaching to incrementally resist the urgency by repeatedly "holding on" for longer and longer time periods, possibly only a few seconds at first but gradually building to enough minutes to be confident that facilities can be reached.[37] A similar program has been found successful in most patients with urge urinary incontinence whether secondary to detrusor instability or overactive bladder syndrome without instability.[38] Although not yet formally evaluated as a single treatment for FI, such training has been incorporated in some biofeedback programs, where it may be combined with dietary or medication measures to firm the stool.[39]

Medication

There is good evidence that loperamide (Imodium) can reduce frequency and firm the stool for people with FI related to loose stool.[40,41] It has been found beneficial in patients with FI secondary to diarrhea-inducing medication, such as orlistat.[42] Once constipation has been excluded as an underlying factor for FI, loperamide is often the first treatment option tried for FI. Patients do need careful teaching, however, on the mechanism of action and how to use loperamide. If used in doses recommended for frank diarrhea, constipation likely occurs. Because it dampens the gastrocolonic response, it is often best to take the medication approximately 30 to 60 minutes before a meal. Onset of action is rapid and a half-life of approximately 8 hours means that as-needed use (as opposed to routine dosage) can be useful. A syrup formulation enables fine titration of dose to individual response and gives the patient a useful sense of control.

Codeine phosphate, diphenoxylate, or low-dose amitriptyline (the latter particularly if there are symptoms of IBS) are alternatives,[1,41] but tend to have more side effects than loperamide. Stool bulking agents may help to form loose stool. There is also a suggestion from a nonrandomized study that low-dose cholestyramine may be useful in patients with FI secondary to loose stool.[43] The anorectum and pelvic floor have estrogen receptors and a small study has suggested benefit of postmenopausal hormone therapy for FI.[44] Medications specifically to modify anal sphincter function have been reported but have yet to reach the market.[45,46]

Pelvic Floor Muscle Training

In contrast to the large literature on urinary incontinence,[38] there has been relatively little attention given to the option of exercises alone, without additional biofeedback for FI. The reason for this is unclear. The few studies that have been reported have given no pointers as to the optimum regimen of exercises (mode of teaching, number and type of exercises, or frequency of practice). Evidence is also lacking or conflicting as to efficacy. One RCT study found that exercises plus conservative management advice was no more effective than the advice alone;[23] two studies have found digitally taught exercises as effective as biofeedback.[23,47] Another small study has found equivalent outcomes comparing verbally taught exercises with biofeedback.[48]

Because exercises are a relatively low-cost and possibly self-directed treatment, it may be worth trying before formal biofeedback training.

BIOFEEDBACK FOR FECAL INCONTINENCE

For many years case series and expert opinion proposed "biofeedback" as the treatment option of first choice in the treatment of FI.[49,50] Case series almost unanimously reported positive patient outcomes, often in over 70% of patients.[51,52] Case series methodology, however, has widely acknowledged weaknesses (it was difficult to know if the biofeedback was the crucial element in an often complex package of care including many of the measures outlined previously). In addition, outcome measurements were often poor, or proxy measures, such as anal sphincter pressures.

DIFFERENT METHODS OF BIOFEEDBACK

There is no standard method of biofeedback for FI and some authors have failed to describe the makeup of their intervention. Most include one-to-one sessions with a therapist (doctor, nurse, physical therapist, clinical scientist, or other) of different durations (typically 30–60 minutes) at variable time intervals (from more than once daily to once per month or less frequently) and some have admitted patients to hospital for intensive treatment.[53] All involve some type of anorectal instrumentation to enable the patient to become aware of voluntary or autonomic functions and modify those functions, but the proportion of each session devoted to this activity is seldom stated, because presumably most therapists also interact socially and review symptoms and incorporate other advice and education. The impression is that some authors have used sessions for multiple repeated attempts to modify function, whereas others have used instruments as a quick check on progress and spent most of each session concentrating on the education elements. The main modalities of instrumented biofeedback are discussed next.

Measures of Voluntary Squeeze

This has been displayed to the patient using electromyography (EMG), manometry, and anal or perineal ultrasound. The patient may lie or sit with direct views of the computer or imaging monitor and attempt squeezing with real-time feedback (usually visual but occasional auditory) of the success of each attempt. The therapist can coach the patient to improve performance. Some equipment sets goals for patients, such as grid lines to follow for the pressure of each squeeze. The aim is usually to demonstrate the correct action to the patient and then to monitor progress of a structured pelvic floor muscle exercise program conducted by the patient at home between visits. Some authors have included abdominal EMG to enable the patient to isolate anal contraction from abdominal effort, avoiding any counterproductive straining effect during exercises.

Modification of Anorectal Sensation

Typically, a rectal balloon is inserted and gradually filled with air or water. Depending on the assessed problem, this may be used to raise or lower sensory thresholds or tolerated volumes. Patients found to have a high threshold of sensation to rectal filling have been reported to experience improved symptoms if their threshold can be lowered,[54] presumably by allowing earlier perception of stool and the possibility of responding by anal contraction or finding toilet facilities promptly. This is usually achieved by finding the volume that can be reliably detected and then repeatedly filling at volumes below this threshold until the patient learns to perceive this. Conversely, patients with an oversensitive rectum may learn that if this sensation is ignored or resisted, then it diminishes and larger volumes can be tolerated.[37,55]

Co-ordination Training

A two- or three-balloon system is used to simulate the rectoanal inhibitory reflex and train the patient to increase speed of reaction and voluntary squeeze increment in response. The rectal balloon is inflated with air or water. One or two balloons in the anal canal record the consequent fall in anal pressure and the patient is asked to counteract this fall by a voluntary contraction of the external anal sphincter. Repeated trials may be conducted until the patient is successful in achieving no fall in anal pressure. Alternatively, the patient is taught to squeeze in response to successively weaker rectal stimuli.[54] The patient may also be instructed to practice the same maneuver in response to each urge to defecate. This "urge resistance" has also been described as an instruction to the patient in the absence of any biofeedback to assist in learning the technique.

Biofeedback protocols have varied greatly in terms of number and frequency of sessions, length of sessions, and therapist training. It has been reported in a nonrandomized study that less intensive telephone follow-up may be as effective as face-to-face contact,[56] suggesting that the instrumental elements of biofeedback may not be the most crucial element.

Evidence for the Efficacy of Biofeedback

Given the possible complexity of an individual patient care plan during biofeedback (which might include any or all of the modalities of biofeedback and adjunctive therapies listed previously), it has been difficult to determine whether biofeedback per se is the effective element of any intervention. Trials comparing different methods of biofeedback, including home practice machines, EMG, pressure, and ultrasound biofeedback, have failed to find any difference in outcomes.[23,47,57] The addition of biofeedback and exercises after sphincter repair made little difference compared with sphincter repair alone.[58] A Cochrane review of 11 RCTs has concluded that there is no evidence at present of one method of biofeedback giving any benefit over any other method, or that exercises or biofeedback offer any advantage over other conservative care.[59] The evidence from RCTs to 2008 is summarized in **Table 2**.

It does seem that the effect of biofeedback interventions is largely maintained at 1 year.[23,60] Some specific patient groups have been studied in uncontrolled trials with suggestion of benefit, such as patients with FI after anterior rectal resection with or without radiotherapy.[53] Controlled studies of the preventive value of pelvic floor muscle training have failed to show a difference in postnatal FI compared with controls.[61–63]

Loose stool, symptom of passive (as compared with urge) FI, and previous third-degree tear have been found to predict poorer outcomes from exercises or biofeedback, as may more severe initial symptoms, whereas baseline tests have little predictive value.[64] Other authors, however, have reported that more severe symptoms may predict better results.[65] Men may do less well than women, for reasons as yet undetermined.[65]

Electrical Stimulation

Stimulation of striated muscle at a frequency sufficient to produce a tonic involuntary contraction (usually 30–50 Hz) can increase muscle strength, increase conduction rate of the pudendal nerve, increase the size of motor units, encourage neuronal sprouting, and promote local blood flow. This has been used to enhance the squeeze pressure of the external anal sphincter. Stimulation at lower frequencies (typically 5–10 Hz) can modulate autonomic function including both sensation and overactivity. This has been used successfully in patients with overactive bladder but has received little attention in FI.

Studies of electrical stimulation for FI have to date been largely small and uncontrolled or with confounding effects of exercises, biofeedback, or other interventions.[66,67] A recent Cochrane review found only four RCT studies with 260 participants in the world literature.[68] One study found that anal electrical stimulation with anal biofeedback produced more short-term benefits than vaginal biofeedback alone in women with postnatal FI (n = 40).[69] Another study found no additional benefit of exercises, biofeedback, and electrical stimulation over exercises and biofeedback alone in a similar group of 60 women, many of them with evidence of sphincter disruption.[70] One study found that patients (n = 90) improved equally using stimulation at 1 Hz and 35 Hz over an 8-week period with no adjunctive therapies, suggesting that any effect may be by enhancing sensation rather than muscle strengthening.[71] It is difficult to be sure that it is electrical stimulation itself that produces any reported effect. The final RCT in the review compared conservative treatment (daily anal electrical stimulation) with levatorplasty surgery over 2 years in 70 patients and found the surgery intervention to be superior in terms of continence outcome, although physiologic parameters were similar.[72] The authors of the Cochrane review concluded that there is a suggestion that electrical stimulation may have an effect and that further and larger studies are needed.[68]

Subsequent to the Cochrane review two new RCTs have been published. One study (n = 48) has found no difference between daily home stimulation and weekly biofeedback alternating with electrical stimulation in the clinic, with both groups reporting improvement and improved manometry.[73] A second study compared twice-daily 30-minute home sessions of electrical stimulation or biofeedback in 40 women after obstetric injury for 8 weeks. There was no difference between the groups at the end of treatment. Both groups improved their satisfaction and subjective symptoms, but there were no changes in continence scores or quality of life measures.[74]

WHEN BIOFEEDBACK DOES NOT WORK

Few other options have been described for conservative management of FI. Surgery is discussed elsewhere in this issue.

Rectal Irrigation

Rectal irrigation with tap water has been found to improve bowel management, constipation, and FI in patients with problematic bowel management following spinal cord injury.[75] This warrants further evaluation in other populations because uncontrolled case series report possible efficacy in FI.[76–78]

Products to Manage Fecal Incontinence

There are few purpose-designed products that target FI. Absorbent diapers are generally held to be unsatisfactory in providing security and comfort, protecting the skin, or disguising odor. Many people with FI choose not to wear pads.[4] Small anal dressings may be useful for people with minor soiling contained between the buttocks,[79] but can become costly if several are needed each day.

An anal plug contains FI for some patients,[80] with a recommended wear time of up to 12 hours. If rectal and anal sensation is intact, however, many patients find the plug difficult to tolerate because of discomfort or a desire to defecate.[81] Some patients anecdotally report being able gradually to increase tolerance and wear time for an anal plug, but generally use is confined to those with neurologic impairment.

Other products helpful to individual patients include skin care and barrier products,[82,83] and odor control. Again, there is little research in FI, but in clinical practice many ostomy products are useful.

SUMMARY

Biofeedback as delivered in most clinical settings in Western medicine has been consistently reported to improve symptoms of FI. Numerous case series attest to efficacy. Closer scrutiny of the elements of the intervention and controlled studies have consistently failed, however, to find any benefit of the biofeedback element of this complex package of care, with one exception reported only in abstract;[84] nor has any superiority been found for one modality over another. There is certainly a need for further well-designed and adequately powered RCTs.[49,59] Labeling an intervention "biofeedback" certainly assists with reimbursement and billing issues in some health care environments, but from a scientific viewpoint the added benefit of adding biofeedback to other elements of care has yet to be convincingly demonstrated. As ever, absence of evidence is not the same thing as evidence of absence,

Table 2
Randomized controlled trials of biofeedback or exercises for fecal incontinence in adults

Author, Year, Country	Population	Intervention	Control	Outcome	Comments
Davis 2004 UK	38 women undergoing anal sphincter repair. Mean age 60 (range, 26–78).	Manometric BFB starting 3 months after surgery: 1 h/wk for 6 weeks (exercise and sensory training). N = 14 completed.	Usual care. N = 17 completed.	31 completed at 12 months after surgery. VAS for subjective outcome: NSD. QoL: NSD. Score: NSD. Manometry: NSD.	No ITT analysis. Scores, satisfaction, and manometry improved in both groups compared with 3 months postsurgery. Paper focuses on before-after changes within groups and does not report detailed differences between groups.
Fynes 1999 Ireland	40 women with obstetric-related FI. Mean age 32 years (range, 18–48).	Weekly anal EMG BFB plus electrical stimulation (20 Hz and 50 Hz) with physiotherapist (augmented BFB).	Weekly vaginal manometric BFB with nurse specialist.	At end of 12 weeks treatment score improved more in augmented group (P = <0.001)	No ITT analysis. Paper focuses on before-after changes within groups and does not report detailed differences between groups.
Heymen 2007 USA	108 patients, 25 men. Failed previous maximal medical management.	61-h sessions alternate weeks. EMG BFB plus PFMT (N = 44). Plus sensory training?	61-h sessions alternate weeks. PFMT (N = 64).	"Adequate relief": yes/no at 3 months after treatment: BFB: 77% yes. PFMT: 41% yes (P = .001). FISI: BFB > PFMT (P = .001). Diary: trend to BFB >PFMT (P = .07). Per protocol: 66 BFB versus 48% controls fully continent.	Abstract only. ITT analysis performed.

Heymen 2000 USA	40 patients with FI not suitable for surgery. Mean age 74 years (range, 36–88), 11 men.	Four groups: 1. Anal clinic EMG 2. Anal clinic EMG plus sensory balloon training 3. Anal clinic plus home trainer EMG 4. Anal clinic EMG plus sensory balloon training plus home trainer	See four intervention groups.	34 patients completed. Diary (days with FI episode): NSD.	No ITT analysis. All groups significantly reduced incontinence frequency.
Ilnyckyj 2005 Canada	23 women with regular and frequent FI. Mean age 59 years (range, 26–75). Excluded irritable bowel syndrome.	Education plus manometric BFB. N = 7 completed.	Education plus PFMT. N = 11 completed.	18 completed. Success = no FI in last week of study: BFB 6/7 (86%) PFMT 5/11 (45%) P = .2.	No ITT analysis. Underpowered to detect a difference?
Latimer 1984 Canada	8 subjects (four children) range, 8–72 years.	Four phases: 1. 1 month diary 2. PFMT with balloon and verbal feedback 3. Rectal sensory training 4. Three balloon BFB	Varied order of phases.	—	Complex design. Underpowered to detect a difference.
Mahony 2004 Ireland	60 consecutive women with FI after obstetric injury in perineal clinic (range, 22–42 years).	Anal EMG BFB weekly for 12 weeks (26 completed).	Anal EMG BFB weekly for 12 weeks plus 20 minute electrical stimulation at 35 Hz (28 completed).	54 completed. Score: NSD. Manometry: NSD.	No ITT analysis. Both groups improved equally. Most results reported by group before-after.
McHugh 1986 Canada	23 women with regular FI.	Three sessions "standard" BFB over 2 months (no details given).	Home manometry. BFB daily.	13 completed. Diary: insufficient information to judge.	Abstract only.

(*continued on next page*)

Table 2
(continued)

Author, Year, Country	Population	Intervention	Control	Outcome	Comments
Miner 1990 UK	25 consecutive patients with FI, 8 men. Age range, 17–76 years.	1. Rectal sensation training. 2. Strength or coordination training (crossed over).	1. Sham rectal sensation training. 2. Coordination or strength training (crossed over).	End of active versus sham: active reduced FI.	No ITT analysis. Complex crossover design and small sample size. Both groups improved: plus 24-month follow-up: improvement maintained.
Naimy 2007 Norway	49 women after third or fourth degree obstetric tear (referred or identified by survey). Mean age 36 (range, 22–44).	BFB: EMG, anal probe, home exercises (fast, 10 second and endurance squeezes). 20 minutes, twice daily at home for 8 weeks plus two sessions with therapist.	Electrical stimulation at 30–40 Hz, pulse width 200 μs, limit at 80 mA, anal probe 20 minutes, twice daily at home for 8 weeks plus two sessions with therapist.	40 completed. Score: NSD. QoL: NSD. Both groups subjectively improved.	No ITT analysis. Compared median changes pretreatment and posttreatment between groups rather than direct comparison. Both groups improved subjective perception of control, but no changes shown in other parameters. Mostly mild FI: limits potential to benefit?
Norton 2003 UK	171 patients referred for BFB. Mean age 56 (range 26–85), 12 men.	Four groups, all up to 61-hour sessions: 1. Education, advice, plus urge resistance. 2. As group 1 plus PFMT taught digitally. 3. As group 2 plus clinic manometric BFB. 4. As group 3 plus home EMG BFB.	See four intervention groups.	140 completed. Immediate plus 12 months: Subjective: NSD. Satisfaction: NSD. Score: NSD. QoL: NSD. Manometry: NSD. Anxiety and depression: NSD. Diary: NSD.	Performed ITT analysis. Global improvement across all groups.

Solomon 2003 Australia	120 patients who had failed diet and medical management. Mean age 62 years, 13 men.	Five monthly 30-minute sessions. Three groups: 1. PFMT taught digitally. 2. PFMT plus anal ultrasound BFB. 3. PFMT plus manometric BFB.	See groups.	102 completed. End of treatment: score: NSD. QoL: NSD. Manometry: NSD. Subjective: NSD.	No ITT analysis. All groups improved equally and significantly.
Whitehead 1985 USA	18 older patients recruited from clinics or newspaper advertisement. Mean age 73 years (range, 65–92), three men, six double incontinence.	4 weeks habit training plus PFMT (50 squeezes per day for 10 seconds).	4 weeks habit training alone.	End of treatment: No statistical analysis given of difference between groups.	No ITT analysis. If still incontinent after 4 weeks, all received BFB.

Abbreviations: BFB; EMG, electromyography; FI, fecal incontinence; FISI, fecal incontinence severity index; ITT, intention to treat; NSD, no significant difference; PFMT, pelvic floor muscle training; QoL, quality of life; VAS, visual analogue scale.

and it may be in the future that additional efficacy will be demonstrated. Meanwhile, there can be little doubt that conservative interventions improve many patients with FI to the point where most report satisfaction with treatment and do not wish to consider more invasive options, such as surgery.

REFERENCES

1. Norton C, Whitehead WE, Bliss DZ, et al. Conservative and pharmacological management of faecal incontinence in adults. In: Abrams P, Cardozo L, Khoury S, editors. Incontinence. Plymouth (UK): Health Publications; 2005. p. 1521–63.
2. Perry S, Shaw C, McGrother C, et al. The prevalence of faecal incontinence in adults aged 40 years or more living in the community. Gut 2002;50:480–4.
3. Macmillan AK, Merrie AEH, Marshall RJ, et al. The prevalence of fecal incontinence in community-dwelling adults: a systematic review of the literature. Dis Colon Rectum 2004;47:1341–9.
4. Bharucha AE, Zinsmeister AR, Locke GR, et al. Prevalence and burden of fecal incontinence: a population-based study in women. Gastroenterology 2005;129: 42–9.
5. Fritel X, Ringa V, Varnoux N, et al. Mode of delivery and fecal incontinence at midlife: a study of 2,640 women in the Gazel cohort. Obstet Gynecol 2007; 110(1):31–8.
6. Norton C. Nurses, bowel continence, stigma and taboos. J Wound Ostomy Continence Nurs 2004;31(2):85–94.
7. Norton N. The perspective of the patient. Gastroenterology 2004;126:S175–179.
8. Wilson M. The impact of faecal incontinence on the quality of life. Br J Nurs 2007; 16(4):204–7.
9. Rockwood TH, Church JM, Fleshman JW, et al. Fecal incontinence quality of life scale. Dis Colon Rectum 2000;43:9–17.
10. Cotterill N, Norton C, Avery K, et al. A patient-centred approach to developing a comprehensive symptom and quality of life assessment of anal incontinence. Dis Colon Rectum 2008;51:82–7.
11. Bharucha AE, Locke GR, Seide BM, et al. A new questionnaire for constipation and faecal incontinence. Aliment Pharmacol Ther 2004;20:355–64.
12. Vaizey CJ, Carapeti EA, Cahill JA, et al. Prospective comparison of faecal incontinence grading systems. Gut 1999;44:77–80.
13. Maeda Y, Pares D, Norton C, et al. Does the St. Mark's incontinence score reflect patients' perceptions? A review of 390 patients. Dis Colon Rectum 2008;51: 436–42.
14. Engel AF, Kamm MA, Bartram CI, et al. Relationship of symptoms in faecal incontinence to specific sphincter abnormalities. Int J Colorectal Dis 1995;10: 152–5.
15. Vaizey CJ, Kamm MA, Bartram CI. Primary degeneration of the internal anal sphincter as a cause of passive faecal incontinence. Lancet 1997;349:612–5.
16. Norton C, Thomas L, Hill J. Management of faecal incontinence in adults: summary of NICE guidance. Br Med J 2007;334:1370–1.
17. Bharucha AE. Fecal incontinence. Gastroenterology 2003;124:1672–85.
18. Wald A. Fecal incontinence in adults. N Engl J Med 2007;356(16):1648–55.
19. National Institute of Clinical Excellence. Management of faecal incontinence in adults. London: National Institute of Clinical Excellence; 2007.

20. Norton C, Chelvanayagam S. A nursing assessment tool for adults with fecal incontinence. J Wound Ostomy Continence Nurs 2000;27:279–91.
21. Norton C. Faecal incontinence. In: Haslam J, Laycock J, editors. Therapeutic management of incontinence and pelvic pain. 2nd edition. London: Springer; 2008. p. 199–211.
22. Heymen S, Jones KR, Ringel Y, et al. Biofeedback for fecal incontinence and constipation: the role of medical management and education. Gastroenterology 2001;120(Suppl 1):A397.
23. Norton C, Chelvanayagam S, Wilson-Barnett J, et al. Randomized controlled trial of biofeedback for fecal incontinence. Gastroenterology 2003;125:1320–9.
24. Bliss DZ, Fischer LR, Savik K. Self-care practices of the elderly to manage fecal incontinence. J Gerontol Nurs 2005;31(7):35–44.
25. Norton C, Kamm MA. Bowel control: information and practical advice. Beaconsfield (UK): Beaconsfield Publishers; 1999.
26. Bliss DZ, Jung H, Savik K, et al. Supplementation with dietary fiber improves fecal incontinence. Nurs Res 2001;50(4):203–13.
27. Lauti M, Scott D, Thompson-Fawcett W. Fibre supplementation in addition to loperamide for faecal incontinence in adults: a randomized trial. Colorectal Dis 2008;10(6):553–62.
28. National Institute of Clinical Excellence. Irritable bowel syndrome: NICE guidance; CG 61. London: National Institute of Clinical Excellence; 2008.
29. Choi YK, Kraft N, Zimmerman B, et al. Fructose intolerance in IBS and utility of frustose-restricted diet. J Clin Gastroenterol 2008;42(3):233–7.
30. Abramov Y, Sand PK, Botros SM, et al. Risk factors for female anal incontinence: new insight through the Evanston-Northwestern Twin Sisters Study. Obstet Gynecol 2005;106(4):726–32.
31. Richter HE, Burgio KL, Clements RH, et al. Urinary and anal incontinence in morbidly obese women considering weight loss surgery. Obstet Gynecol 2005; 106(6):1272–7.
32. Fornell EU, Wingren G, Kjolhede P. Factors associated with pelvic floor dysfunction with emphasis on urinary and fecal incontinence and genital prolapse: an epidemiological study. Acta Obstet Gynecol Scand 2004;83:383–9.
33. Wasserberg N, Haney M, Petrone P, et al. Fecal incontinence among morbid obese women seeking for weight loss surgery: an underappreciated association with adverse impact on quality of life. Int J Colorectal Dis 2008;23:493–7.
34. Fox M, Schwizer W, Menne D, et al. The physical properties of rectal contents have effects on anorectal continence: insights from a study into the cause of fecal spotting on orlistat. Dis Colon Rectum 2004;47(12):2147–56.
35. Chelvanayagam S, Stern J. Using therapeutic groups to support women with faecal incontinence. Br J Nurs 2007;16(4):214–8.
36. Rausch T, Beglinger C, Alam N, et al. Effect of transdermal application of nicotine on colonic transit in healthy nonsmoking volunteers. Neurogastroenterol Motil 1998;10:263–70.
37. Norton C, Chelvanayagam S. Methodology of biofeedback for adults with fecal incontinence: a program of care. J Wound Ostomy Continence Nurs 2001;28. 156–68.
38. Wilson PD, Berghmans B, Hagen S, et al. Adult conservative management. In: Abrams P, Cardozo L, Khoury S, et al, editors. Incontinence. Plymouth (UK): Health Books; 2005. p. 855–964.
39. Norton C, Chelvanayagam S, Kamm MA. Randomised controlled trial of biofeedback for faecal incontinence. [abstract]. Gut 2002;50(Suppl 11):A61.

40. Cheetham M, Brazzelli M, Norton C, et al. Drug treatment for faecal incontinence in adults (Cochrane review). Cochrane database of systematic reviews, the Cochrane library. Chichester (UK): John Wiley & Sons; 2002. 10.1002/14651858.CD002116 [Issue 3. Art. No.: CD002116].
41. Ehrenpreis ED, Chang D, Eichenwald E. Pharmacotherapy for fecal incontinence: a review. Dis Colon Rectum 2007;50(5):641–9.
42. Fox M, Stutz B, Menne D, et al. The effects of loperamide on continence problems and anorectal function in obese subjects taking orlistat. Dig Dis Sci 2005;50(9): 1576–83.
43. Remes-Troche JM, Ozturk R, Philips C, et al. Cholestyramine: a useful adjunct for the treatment of patients with fecal incontinence. Int J Colorectal Dis 2008;23(2): 189–94.
44. Donnelly V, O'Connell PR, O'Herlihy C. The influence of oestrogen replacement on faecal incontinence in postmenopausal women. Br J Obstet Gynaecol 1997; 104:311–5.
45. Carapeti EA, Kamm MA, Evans BK, et al. Topical phenylephrine increases anal sphincter resting pressure. Br J Surg 1999;86(2):267–70.
46. Carapeti EA, Kamm MA, Phillips RK. Randomized controlled trial of topical phenylephrine in the treatment of faecal incontinence. Br J Surg 2000;87: 38–42.
47. Solomon MJ, Pager CK, Rex J, et al. Randomised, controlled trial of biofeedback with anal manometry, transanal ultrasound, or pelvic floor retraining with digital guidance alone in the treatment of mild to moderate fecal incontinence. Dis Colon Rectum 2003;46(6):703–10.
48. Ilnyckyj A, Fachnie E, Tougas G. A randomized controlled trial comparing an educational intervention alone vs education and biofeedback in the management of faecal incontinence in women. Neurogastroenterol Motil 2005;17:58–63.
49. Chiarioni G, Ferri B, Morelli A, et al. Bio-feedback treatment of fecal incontinence: where are we, and where are we going? World J Gastroenterol 2005;11(31): 4771–5.
50. Whitehead WE, Wald A, Norton N. Treatment options for fecal incontinence: consensus conference report. Dis Colon Rectum 2001;44:131–44.
51. Heymen S, Jones KR, Ringel Y, et al. Biofeedback treatment of fecal incontinence: a critical review. Dis Colon Rectum 2001;44:728–36.
52. Norton C, Kamm MA. Anal sphincter biofeedback and pelvic floor exercises for faecal incontinence in adults: a systematic review. Aliment Pharmacol Ther 2001;15:1147–54.
53. Allgayer H, Dietrich CF, Rohde W, et al. Prospective comparison of short- and long-term effects of pelvic floor exercise/biofeedback training in patients with fecal incontinence after surgery plus irradiation versus surgery alone for colorectal cancer: clinical, functional and endoscopic/endosonographic findings. Scand J Gastroenterol 2005;40(10):1168–75.
54. Chiarioni G, Bassotti G, Stranganini S, et al. Sensory retraining is key to biofeedback therapy for formed stool incontinence. Am J Gastroenterol 2002; 97:109–17.
55. Schiller LR, Santa Ana C, Davis GR, et al. Faecal incontinence in chronic diarrhoea: report of a case with improvement after training with rectally infused saline. Gastroenterology 1979;77:751–3.
56. Byrne CM, Solomon MJ, Rex J, et al. Telephone vs. face-to-face biofeedback for fecal incontinence: comparison of two techniques in 239 patients. Dis Colon Rectum 2005;48:2281–8.

57. Heymen S, Pikarsky AJ, Weiss EG, et al. A prospective randomised trial comparing four biofeedback techniques for patients with faecal incontinence. Colorectal Dis 2000;2(2):88–92.
58. Davis KJ, Kumar D, Poloniecki J. Adjunctive biofeedback following anal sphincter repair: a randomised study. Aliment Pharmacol Ther 2004;20:539–49.
59. Norton C, Cody JD, Hosker G. Biofeedback and/or sphincter exercises for the treatment of faecal incontinence in adults. Cochrane database of systematic reviews, Cochrane library. Chichester (UK): John Wiley & Sons; 2006. 10.1002/14651858.CD002111.pub2 [Issue 3. Art. No.: CD002111].
60. Ozturk R, Niazi S, Stessman M, et al. Long-term outcome and objective changes of anorectal function after biofeedback therapy for faecal incontinence. Aliment Pharmacol Ther 2004;20:667–74.
61. Dannecker C, Baur C, Ruckhaberle E, et al. The effect of the pelvic floor training device Epi-No on the maternal pelvic floor function six months after childbirth: follow-up study of a randomised controlled trial. Geburtshilfe Frauenheilkd 2004;64(11):1192–8.
62. Sleep J, Grant A. Pelvic floor exercises in postnatal care. Midwifery 1987;3(4):158–64.
63. Meyer S, Hohlfield P, Achtari C, et al. Pelvic floor education after vaginal delivery. Obstet Gynecol 2001;97(5):673–7.
64. Terra MP, Deutekom M, Dobben AC, et al. Can the outcome of pelvic-floor rehabilitation in patients with fecal incontinence be predicted? International Journal of Colorectal Disease 2008;23:503–11.
65. Byrne CM, Solomon MJ, Young JM, et al. Biofeedback for fecal incontinence: short-term outcomes of 513 consecutive patients and predictors of successful treatment. Dis Colon Rectum 2007;50(4):417–27.
66. Osterberg A, Graf W, Eeg-Olofsson K, et al. Is electrostimulation of the pelvic floor an effective treatment for neurogenic faecal incontinence? Scand J Gastroenterol 1999;34(3):319–24.
67. Terra MP, Dobben AC, Berghmans B, et al. Electrical stimulation and pelvic floor muscle training with biofeedback in patients with fecal incontinence: a cohort study of 281 patients. Dis Colon Rectum 2006;49(8):1149–59.
68. Hosker G, Cody JD, Norton C. Electrical stimulation for faecal incontinence in adults (Cochrane review). Cochrane Database Syst Rev 2007;(2): CD001310. 10 1002/14651858. CD001310 pub2 2007
69. Fynes MM, Marshall K, Cassidy M, et al. A prospective, randomized study comparing the effect of augmented biofeedback with sensory biofeedback alone on fecal incontinence after obstetric trauma. Dis Colon Rectum 1999;42(6):753–8.
70. Mahony RT, Malone P, Nalty J, et al. Randomized clinical trial of intra-anal electromyographic biofeedback physiotherapy with intra-anal electromyographic biofeedback augmented with electrical stimulation of the anal sphincter in the early treatment of postpartum fecal incontinence. Am J Obstet Gynecol 2004;191:885–90.
71. Norton C, Gibbs A, Kamm MA. Randomised trial of electrical stimulation for faecal incontinence. Dis Colon Rectum 2005;49(6):190–6.
72. Osterberg A, Eeg-Olofsson K, Hallden M, et al. Randomized controlled clinical trial comparing conservative and surgical treatment of neurogenic faecal incontinence. Br J Surg 2004;91:1131–7.
73. Healy CF, Brannigan AE, Connolly EM, et al. The effects of low-frequency endo-anal electrical stimulation on faecal incontinence: a prospective study. Int J Colorectal Dis 2006;21(8):802–6.

74. Naimy N, Lindam AT, Bakka A, et al. Biofeedback vs. electrostimulation in the treatment of postdelivery anal incontinence: a randomized, clinical trial. Dis Colon Rectum 2007;50(12):2040–6.
75. Christensen P, Bazzocchi G, Coggrave M, et al. A randomized, controlled trial of transanal irrigation versus conservative bowel management in spinal cord-injured patients. Gastroenterology 2006;131:738–47.
76. Briel JW, Schouten WR, Vlot EA, et al. Clinical value of colonic irrigation in patients with continence disturbances. Dis Colon Rectum 1997;40(7):802–5.
77. Gardiner A, Marshall J, Duthie GS. Rectal irrigation for relief of functional bowel disorders. Nurs Stand 2004;19(9):39–42.
78. Crawshaw A. How to establish a rectal irrigation service. Gastrointestinal Nursing 2004;2(2):29–31.
79. Bliss DZ, Savik K. Use of an absorbent dressing specifically for fecal incontinence. J Wound Ostomy Continence Nurs 2008;35(2):221–8.
80. Deutekom M, Dobben AC. Plugs for containing faecal incontinence. Cochrane Database Syst Rev 2005;(3):CD005086:10.1002/1465.1858.CD005086.pub2.
81. Norton C, Kamm MA. Anal plug for faecal incontinence. Colorectal Dis 2001;3:323–7.
82. Gray M. Preventing and managing perineal dermatitis: a shared goal for wound and continence care. J Wound Ostomy Continence Nurs 2004;31(Suppl 1):S2–9.
83. Bliss DZ, Zehrer CL, Savik K, et al. An economic evaluation of four skin damage prevention regimens among nursing home residents with incontinence. J Wound Ostomy Continence Nurs 2007;34(2):143–52.
84. Heymen S, Scarlett Y, Jones KR, et al. Randomized controlled trial shows biofeedback to be superior to alternative treatments for patients with fecal incontinence. [abstract]. Gastroenterology 2007;132(4):A83.

Surgical Treatment of Patients with Constipation and Fecal Incontinence

Marc A. Gladman, MBBS, PhD, MRCOG, FRCS (Gen Surg),
Charles H. Knowles, MBBChir, PhD, FRCS (Gen Surg)*

KEYWORDS

• Surgery • Constipation • Fecal incontinence

Constipation and fecal incontinence (FI) both represent symptom complexes that in clinical practice present to health care providers when symptoms are sufficiently severe, and to surgeons when first-line, conservative measures have failed. It is important to consider, especially when surgical intervention is being contemplated, that patients with constipation or FI represent heterogeneous populations both in terms of reported symptoms and underlying pathophysiology. Accordingly, detailed assessment of clinical symptoms and their severity and full characterization of underlying physiologic abnormalities are required in individual patients before embarking on potentially irreversible interventions. With such information to hand, the surgeon is then able to tailor the procedure to specific underlying abnormalities to restore normal physiology and it is hoped function. Unfortunately, this is not always possible and, in such cases, treatment is frequently empiric (ie, aimed at reducing symptom severity, rather than restoring normal function).

For the purposes of the following discussion, surgical treatment of constipation and FI are considered separately, although it should be acknowledged, as is being increasingly recognized, that both conditions may coexist in individual patients (eg, outlet obstruction and passive FI).[1] Some procedures may treat FI by improving evacuation.[2] Classically, surgery is considered as a branch of medicine that treats diseases, injuries, and deformities by manual or operative methods. This article includes some therapeutic procedures that are perceived to be less invasive (eg, sacral nerve

Marc A. Gladman is supported by the Frances and Augustus Newman Foundation Research Fellowship of the Royal College of Surgeons of England. Charles H. Knowles is funded by the Higher Education Funding Council for England.
Centre for Academic Surgery, Institute of Cell and Molecular Science, Barts and The London School of Medicine and Dentistry, Whitechapel, London E1 1BB, UK
* Corresponding author. Centre for Academic Surgery, Third Floor Alexandra Wing, Royal London Hospital, Whitechapel, London E1 1BB, UK.
E-mail address: c.h.knowles@qmul.ac.uk (C.H. Knowles).

Gastroenterol Clin N Am 37 (2008) 605–625
doi:10.1016/j.gtc.2008.06.009
0889-8553/08/$ – see front matter

stimulation [SNS] and injection of biomaterials) but does not include purely diagnostic interventions, such as full-thickness rectal biopsies. For both constipation and FI, the reader is guided by dividing surgical interventions into those regarded as historical, contemporary, or evolving. Provided for each are the (1) rationale; (2) indications (including patient selection); (3) results including complications; and (4) the current position of the procedure in the management armamentarium, especially including controversies. The published success rates, outcome measures, and grades of evidence[3] are summarized for each of these procedures in **Tables 1** and **2**. In the most part, the treatment refers to that of adults unless specified. Throughout, it is assumed that organic causes have been excluded.

SURGICAL TREATMENT OF CONSTIPATION

Introduction

Patients with constipation usually present to the surgeon when nonsurgical therapies (laxatives, behavioral therapies including biofeedback) have already failed. In practice, this group has a strong female predominance and includes patients who on specialist physiologic investigation commonly have slow colonic transit, severe outlet obstruction, or both.[4] Aside from such interventions as manual evacuation, the mainstay of surgical treatment for slow transit constipation (STC) has been colectomy, whereas outlet obstruction has less clearly defined effective therapies. In respect of the latter, although they may be pathophysiologically associated, the numerous therapies for rectal prolapse and rectocele are not addressed. **Table 1** summarizes the procedures that are discussed in detail.

Historical Surgical Treatments

Colectomy, first described for constipation 100 years ago,[5] is still performed and is discussed next. In contrast, a variety of anorectal procedures (eg, anal dilatation, anorectal myectomy, partial division of puborectalis) had been performed with the

Table 1
Surgical interventions for patients with constipation

Procedure	Success Rate	Outcome Measures	Grade of Evidence
Historical			
Pelvic floor procedures	<50% (17%–48%)	Spontaneous defecation	D
Contemporary			
Colectomy	86% (39%–100%)	Satisfaction ratings, QOLclinical, physiologic	D
Anterograde colonic enema	47%	Satisfaction	D
Fecal diversion	No valid data	N/A	N/A
Evolving			
Sacral nerve stimulation	42%–66%	50% symptom improvement	D
STARR procedure	50%–90%	Overall satisfaction	B/D[a]
Vertical reduction rectoplasty	70%	Satisfaction, clinical (CCS), physiologic	D

Abbreviations: CCS, Cleveland Clinic Constipation score; QOL, quality of life.
[a] One randomized controlled trial available but comparison with another experimental surgical procedure only.

Table 2
Surgical interventions for patients with fecal incontinence

Procedure	Success Rate	Outcome Measures	Grade of Evidence
Historical			
Pelvic floor procedures	33%–50%	Full continence	B[a]
Contemporary			
Sphincter repair	50%–66%[b]	Clinical, physiologic	B[a]
Sacral nerve stimulation	40%–75% 75%–100%	Complete continence Improved (by 50%) continence	A
Dynamic gracilis neosphincter	42%–85%	Restoration of continence	D[c]
Artificial bowel sphincter	50%–100%[d]	Full continence	B[a]
Fecal diversion	No valid data	N/A	N/A
Evolving			
Injection of biomaterials	66% short term[e]	Cessation leakage and improved continence	D
SECCA procedure	84%	50% improvement	D
Rectal augmentation	64%	Avoidance of stoma	D

[a] Derived from Cochrane review but in some instances data extrapolated from only one study.
[b] 5-year success rates fall to 50%.
[c] Systematic review available but only of case series with no comparative studies.
[d] Explantation rates in case series approximately 50%.
[e] No change in continence scores compared with preoperatively at long-term follow-up.

primary aim of alleviating outlet obstruction in children and adults on the basis that this was caused by sphincter–pelvic floor hypertonia. Despite short-term improvement in up to 60% of patients, long-term results of pelvic floor procedures are disappointing, with success rates of only 48%.[6] In recent years, the concept of paradoxical contraction of the pelvic floor musculature as a cause of constipation has been seriously questioned.[7] Furthermore, there is a risk of incontinence following such interventions.

Contemporary Surgical Treatments

Colonic resection

Resection of all or part of the colon has been described as a treatment for severe constipation since 1908[5] and for patients with proved slow colonic transit since 1984.[8] Having peaked in popularity in the early 1990s, some more disappointing European long-term results and high complication rates have led to its more cautious application in the twenty-first century. Nevertheless, it continues to be used.

Rationale The shortened colon reduces colonic transit time and delivers less solid (more easily evacuated) stool to the rectum.

Indications and patient selection It is now widely accepted that the procedure should be reserved for those with documented slow transit in whom nonsurgical interventions have failed to ameliorate symptoms that are sufficiently severe to affect adversely quality of life. Furthermore, expectations should be clearly defined in relation to outcomes and complications, particularly in respect of the relative lack of efficacy of this procedure in treating abdominal pain and bloating, body image, or psychologic complaints.[9,10] **Fig. 1** demonstrates the factors to be consideration when contemplating surgical intervention. Specific clinical and physiologic findings in relation to patient selection are discussed next.

Results and complications These were systematically reviewed in 1999.[11] Overall, 32 case series (1981–1998) provided outcome data in 12 to 106 patients. Mortality rates were documented in 23 series, and varied from 0% to 6%. The commonest postoperative morbidity was small bowel obstruction occurring in 2% to 71% patients (median, 18%), and resulted in reoperation in 0% to 50% (median, 14%).[11] Overall documented patient satisfaction rates varied from 39% to 100% (median, 86%). Postoperative bowel habit was only numerically quantified in 20 series, with median or mean bowel habit figures available in only 14 series (range of medians/means, 1.3–5 times per day; median, 2.9).[11] Other functional outcome measures included diarrhea (range, 0%–46%; median, 14%); incontinence (range, 0%–52%; median, 14%); and recurrent constipation (range, 0%–33%; median, 9%). The percentage of patients still experiencing abdominal pain was documented in 14 series (range, 0%–90%; median, 41%).[11] As a result of poor functional outcome, in particular diarrhea and incontinence or recurrent constipation, permanent ileostomy was formed in up to 28% of patients (median, 5%; range, 0%–28%). Success rates were higher in United States series (n = 11: 75%–100%, median, 94% versus Europe [65%]).[11]

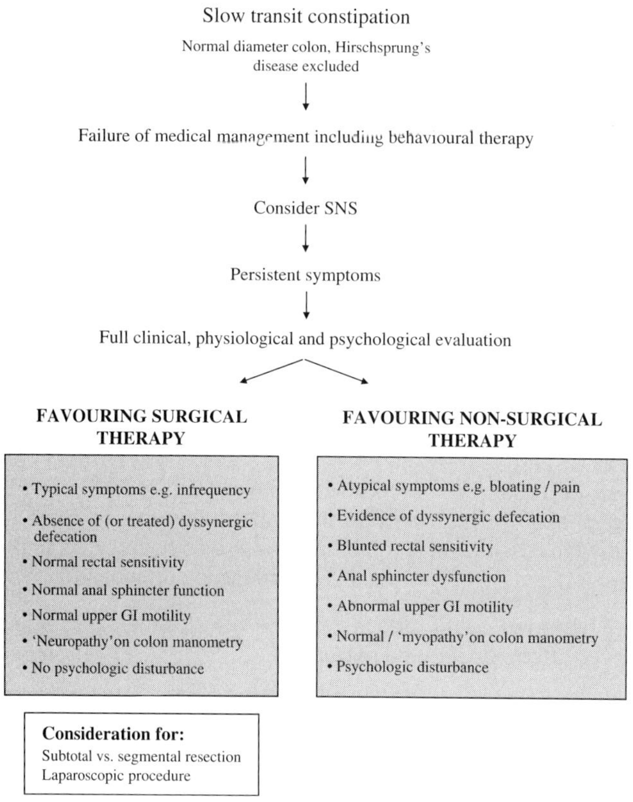

Fig. 1. Factors guiding selection of patients with slow-transit constipation for surgical intervention. GI, gastrointestinal; SNS, sacral nerve stimulation.

Although there was no overall direct effect of length of follow-up, for study groups with results at two or more time points, successful outcomes seemed to fall off with time. Prospective studies had superior outcomes (n = 16; median, 90%; range, 50%–100%) versus retrospective studies (n = 13; median, 67%; range, 39%–100%) that may in part have been caused by more rigorous patient selection. In studies that performed anorectal physiology and transit studies, the median satisfaction rate was 89% (range, 63%–100%) versus incomplete physiology, where the median satisfaction rate was 80% (range, 39%–100%). Studies in which all patients had proved slow transit had superior outcomes to those without (median outcome, 90% versus 67%, respectively).[11]

Since this review, several studies have continued to demonstrate similar complication rates[12,13] and long-term results that vary from the very good (>80% success) [14,15] to the more modest (50% success),[12] the latter despite rigorous selection criteria. Quality of life has now also been assessed by one study using validated tools and has been shown to increase in accord with functional results.[15]

Current position controversies

Role of segmental resection Where selection for extent of colectomy has not been based on segmental transit studies, results for limited subtotal resections (either subtotal colectomy with cecorectal anastomosis[8] or ileosigmoid anastomosis)[16] have proved generally inferior to subtotal colectomy with ileorectal anastomosis. The results of segmental resection (hemicolectomy) have proved even more disappointing.[8] Although subtotal colectomy with ileorectal anastomosis offers the best success rates, there is a perception, born out to some extent in the literature, that complications, including leakage, are more common following this anastomosis.[17] The indication for surgery in most patients was polyposis coli or Crohn's disease,[18] however, and whether these results can be extrapolated to patients with constipation is unclear. In addition, functional complications, including diarrhea and urgency of defecation, may complicate this procedure and are frequently difficult to manage in clinical practice. Suboptimal function is far less problematic in patients undergoing this procedure for constipation, however, than for Crohn's disease.

Several groups have attempted to tailor segmental surgery to pattern of transit with the use of more complex serial radiopaque marker or scintigraphic transit studies and avoid ileorectal anastomosis. De Graaf and colleagues[19] measured segmental transit using radiopaque marker studies to select patients for partial left-sided colectomy or subtotal colectomy. Although results as a whole were disappointing, the study concluded that in terms of complications and functional outcome, there was little difference between procedures, and that a more limited resection was a reasonable option in this selected group.[19] More recently, two studies of 40 and 28 patients [20,21] have reported the use of left, right, or subtotal colectomy based on segmental transit time measurements (the latter using scintigraphy) with excellent results (82/93%). In cases where constipation recurred following segmental resection, a subtotal colectomy was undertaken successfully at a later date. Finally, the results of colonic manometry by prior colonic diversion have been used as a successful guide to surgery in 10 of 12 children.[22] A variation on this theme has been the use of colonic manometry to select patients for subtotal colectomy, based on findings said to be consistent with colonic neuropathy.[23]

Effect of coexistent outlet obstruction Some studies have demonstrated a deleterious effect of untreated disorders of rectal evacuation,[24] whereas others have not.[9] Some groups have treated coexistent abnormalities of the pelvic floor preoperatively.

A recent study of 106 patients demonstrated that despite preoperative biofeedback training, patients with nonrelaxing pelvic floor (n = 16) had significantly higher rates of recurrent defecatory difficulty, and lower rates of satisfaction after colectomy.[25] Postoperative biofeedback has been used by others.[26] Rectal hyposensation seems to confer a significant detrimental effect on outcome.[21,27]

The effect of coexistent upper gastrointestinal dysmotility It is generally accepted that patients with small bowel dysmotility have poor outcomes after colectomy.[24,28,29] A fall in long-term success rate (as a result of recurrent constipation or intractable diarrhea) was demonstrated by a long-term prospective study by Redmond and coworkers [28] (successful outcome 90%: no gastrointestinal dysmotility versus 13% gastrointestinal dysmotility) and one from Stockholm (no gastrointestinal dysmotility: 100% versus 55% with gastrointestinal dysmotility including two deaths).[14] A high postoperative morbidity from recurrent small bowel obstruction (70%) has also been shown in such patients.[29]

The role of laparoscopic surgery With the safe use of laparoscopy to other areas of colorectal surgery and the disproportionately high adhesional obstruction rates after colectomy for constipation, laparoscopic colectomy has been reported in several very small case series.[30] Only one retrospective study compared laparoscopic with open colectomy for STC with 17 patients undergoing an open and 7 a laparoscopic procedure.[31] The laparoscopic colectomy group were more satisfied with the cosmetic outcome but had longer operation times (mean increase of 74 minutes) and increased complications.[31] In the future, the combination of laparoscopy with tailored segmental rather than subtotal resection would have the advantage of not requiring the acknowledged technical challenges of mobilizing both colonic flexures laparoscopically.

Special considerations: idiopathic megabowel A proportion of patients with dilatation of colon or rectum are forced to seek a surgical solution to their symptoms when conservative therapy is ineffective, is poorly tolerated, or because of complications.[32] Numerous surgical procedures have been attempted in patients with idiopathic megabowel, including subtotal or segmental colonic resection, rectal and pelvic floor procedures, and fecal diversion. The results of these have recently undergone systematic review.[33] In brief, colonic procedures either address the dilated bowel or have as their rationale the presentation of liquid stool to a dysfunctional rectum, which itself is not addressed (subtotal colectomy). The lower morbidity and mortality of these procedures make them attractive but functional results can be poor. Rectal procedures have higher success rates but are associated with significant morbidity and mortality (principally from intraoperative hemorrhage and pelvic sepsis). Fecal diversion remains a possibility but is an unattractive prospect in young patients. Two procedures that are gaining greater recognition are restorative proctocolectomy with ileal pouch formation (outcome reported in 22 patients in the literature, being successful in 73% [range, 57%–100%] [33]) and a novel procedure, the vertical reduction rectoplasty.[34] The latter, at medium-term (5-year) follow-up, was successful in achieving and maintaining correction of rectal diameter, compliance, and sensory function in most of 10 patients, and this was translated into clinical benefit with no operative mortality and minimal morbidity.[2]

Anterograde colonic enema

The anterograde colonic enema technique was first described by Malone and coworkers[35] in 1990 using the appendix as a conduit in children with neuropathic constipation. Various modifications have subsequently been described.

Rationale The purpose is to maintain efficient emptying of the lower bowel through regular irrigation of water or saline, with or without aperients, by a catheter inserted into the proximal colon.

Indications and patient selection The use of anterograde colonic enema should be considered as an alternative to colectomy or stoma when conservative methods of laxatives have failed and more radical surgery is to be avoided because of recognized lack of efficacy (particularly severe outlet obstruction) or unacceptability (eg, in children). In patients with previous appendicectomy or in whom the appendix cannot be satisfactorily used, cecostomy may be effected using a percutaneously placed Chait tube[36] or surgically by more complex techniques, such as stapled tubularized cecal neoappendicostomy[37] or continent colonic conduit.[38]

Results and complications In general, success rates have been lower in adults[37] than in children.[35,39] Despite early functional success, in the long term, such complications as stomal stenosis and leakage, or failure effectively to treat symptoms, commonly (>50% at 3 years) lead to revision, reversal, or conversion to stoma.[37]

Current position controversies The role of anterograde colonic enema in adults is less clear than in children. There are no trials comparing anterograde colonic enema with other therapies for constipation in any group of patients.

Stoma

A stoma may be used as a definitive procedure, as a guide to further treatment, or as salvage from failed or complicated prior surgical intervention. There are little published data to support an evidence-based use; however, the suggestion that an ileostomy can guide the use of colectomy is an approach used by the authors and others[40] when subsequent colectomy would be avoided if the ileostomy output is unsatisfactorily high or symptoms, such as pain and bloating untouched by diversion. As a definitive procedure both colostomy and ileostomy have been described for a diversity of adult and childhood disorders characterized by constipation including spinal cord injury, megacolon, and outlet obstruction.[41] There is little evidence to guide choice of ileostomy or colostomy[42]; however, some report high complication rates of ileostomy[43] and STC may be unsatisfactorily treated by colostomy.[44]

Evolving Surgical Treatments

Sacral nerve stimulation

First applied in urology and thence FI[45] (see later), SNS is increasingly being considered as the first-line procedural intervention in constipation after failure of conservative measures.

Rationale As in FI, the mechanism of action of SNS is not conclusively proved and may involve direct effects on colorectal sensory or motor function or central effects at the level of spinal cord or brain.[46]

Indications Although yet to be clearly established, SNS will probably come to have a role in idiopathic constipation (with or without proved transit disturbance) that is resistant to conservative treatment (laxatives, behavioral modification) before more radical measures, such as resectional surgery or anterograde enema, are considered.

Results Although sacral root (parasympathetic) Brindley stimulation was described for neurogenic constipation in 1991,[47] it was not until 2002 that the St. Mark's group first described the application of SNS in its current form in three pilots of small numbers of patients with severe idiopathic constipation, some of whom had STC.[48–50] From a clinical perspective, these demonstrated (1) symptomatic benefit of temporary stimulation for a 3-week period in two of eight patients with STC;[50] (2) symptomatic and quality-of-life benefits of permanent stimulation in three of four patients (two with STC);[49] and (3) demonstration of efficacy with a crossover design of two patients with stimulation "on" and "off".[48] A recent multicenter European study of 65 patients with normal or STC has subsequently built on these results with 43 (66%) patients going on to permanent stimulation on the basis of 50% symptom improvement.[51] In this group, there were significant improvements in nearly all symptoms and quality-of-life measures.[51] The relatively high success rate in this study should be tempered by a very recent study of 19 patients with mixed STC and outlet obstruction that demonstrated a more modest success rate of 42%.[52]

From a mechanistic perspective, the earlier temporary stimulation study of Malouf and colleagues,[50] which comprised eight patients with STC, showed no effect on colonic transit times even in the two patients with improved symptoms. This contrasted with another mechanistic study, in which six of eight patients with STC benefited from SNS.[53] In this study, stimulation caused significant alterations in the incidence of colonic high-amplitude propagating contractions,[53] the main functional correlate of which is thought to be mass movements of stool, and whose incidence has been shown to be reduced in patients with STC compared with control subjects. In the larger European study, transit times were normalized in one half of patients with STC at baseline.[51] More consistent is the effect of SNS to improve rectal sensory function.[50,51] This has been well reported for FI [46] and is also of interest mechanistically given that a significant proportion of patients with STC or outlet obstruction have reduced perception of rectal filling often with accompanying loss of defecatory urge (ie, rectal hyposensitivity).[54]

Current position controversies Common to both studies of FI and constipation is the rather arbitrary definition of success as a 50% improvement in symptoms and the subsequent failure of study design to incorporate intention-to-treat analysis. Long-term data are still lacking in respect to constipation. Nevertheless, as suggested by a recent Cochrane review,[55] the limited evidence suggests that the procedure holds promise for selected patients. The effects on reducing bloating and abdominal pain (poorly addressed by other modalities of treatment) in most studies [50,51] suggest that patients in which these symptoms predominate may perhaps be benefited most (although this requires confirmation).

Stapled transanal rectal resection: STARR

Following the introduction of stapled hemorrhoidopexy in the 1980s, there has been recent interest in using circular staplers in the management of obstructed defecation.[56] This procedure, although perhaps also addressing anatomic abnormalities excluded from this article (eg, rectocele, prolapse, intussusception), is briefly described on the basis that obstructed defecation (with constipation) may be treated in some patients who have no such evident proctologic abnormalities.

Rationale Obstructed defecation encompasses a number of symptoms that in part or whole may relate to a number of clinical and physiologic findings, such as perineal descent, rectocele, and intussusception. The stapled transanal rectal resection procedure resects internally prolapsed rectum with the aim of improved function (perhaps through improved rectal compliance and sensation and volume).

Indications The procedure is indicated for failed prior conservative management in patients with characteristic symptoms and clinical or physiologic findings of obstructed defecation. A number of specific exclusion criteria also exist.[57]

Results In the last 4 years, several publications have attested to the successful results of this procedure in treating obstructed defecation symptoms (eg, 88% in one study).[58] The procedure has the advantage of minimal postoperative pain; however, numerous quite serious complications (eg, fistula) have been described [57] in up to 50% of patients.[59]

Current position controversies There is a requirement to define criteria better for the procedure and long-term results. Complications remain a concern.

SURGICAL TREATMENT OF FECAL INCONTINENCE

Introduction

Most patients with mild to moderate symptoms successfully respond to conservative management, and this must be considered as first-line therapy. Therapeutic strategies comprise pharmacologic, behavioral, and physical modalities. Only patients who fail to respond to such measures (ie, those with severe symptoms or major incontinence) should be referred to a specialist tertiary center for further investigation and consideration for surgical intervention. The surgical management of FI is often complex, and in common with any surgical procedure has its own inherent risks and complications. It should be reserved for patients with severe incontinence with impaired quality of life who have failed, or are deemed unsuitable for nonsurgical management. The management of patients with FI in a specialist surgical unit involves a multidisciplinary team of professionals. Because patient selection is crucial for a successful outcome, the importance of a thorough and comprehensive clinical and physiologic assessment cannot be overstressed. Because no form of surgical intervention offers certainty of cure, preoperatively counseling before surgery is obligatory.

The following description concentrates specifically on the choice of surgical procedure appropriate to the underlying pathophysiology of the incontinence. Detailed, objective assessment yields four broad clinical categories of patients with FI. These include patients with predominantly (1) simple, structural defects of the anal sphincters; (2) weak but intact anal sphincters; (3) complex disruption of the anal sphincter complex; and (4) extrasphincteric abnormalities. The surgical interventions available to address such abnormalities and their outcomes are shown in **Table 2**.

Historical: Correction of Abnormalities of the Pelvic Floor

Traditionally, pelvic floor procedures (postanal repair, anterior levatorplasty, total pelvic floor repair) have been performed for patients without a specific sphincter defect who suffer with idiopathic or neurogenic incontinence. Such procedures involved plication of various components of the pelvic floor musculature (levator ani, puborectalis, and the external anal sphincter [EAS]) to reconstitute the anorectal angle and lengthen the anal canal. Follow-up studies following postanal repair and anterior levatorplasty have revealed disappointing results with typically only one third to one half of patients having improved continence, with no observed difference between the two procedures in comparative studies.[60] Total pelvic floor repair involves a combination of postanal repair with anterior levatorplasty and sphincter plication, but only achieves improved continence and quality of life in approximately one half of all patients.[61] A recent Cochrane review of randomized trials has confirmed no difference in numbers of patients achieving full continence in anterior levatorplasty compared with postanal repair, total pelvic floor repair compared with anterior levatorplasty, and total pelvic floor repair compared with postanal repair.[60] Although once popular in the United Kingdom and Europe, pelvic floor procedures are now far less frequently performed.

Contemporary

Correction of abnormalities and augmentation of the native anal sphincter complex

Sphincteroplasty Surgery to the anal sphincter complex has largely been confined to repair of EAS defects, because repair of isolated internal sphincter defects has not proved successful in patients with passive fecal soiling.[62] Anterior EAS defects usually follow obstetric trauma, and may be repaired immediately if identified at the time of injury. Delayed repair is more frequently performed, however, because of unrecognized injury or failure of primary repair. Such repair may involve direct apposition, or overlapping, of the edges of the disrupted sphincter.

Rationale Sphincteroplasty aims to restore anatomic integrity and function to a disrupted EAS.

Indications and patient selection Direct repair is appropriate in patients with isolated defects affecting one third or less of the circumference of the EAS on endosonography.

Results and complications Most studies addressing the functional outcome of sphincteroplasty report early success rates of 70% to 90%,[63,64] but are generally restricted to short-term follow-up. Reported success rates at 5 years fall to approximately 50%.[65,66] Furthermore, some patients may develop problematic evacuation disorders.[66]

Current position controversies

1. Redo sphincteroplasty following failed repair. Given the 70% to 90% short-term and 50% long-term success rates of sphincteroplasty, it is clear that some patients have persistent FI after surgery. Because many of these patients have residual anterior sphincter defects, it is possible to perform a repeat sphincter repair. The outcome of repeat sphincter repair does not seem to be affected by previous surgery, and is associated with significant improvements in patient continence scores.[67]
2. Overlapping versus direct sphincter repair. Previously, sphincter repair was performed by apposition of the separated edges of the external sphincter. More recently, superior results have been suggested if an overlapping repair is performed, which is now largely considered the operation of choice for definable sphincter defects. A recent Cochrane review has revealed that outcome is the same, however, regardless of whether the sphincter repair is direct or overlapping.[60]
3. Influence of clinical and physiologic factors on outcome of repair. It has been suggested that certain factors, such as patient age and pudendal nerve function, may be important in predicting outcome following surgery, although the literature is largely contradictory in this regard. Some studies have reported increasing age (especially in those >50 years) as a predictor of failure.[68] In contrast, others have found no influence of age on functional outcome[64] or even a superior functional outcome in patients older than 50 years compared with their younger counterparts.[69] Controversy also exists relating to pudendal nerve function. Several studies have implicated pudendal neuropathy as a predictor of failure following sphincteroplasty.[65] Other studies have failed to identify any relationship[68] and conclude that repair of anatomic sphincter defects should still be considered in the presence of pudendal neuropathy.[70]

Sacral nerve stimulation

Rationale The exact mechanism of action of SNS remains unclear [55] with the initial, and intuitive, premise that SNS would directly augment anal sphincter function and improve FI now questioned by more detailed physiologic studies. Indeed, the observation that improved continence occurred without change in anal sphincter function has led to the suggestion that SNS has predominantly suprasphincteric effects. The mechanism of action of SNS is not conclusively proved and may involve direct effects peripherally on colorectal sensory or motor function, or central effects at the level of spinal cord or brain.[46]

Indications and patient selection Early studies of SNS in FI restricted inclusion of patients to those with a functionally deficient but morphologically intact anal sphincter. With increasing experience of the technique the inclusion criteria have extended to include patients with EAS defects;[71] internal anal sphincter (IAS) defects;[72] and FI secondary to cauda equina syndrome[73] and (partial) spinal injuries.[74]

Results and complications Initial reports of SNS detailed successful short-term results in small numbers of patients, with marked improvements in clinical symptoms associated with improvement of physiologic parameters, such as anal canal pressures and rectal sensory function.[75,76] Significant improvements in quality of life have been demonstrated using both generic and incontinence-specific measures.[77] The results of multicenter studies of SNS also support these findings, with a marked, unequivocal improvement in FI and patient quality of life,[78,79] with such improvements being sustained in the medium term (24 months).[80]

A recent systematic review of the published outcomes of trials investigating SNS revealed that 40% to 75% of patients achieved complete fecal continence and 75% to 100% experienced improvement in episodes of incontinence, with a low (10%) incidence of adverse events.[55] Further confirmation of the effectiveness of SNS in the treatment of FI was recently demonstrated in a randomized, controlled trial where it was found to be superior to treatment with best supportive therapy (pelvic floor exercises, bulking agents, and dietary manipulation) in terms of improvement in fecal continence and the FI quality-of-life scores.[81] The availability of this level 1 evidence, which is lacking for most surgical procedures for FI, allows SNS to be considered as a contemporary treatment option for FI rather than one that is evolving.

Current position controversies

1. Reporting of outcomes and definition of success. As noted in the constipation section, the arbitrary definition of success as being a 50% reduction in incontinence episodes, while satisfying the indications for permanent stimulation, is of little comfort to the patient who may still have significant, albeit reduced, episodes of FI. Again, the failure to account for drop-outs (ie, those patients not going on to permanent stimulation) in the reporting of outcomes (ignoring the convention of clinical trials to use intention-to-treat analyses) should be noted.
2. Long-term results. Current outcome studies of SNS are limited to medium-term follow-up, and whether such benefit is maintained in the longer-term is currently unknown. Accordingly, patients should be counseled appropriately until long-term data are available.
3. Range of indications for SNS in FI. There are some preliminary data suggesting that SNS can be successfully applied to patients with FI secondary to neurologic conditions[73,74] and those with anal sphincter defects.[71,72] Indeed, there is a growing body of evidence that suggests that patients with de novo EAS defects or defects after unsuccessful previous sphincter repair receive benefit from SNS[71] and that there is no difference in medium-term outcome between patients with EAS defects and patients with intact anal sphincter muscles.[82] The contemporary view is that

a morphologically intact anal sphincter is not a prerequisite for success in the treatment of FI with SNS and that EAS defects of less than 33% of the circumference can be effectively treated primarily without repair.[71]

Creation of a new anal sphincter (neosphincter)

Electrically stimulated (dynamic) graciloplasty Encirclement procedures involving transposition of skeletal muscle around the anus to create a neosphincter have been performed for many years. The gluteus maximus, adductor longus, and obturator internus muscles have all been used, although the gracilis muscle is the favored option, being the most superficial medial adductor muscle with a sufficiently plastic neurovascular supply.[83]

Rationale Gracilioplasty involves reconstruction of the anal sphincter using native skeletal muscle. When first performed, improvements in continence were dependent on causing a degree of anal canal obstruction and the results were generally poor. The procedure gained popularity following description of the dynamic graciloplasty, however, which involved the application of chronic low-frequency electrical stimulation to the muscle by a subcutaneously placed generator, transforming it to a slow-twitch nonfatigable muscle capable of a tonic state of contraction.[84,85] The electrode lead is connected to the stimulator, which is implanted subcutaneously. On-off function of the stimulator, allowing defecation to take place, is governed by a hand-held magnet.

Indications and patient selection The procedure is reserved for carefully selected patients in whom the anal sphincter musculature is irreparable and who are desperate to avoid a stoma. This includes those with disrupted anal sphincters that are unsuitable for or have already failed the procedures discussed previously, together with those who have a damaged or absent (often as a result of congenital defects) IAS resulting in severe passive leakage, refractory to all other treatments.

Results and complications In prospective multicenter trials, between 56% and 72% of patients undergoing dynamic graciloplasty have achieved and maintained a successful outcome, with the best outcomes observed in those with traumatic incontinence,[86,87] with similar success rates (42%–85%) observed in a recent systematic review.[88] The only outcomes have thus far been reported by centers with a particular interest in the procedure, where continence to at least solid and liquid stool has been reported in approximately 70% of all patients at median-term follow-up.[89,90] It should be noted, however, that this procedure has never been the subject of controlled or comparative trials.[60]

Dynamic graciloplasty operations are technically demanding and may be associated with high morbidity, with infection reported in up to one third of cases.[87] In addition, postoperative evacuatory disorders occur in up to one quarter of patients and are more difficult to resolve.[86] It seems likely that the procedure should be confined to specialist colorectal centers, and reserved for carefully selected patients.

Artificial bowel sphincter Anal sphincter reconstruction can also be performed using a synthetic sphincter device. Having been used for many years in the treatment of urinary incontinence, the first successful use of an artificial sphincter for the treatment of FI was in 1987.[91]

Rationale The contemporary device consists of an inflatable silicon cuff, which is implanted around the anal canal and controlled by the patient by a pump located in the scrotum or labium majus. Activation of the pump forces fluid from the cuff into a reservoir implanted suprapubically in the space of Retzius, deflating the cuff and allowing defecation. Subsequently, the cuff automatically reinflates slowly to maintain continence until the next evacuation.[91]

Indications and patient selection The indications for use of this procedure are broadly the same as for dynamic graciloplasty. It may additionally be used in FI of neuromuscular origin (eg, myasthenia gravis and neuropathy secondary to diabetes mellitus).

Results and complications Several groups have reported their experiences with the artificial bowel sphincter in small numbers of patients with overall improvements in continence in approximately one half to three quarters of patients.[92,93] Further, artificial bowel sphincter, unlike dynamic graciloplasty, has been the subject of a prospective, randomized, controlled trial where it was demonstrated to be better than conservative treatment in improving continence.[94] Long-term outcome seems less encouraging, however, with two studies with a median follow-up of approximately 7 years documenting success rates of less than 50%, explantation rates as high as 49%,[95,96] and infection in up to one third of cases.[96] As with dynamic gracilioplasty, there seems to be a high incidence of postoperative evacuatory difficulties, which are present in up to one half of patients.[92,93]

End-stage and refractory fecal incontinence

Permanent end stoma As for constipation, fecal diversion usually by colostomy is an option in end-stage, devastating FI affecting quality of life. Most patients (83%) who have a permanent end colostomy fashioned for FI report that the stoma restricted their life "a little" or "not at all" and would "probably" or "definitely" choose to have the stoma again, although overall quality of life, assessed using generic measures, was poor.[97] A few had not adapted, however, and disliked the stoma intensely.[97] Furthermore, there may be a high rate of stoma complications.[43]

Evolving

Correction of abnormalities and augmentation of the native anal sphincter complex

Perianal injection of biomaterials Perianal injection of various bulking agents has been performed in patients with FI. Numerous biomaterials have been injected, details of which can be found in a recent review article;[98] most experience and success has been achieved with silicone.[99,100]

Rationale The injection of biomaterials physically augments the (internal) anal sphincter.

Indications and patient selection It is indicated in FI caused by a weak or disrupted IAS or patients with passive fecal soiling.

Results and complications Injection of silicone seems to be associated with an improvement in fecal continence and quality of life in patients with internal sphincter dysfunction, with approximately two thirds of patients showing either marked improvement or complete cessation of leakage in the short term.[99] Longer term (5 years) revealed little change in their incontinence score compared with before the procedure, however, with one of six patients requiring a colostomy for FI and another for a rectovaginal fistula.[100] The considerable morbidity of this procedure has cast serious doubts on the use of this intervention in patients with FI, although it may be considered in carefully counseled patients with passive FI secondary to IAS dysfunction or defects in whom treatment options are otherwise limited.

Radiofrequency energy delivery to the anal canal (SECCA procedure) Temperature-controlled radiofrequency energy has been delivered deep to the mucosa of the anal canal by multiple needle electrodes using a specially designed anoscopic handpiece inserted into the anal canal in patients with FI.[101]

Rationale The proposed mechanism of action is by heat-induced tissue contraction and remodeling of the anal canal and distal rectum.[102]

Indications and patient selection Recruitment of patients into studies to date has included those with FI refractory to standard medical therapy from varying causes.[101,103]

Results and complications In the first reported case series, 8 of 10 patients responded to the treatment and the modality was found to be safe and associated with improved continence and quality of life scores.[101] Symptomatic improvement was sustained at 2 years[102] and recently published medium-term data reveal significant and sustained improvements in symptoms of FI and quality of life are seen at 5 years after treatment.[104] A multicenter trial also confirms the improvements in FI and quality of life[103] at least in the short term (at 6-month follow-up). Complications included ulceration of the mucosa and delayed bleeding.[103] There were no changes in the results of anal manometry pudendal nerve terminal motor latencies or endoanal ultrasound.[103] A randomized trial to determine its role in the treatment of FI has been recently completed in the United States, and the data should be available soon. Further studies of greater numbers of patients are required before its widespread use can be recommended.

Correction of extrasphincteric physiologic abnormalities: dysfunction rectal reservoir In addition to occurring secondary to anal sphincter dysfunction, there is increasing awareness that FI may also result from suprasphincteric causes, such as dysfunction of the rectal reservoir. This dysfunction may manifest as an impaired ability to store[105,106] or evacuate feces.[4,34] Reservoir dysfunction may occur in isolation, or combination with other pathophysiologic abnormalities, and may complicate surgical procedures designed to improve continence.[66,86,92] The anterograde colonic enema may also be used to overcome reservoir dysfunction in patients with (overflow) FI secondary to impaired rectal evacuation.

Rectal augmentation for storage dysfunction Rectal augmentation is a novel approach to correct physiologic abnormalities in a subgroup of patients with intractable FI secondary to reservoir dysfunction (akin to the clam enterocystoplasty for the treatment of the overactive bladder). Even in the absence of anal sphincter dysfunction, patients may still suffer with severe urgency of defecation and urge incontinence secondary to derangements of rectal sensorimotor function.[106] Such patients have low rectal compliance and heightened rectal sensation (rectal hypersensitivity).[106] Management is problematic, because correction of the sphincter defect does not abolish the incapacitating urgency or incontinence.

Rationale A novel procedure was developed to treat selected patients presenting with incapacitating urgency and FI by specifically addressing the underlying pathophysiologic abnormalities. The procedure involves the creation of a side-to-side ileorectal pouch, or ileorectoplasty, which involves incorporating a 10-cm patch of ileum on its vascular pedicle into the anterior rectal wall (**Fig. 2**) to increase its capacity and compliance and restore rectal sensitivity to normal.[105]

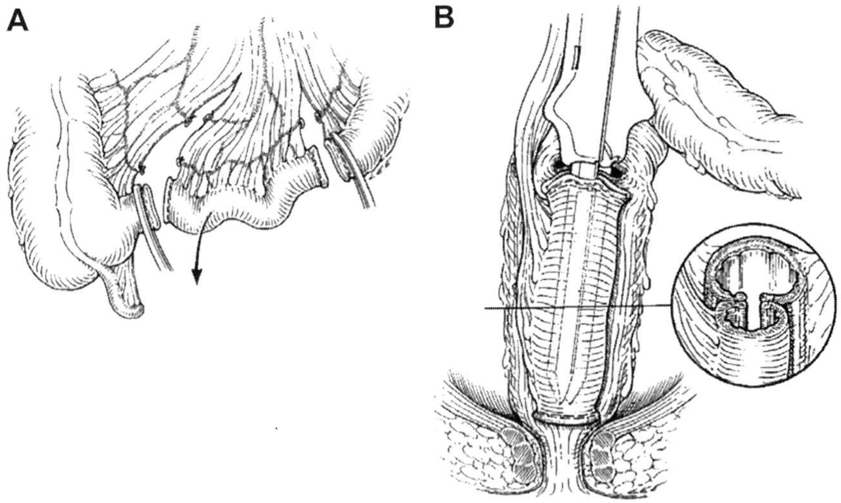

Fig. 2. Rectal augmentation procedure. A segment of terminal ileum is isolated on its vascular pedicle (*A*) and a side-to-side ileorectoplasty is fashioned using a linear stapler to increase the capacity and compliance of the rectum (*B*) (*From* Williams NS, Ogunbiyi OA, Scott SM, et al. Rectal augmentation and stimulated gracilis anal neosphincter: a new approach in the management of fecal urgency and incontinence. Dis Colon Rectum 2001;44:192–8; with permission.)

Indications and patient selection This procedure is intended for patients with severe, incapacitating fecal urgency and incontinence with evidence of reduced rectal wall compliance, hypersensitivity to distention, and hypercontractility on prolonged manometric investigation.[105,106]

Results and complications Initial experience revealed that urgency was abolished and continence restored in three individuals and that postoperative physiologic investigation revealed elevated thresholds to rectal distention and a reduction in the number of high-amplitude rectal pressure waves in all cases.[105] At medium-term follow-up (4.5 years), there was a sustained increase in rectal capacity, as demonstrated by restoration of sensory threshold volumes and rectal compliance to normal limits in all 11 subjects, associated with a concomitant improvement in clinical symptoms (increased ability to defer defecation and reduced frequency of episodes of incontinence) and quality of life.[107]

SUMMARY

With the advent of anorectal physiologic investigations, a detailed understanding of the pathophysiologic mechanisms underlying constipation and FI is evolving. The results of tests of anorectal physiologic function help to suggest appropriate rather than empiric management, particularly when surgical intervention is contemplated. In those patients referred for surgical amelioration of their symptoms, the integration of the findings from clinical history, physical examination, and investigations enables the choice of suitable procedure to be tailored on an individual basis, and to be directed specifically to the underlying abnormalities.

It should be emphasized that the reported surgical outcome data must be interpreted with considerable caution because most available evidence was of low quality, being frequently obtained from case series and very often without any control group data (and when controlled without random allocation to different interventions).[11,33,60] Comparison of different procedures is problematic, and dictates that no firm recommendations can be made about the selection of the most appropriate surgical intervention for individual patients. Such difficulties imply that didactic "patient pathways" cannot be prescribed in this article. Some tentative observations can be made on the basis of the published results, however, which in part also reflect the authors' opinion. In constipation, surgery should probably be avoided. Where deemed necessary, because of the lesser morbidity and reversibility of the procedure, SNS should be considered before colectomy. In FI, probably all patients in whom surgical intervention is contemplated should undergo a trial of SNS, regardless of sphincter integrity. In those with significant isolated sphincter defect and unsatisfactory response to SNS, a direct or overlapping repair based on the surgeon's preference should be performed. This recommendation is in contrast to that of Tan and colleagues,[108] who in their recent review suggested that patients with FI should only undergo SNS if sphincteroplasty or injection of biomaterials fails. The level 1 evidence for the efficacy of SNS in the treatment of FI, together with its extremely low morbidity, make it more attractive than these other options, both of which lack this quality of evidence and both of which have (considerable) associated morbidity. Lack of available data and variability in outcomes in morbidity mean that one cannot be prescriptive about the role of the other procedures for FI discussed in this article, although they may be considered in end-stage cases. The need for better designed and conducted surgical trials in these areas cannot be overstated.

REFERENCES

1. Rao SS, Ozturk R, Stessman M. Investigation of the pathophysiology of fecal seepage. Am J Gastroenterol 2004;99:2204–9.
2. Gladman MA, Williams NS, Scott SM, et al. Medium-term results of vertical reduction rectoplasty and sigmoid colectomy for idiopathic megarectum. Br J Surg 2005;92(5):624–30.
3. Harbour R, Miller J. A new system for grading recommendations in evidence based guidelines. BMJ 2001;323(7308):334–6.
4. Rao SS. Constipation: evaluation and treatment of colonic and anorectal motility disorders. Gastroenterol Clin North Am. 2007;36(3):687–711.
5. Arbuthnot Lane W. The results of operative treatment of chronic constipation. BMJ 1908;1:126–30.
6. Coremans GE. Surgical aspects of severe chronic non-Hirschsprung constipation. Hepatogastroenterology 1990;37(6):588–95.
7. Schouten WR, Briel JW, Auwerda JJ, et al. Anismus: fact or fiction? Dis Colon Rectum 1997;40(9):1033–41.
8. Preston DM, Hawley PR, Lennard-Jones JE, et al. Results of colectomy for severe idiopathic constipation in women (Arbuthnot Lane's disease). Br J Surg 1984;71(7):547–52.
9. Kamm MA, Hawley PR, Lennard-Jones JE. Outcome of colectomy for severe idiopathic constipation. Gut 1988;29(7):969–73.
10. Pluta H, Bowes KL, Jewell LD. Long-term results of total abdominal colectomy for chronic idiopathic constipation: value of preoperative assessment. Dis Colon Rectum 1996;39(2):160–6.
11. Knowles CH, Scott M, Lunniss PJ. Outcome of colectomy for slow transit constipation. Ann Surg 1999;230(5):627–38.

12. Mollen RM, Kuijpers HC, Claassen AT. Colectomy for slow-transit constipation: preoperative functional evaluation is important but not a guarantee for a successful outcome. Dis Colon Rectum 2001;44(4):577–80.
13. Zutshi M, Hull TL, Trzcinski R, et al. Surgery for slow transit constipation: are we helping patients? Int J Colorectal Dis 2007;22(3):265–9.
14. Glia A, Akerlund JE, Lindberg G. Outcome of colectomy for slow-transit constipation in relation to presence of small-bowel dysmotility. Dis Colon Rectum 2004;47(1):96–102.
15. Hassan I, Pemberton JH, Young-Fadok TM, et al. Ileorectal anastomosis for slow transit constipation: long-term functional and quality of life results. J Gastrointest Surg 2006;10(10):1330–6.
16. Pemberton JH, Rath DM, Ilstrup DM. Evaluation and surgical treatment of severe chronic constipation. Ann Surg. 1991;214(4):403–11.
17. Hyman N, Manchester TL, Osler T, et al. Anastomotic leaks after intestinal anastomosis: it's later than you think. Ann Surg 2007;245(2):254–8.
18. Elton C, Makin G, Hitos K, et al. Mortality, morbidity and functional outcome after ileorectal anastomosis. Br J Surg 2003;90(1):59–65.
19. de Graaf EJ, Gilberts EC, Schouten WR. Role of segmental colonic transit time studies to select patients with slow transit constipation for partial left-sided or subtotal colectomy. Br J Surg 1996;83(5):648–51.
20. You Y-T, Wang J-Y, Changchien C-R, et al. Segmental colectomy in the management of colonic inertia. Am Surg 1998;64(8):775–7.
21. Lundin E, Karlbom U, Påhlman L, et al. Outcome of segmental colonic resection for slow-transit constipation. Br J Surg 2002;89(10):1270–4.
22. Villarreal J, Sood M, Zangen T, et al. Colonic diversion for intractable constipation in children: colonic manometry helps guide clinical decisions. J Pediatr Gastroenterol Nutr 2001;33(5):588–91.
23. Rao SS, Sadeghi P, Beaty J, et al. Ambulatory 24-hour colonic manometry in slow-transit constipation. Am J Gastroenterol 2004;99(12):2405–16.
24. Kuijpers HC. Application of the colorectal laboratory in diagnosis and treatment of functional constipation. Dis Colon Rectum 1990;33(1):35–9.
25. Bernini A, Madoff RD, Lowry AC, et al. Should patients with combined colonic inertia and nonrelaxing pelvic floor undergo subtotal colectomy? Dis Colon Rectum 1998;41(11):1363–6.
26. Lubowski DZ, Chen FC, Kennedy ML, et al. Results of colectomy for severe slow transit constipation. Dis Colon Rectum 1996;39(1):23–9.
27. Akervall S, Fasth S, Nordgren S, et al. The functional results after colectomy and ileorectal anastomosis for severe constipation (Arbuthnot Lane's disease) as related to rectal sensory function. Int J Colorectal Dis 1988;3(2):96–101.
28. Redmond JM, Smith GW, Barofsky I, et al. Physiological tests to predict long-term outcome of total abdominal colectomy for intractable constipation. Am J Gastroenterol 1995;90(5):748–53.
29. Ghosh S, Papachrysostomou M, Batool M, et al. Long-term results of subtotal colectomy and evidence of noncolonic involvement in patients with idiopathic slow-transit constipation. Scand J Gastroenterol 1996;31(11):1083–91.
30. Athanasakis H, Tsiaoussis J, Vassilakis JS, et al. Laparoscopically assisted subtotal colectomy for slow-transit constipation. Surg Endosc 2001;15(10):1090–2.
31. Ho YH, Tan M, Eu KW, et al. Laparoscopic-assisted compared with open total colectomy in treating slow transit constipation. Aust N Z J Surg 1997;67(8):562–5.

32. Gladman MA, Knowles CH. Novel concepts in the diagnosis, pathophysiology and management of idiopathic megabowel. Colorectal Dis 2008;10(6):531–8.
33. Gladman MA, Scott SM, Lunniss PJ, et al. Systematic review of surgical options for idiopathic megarectum and megacolon. Ann Surg 2005;241(4):562–74.
34. Williams NS, Fajobi OA, Lunniss PJ, et al. Vertical reduction rectoplasty: a new treatment for idiopathic megarectum. Br J Surg 2000;87:1203–8.
35. Malone PS, Ransley PG, Kiely EM. Preliminary report: the antegrade continence enema. Lancet 1990;336(8725):1217–8.
36. Chait PG, Shandling B, Richards HF. The cecostomy button. J Pediatr Surg 1997;32(6):849–51.
37. Lees NP, Hodson P, Hill J, et al. Long-term results of the antegrade continent enema procedure for constipation in adults. Colorectal Dis 2004;6(5):362–8.
38. Williams NS, Hughes SF, Stuchfield B. Continent colonic conduit for rectal evacuation in severe constipation. Lancet 1994;343(8909):1321–4.
39. Marshall J, Hutson JM, Anticich N, et al. Antegrade continence enemas in the treatment of slow-transit constipation. J Pediatr Surg 2001;36(8):1227–30.
40. Wong SW, Lubowski DZ. Slow-transit constipation: evaluation and treatment. ANZ J Surg 2007;77(5):320–8.
41. Woodward MN, Foley P, Cusick EL. Colostomy for treatment of functional constipation in children: a preliminary report. J Pediatr Gastroenterol Nutr 2004;38(1): 75–8.
42. van der Sijp JR, Kamm MA, Bartram CI, et al. The value of age of onset and rectal emptying in predicting the outcome of colectomy for severe idiopathic constipation. Int J Colorectal Dis 1992;7(1):35–7.
43. Scarpa M, Barollo M, Keighley MR. Ileostomy for constipation: long-term postoperative outcome. Colorectal Dis. 2005;7(3):224–7.
44. Keighley MRB. Constipation. In: Keighley MRB, Williams NS, editors. Surgery of the anus, rectum and colon. 1st edition. London: WB Saunders; 1997. p. 632.
45. Matzel KE, Stadelmaier U, Hohenfellner M, et al. Electrical stimulation of sacral spinal nerves for treatment of faecal incontinence. Lancet 1995;346(8983): 1124–7.
46. Uludag O, Morren GL, Dejong CH, et al. Effect of sacral neuromodulation on the rectum. Br J Surg 2005;92(8):1017–23.
47. Binnie NR, Smith AN, Creasey GH, et al. Constipation associated with spinal cord injury: the effect of pelvic parasympathetic stimulation by the Brindley stimulator. Paraplegia 1991;29:463–9.
48. Kenefick NJ, Vaizey CJ, Cohen CR, et al. Double-blind placebo-controlled crossover study of sacral nerve stimulation for idiopathic constipation. Br J Surg 2002;89(12):1570–1.
49. Kenefick NJ, Nicholls RJ, Cohen RG, et al. Permanent sacral nerve stimulation for treatment of idiopathic constipation. Br J Surg 2002;89(7):882–8.
50. Malouf AJ, Wiesel PH, Nicholls T, et al. Short-term effects of sacral nerve stimulation for idiopathic slow transit constipation. World J Surg 2002;26(2): 166–70.
51. Kamm MA, Dudding TC, Melenhorst J, et al. Sacral nerve stimulation for constipation: an international multi-centre study. Gastroenterology 2007;132(4):A40.
52. Holzer B, Rosen HR, Novi G, et al. Sacral nerve stimulation in patients with severe constipation. Dis Colon Rectum 2008;51(5):524–9.
53. Dinning PG, Fuentealba SE, Kennedy ML, et al. Sacral nerve stimulation induces pan-colonic propagating pressure waves and increases defecation frequency in patients with slow-transit constipation. Colorectal Dis 2007;9(2):123–32.

54. Gladman MA, Lunniss PJ, Scott SM, et al. Rectal hyposensitivity. Am J Gastroenterol 2006;101(5):1140–51.
55. Mowatt G, Glazener C, Jarrett M. Sacral nerve stimulation for faecal incontinence and constipation in adults. Cochrane Database Syst Rev 2007 Jul 18;(3):CD004464.
56. Altomare DF, Rinaldi M, Veglia A, et al. Combined perineal and endorectal repair of rectocele by circular stapler: a novel surgical technique. Dis Colon Rectum 2002;45(11):1549–52.
57. Corman ML, Carriero A, Hager T, et al. Consensus conference on the stapled transanal rectal resection (STARR) for disordered defaecation. Colorectal Dis 2006;8(2):98–101.
58. Boccasanta P, Venturi M, Roviaro G. Stapled transanal rectal resection versus stapled anopexy in the cure of hemorrhoids associated with rectal prolapse: a randomized controlled trial. Int J Colorectal Dis 2007;22(3):245–51.
59. Dodi G, Pietroletti R, Milito G, et al. Bleeding, incontinence, pain and constipation after STARR transanal double stapling rectotomy for obstructed defecation. Tech Coloproctol 2003;7(3):148–53.
60. Brown SR, Nelson RL. Surgery for faecal incontinence in adults. Cochrane Database Syst Rev 2007;(2):CD001757.
61. Korsgen S, Deen KI, Keighley MR. Long-term results of total pelvic floor repair for postobstetric fecal incontinence. Dis Colon Rectum 1997;40(7):835–9.
62. Leroi AM, Kamm MA, Weber J, et al. Internal anal sphincter repair. Int J Colorectal Dis 1997;12(4):243–5.
63. Fang DT, Nivatvongs S, Vermeulen FD, et al. Overlapping sphincteroplasty for acquired anal incontinence. Dis Colon Rectum 1984;27(11):720–2.
64. Oliveira L, Pfeifer J, Wexner SD. Physiological and clinical outcome of anterior sphincteroplasty. Br J Surg 1996;83(4):502–5.
65. Londono-Schimmer EE, Garcia-Duperly R, Nicholls RJ, et al. Overlapping anal sphincter repair for faecal incontinence due to sphincter trauma: five year follow-up functional results. Int J Colorectal Dis 1994;9(2):110–3.
66. Malouf AJ, Norton CS, Engel AF, et al. Long-term results of overlapping anterior anal-sphincter repair for obstetric trauma. Lancet 2000;355(9200):260–5.
67. Giordano P, Renzi A, Efron J, et al. Previous sphincter repair does not affect the outcome of repeat repair. Dis Colon Rectum 2002;45(5):635–40.
68. Nikiteas N, Korsgen S, Kumar D, et al. Audit of sphincter repair: factors associated with poor outcome. Dis Colon Rectum 1996;39(10):1164–70.
69. Ha HT, Fleshman JW, Smith M, et al. Manometric squeeze pressure difference parallels functional outcome after overlapping sphincter reconstruction. Dis Colon Rectum 2001;44(5):655–60.
70. Chen AS, Luchtefeld MA, Senagore AJ, et al. Pudendal nerve latency. Does it predict outcome of anal sphincter repair? Dis Colon Rectum 1998;41(8):1005–9.
71. Melenhorst J, Koch SM, Uludag O, et al. Is a morphologically intact anal sphincter necessary for success with sacral nerve modulation in patients with faecal incontinence? Colorectal Dis 2008;10(3):257–62.
72. Vitton V, Gigout J, Grimaud JC, et al. Sacral nerve stimulation can improve continence in patients with Crohn's disease with internal and external anal sphincter disruption. Dis Colon Rectum 2008 Feb 8;[Epub ahead of print].
73. Gstaltner K, Rosen H, Hufgard J, et al. Sacral nerve stimulation as an option for the treatment of faecal incontinence in patients suffering from cauda equina syndrome. Spinal Cord. 2008 Mar 4;[Epub ahead of print].

74. Jarrett ME, Matzel KE, Christiansen J, et al. Sacral nerve stimulation for faecal incontinence in patients with previous partial spinal injury including disc prolapse. Br J Surg 2005;92(6):734–9.
75. Malouf AJ, Vaizey CJ, Nicholls RJ, et al. Permanent sacral nerve stimulation for fecal incontinence. Ann Surg 2000;232(1):143–8.
76. Ganio E, Masin A, Ratto C, et al. Short-term sacral nerve stimulation for functional anorectal and urinary disturbances: results in 40 patients. Evaluation of a new option for anorectal functional disorders. Dis Colon Rectum 2001;44(9):1261–7.
77. Hetzer FH, Hahnloser D, Clavien PA, et al. Quality of life and morbidity after permanent sacral nerve stimulation for fecal incontinence. Arch Surg 2007; 142(1):8–13.
78. Matzel KE, Kamm MA, Stösser M, et al. Sacral spinal nerve stimulation for faecal incontinence: multicentre study. Lancet 2004;363(9417):1270–6.
79. Leroi AM, Parc Y, Lehur PA, et al. Efficacy of sacral nerve stimulation for fecal incontinence: results of a multicenter double-blind crossover study. Ann Surg 2005;242(5):662–9.
80. Rosen HR, Urbarz C, Holzer B, et al. Sacral nerve stimulation as a treatment for fecal incontinence. Gastroenterology 2001;121(3):536–41.
81. Tjandra JJ, Chan MK, Yeh CH, et al. Sacral nerve stimulation is more effective than optimal medical therapy for severe fecal incontinence: a randomized, controlled study. Dis Colon Rectum. 2008 Feb 16;[Epub ahead of print].
82. Dudding TC, Parés D, Vaizey CJ, et al. Predictive factors for successful sacral nerve stimulation in the treatment of faecal incontinence: a 10-year cohort analysis. Colorectal Dis 2008;10(3):249–56.
83. Keighley MRB. Faecal incontinence. In: Keighley MRB, Williams NS, editors. Surgery of the anus, rectum and colon. 1st edition. London: WB Saunders; 1997. p. 581–94.
84. Williams NS, Hallan RI, Koczc TH, et al. Construction of a neorectum and neoanal sphincter following previous proctocolectomy. Br J Surg 1989;76(11): 1191–4.
85. Baeten C, Spaans F, Fluks A. An implanted neuromuscular stimulator for fecal continence following previously implanted gracilis muscle: report of a case. Dis Colon Rectum 1988;31(2):134–7.
86. Mander BJ, Wexner SD, Williams NS, et al. Preliminary results of a multicentre trial of the electrically stimulated gracilis neoanal sphincter. Br J Surg 1999; 86(12):1543–8.
87. Madoff RD, Rosen HR, Baeten CG, et al. Safety and efficacy of dynamic muscle plasty for anal incontinence: lessons from a prospective, multicenter trial. Gastroenterology 1999;116(3):549–56.
88. Chapman AE, Geerdes B, Hewett P, et al. Systematic review of dynamic graciloplasty in the treatment of faecal incontinence. Br J Surg 2002;89(2):138–53.
89. Rongen MJ, Uludag O, El Naggar K, et al. Long-term follow-up of dynamic graciloplasty for fecal incontinence. Dis Colon Rectum 2003;46(6):716–21.
90. Saunders JR, Darakhshan AA, Eccersley AJ, et al. The colorectal development unit: impact on functional outcome for the electrically stimulated gracilis neoanal sphincter. Colorectal Dis 2006;8(1):46–55.
91. Christiansen J, Lorentzen M. Implantation of artificial sphincter for anal incontinence. Lancet 1987;2(8553):244–5.
92. Altomare DF, Dodi G, La Torre F, et al. Multicentre retrospective analysis of the outcome of artificial anal sphincter implantation for severe faecal incontinence. Br J Surg 2001;88(11):1481–6.

93. Wong WD, Congliosi SM, Spencer MP, et al. The safety and efficacy of the artificial bowel sphincter for fecal incontinence: results from a multicenter cohort study. Dis Colon Rectum 2002;45(9):1139–53.
94. O'Brien PE, Dixon JB, Skinner S, et al. A prospective, randomized, controlled clinical trial of placement of the artificial bowel sphincter (Acticon Neosphincter) for the control of fecal incontinence. Dis Colon Rectum 2004;47(11):1852–60.
95. Christiansen J, Rasmussen OO, Lindorff-Larsen K. Long-term results of artificial anal sphincter implantation for severe anal incontinence. Ann Surg 1999;230(1):45–8.
96. Parker SC, Spencer MP, Madoff RD, et al. Artificial bowel sphincter: long-term experience at a single institution. Dis Colon Rectum 2003;46(6):722–9.
97. Norton C, Burch J, Kamm MA. Patients' views of a colostomy for fecal incontinence. Dis Colon Rectum 2005;48(5):1062–9.
98. Vaizey CJ, Kamm MA. Injectable bulking agents for treating faecal incontinence. Br J Surg 2005;92(5):521–7.
99. Tjandra JJ, Lim JF, Hiscock R, et al. Injectable silicone biomaterial for fecal incontinence caused by internal anal sphincter dysfunction is effective. Dis Colon Rectum 2004;47(12):2138–46.
100. Maeda Y, Vaizey CJ, Kamm MA. Long-term results of perianal silicone injection for faecal incontinence. Colorectal Dis 2007;9(4):357–61.
101. Takahashi T, Garcia-Osogobio S, Valdovinos MA, et al. Radio-frequency energy delivery to the anal canal for the treatment of fecal incontinence. Dis Colon Rectum 2002;45(7):915–22.
102. Takahashi T, Garcia-Osogobio S, Valdovinos MA, et al. Extended two-year results of radio-frequency energy delivery for the treatment of fecal incontinence (the SECCA procedure). Dis Colon Rectum 2003;46(6):711–5.
103. Efron JE, Corman ML, Fleshman J, et al. Safety and effectiveness of temperature-controlled radio-frequency energy delivery to the anal canal (SECCA procedure) for the treatment of fecal incontinence. Dis Colon Rectum 2003;46(12):1606–16.
104. Takahashi-Monroy T, Morales M, Garcia-Osogobio S, et al. SECCA(R) procedure for the treatment of fecal incontinence: results of five-year follow-up. Dis Colon Rectum 2008;51(3):355–9.
105. Williams NS, Ogunbiyi OA, Scott SM, et al. Rectal augmentation and stimulated gracilis anal neosphincter: a new approach in the management of fecal urgency and incontinence. Dis Colon Rectum 2001;44(2):192–8.
106. Chan CL, Lunniss PJ, Wang D, et al. Rectal sensorimotor dysfunction in patients with urge faecal incontinence: evidence from prolonged manometric studies. Gut 2005;54(9):1263–72.
107. Murphy J, Chan CLH, Scott SM, et al. Rectal augmentation: short- and mid-term evaluation of a novel procedure for severe fecal urgency with associated incontinence. Ann Surg 2008;247(3):421–7.
108. Tan JJ, Chan M, Tjandra JJ. Evolving therapy for fecal incontinence. Dis Colon Rectum 2007;50(11):1950–67.

Hemorrhoids and Fissure in Ano

Peter S. Chong, MBChB, BSc (Hons), FRCS[a,b,*],
David C.C. Bartolo, MB, MS, FRCS, FRCSE[a]

KEYWORDS

- Hemorrhoids • Fissure-in-ano • Anorectal pain
- Rectal bleeding • Constipation

Hemorrhoids and anal fissures are common benign anorectal conditions that form a significant part of a colorectal surgeon's workload. In this review we summarize and evaluate the current techniques available in their management.

HEMORRHOIDS

Hemorrhoids are enlarged vascular cushions within the anal canal. They are usually found in three classical locations: left lateral, right anterior, and right posterior (3, 7, and 11 o'clock). They lie beneath the epithelial lining of the anal canal and consist of direct arteriovenous communications and surrounding connective tissue. These vascular cushions are a normal part of human anorectal anatomy, participating in the venous drainage of the anal canal. They also appear to have a role in the maintenance of continence, contributing to resting anal pressure.

Epidemiology

The exact incidence of this common condition is difficult to estimate because many patients are reluctant to seek medical advice for various personal, cultural, and socioeconomic reasons. Epidemiologic studies report a prevalence ranging from 4.4% in adults in the United States to over 30% in general practice in London. A peak in prevalence is seen between 45 and 65 years of age and the development of hemorrhoids before the age of 20 is unusual.[1–3]

Etiology

The main theories regarding the pathophysiology of hemorrhoidal disease are centered on abnormal dilatation of veins of the internal hemorrhoidal venous plexus,

[a] Department of Colorectal Surgery, Western General Hospital, Edinburgh EH4 2XU, UK
[b] Department of Surgery, Gartnavel General Hospital, 1053 Great Western Road, Glasgow G12 0YN, UK
* Corresponding author. Department of Surgery, Gartnavel General Hospital, 1053 Great Western Road, Glasgow G12 0YN, UK.
E-mail address: petechong@tiscali.co.uk (P.S. Chong).

Gastroenterol Clin N Am 37 (2008) 627–644
doi:10.1016/j.gtc.2008.07.001 gastro.theclinics.com
0889-8553/08/$ – see front matter.

abnormal distention of the arteriovenous anastomosis, and prolapse of the cushions and the surrounding connective tissue. Increased anal sphincter pressure is also described as an etiological factor and is a reasonably consistent finding, but it is unclear if this is cause or effect.[4]

The role of mucosal prolapse in hemorrhoidal disease is uncertain. Some regard this as a completely different process, while others consider it an integral part of the hemorrhoidal disease.[5] Straining, inadequate fiber intake, prolonged lavatory sitting, constipation, diarrhea, and such conditions as pregnancy, ascites, and pelvic space-occupying lesions may contribute to development of the disease. The common factor appears to be the association with elevated intra-abdominal pressure. A family history of hemorrhoidal disease has also been suggested to be relevant, but there is no direct evidence of a hereditary predisposition and these observations are probably more related to environment.[6–8]

Classification

The dentate line gives rise to the simplest classification of hemorrhoidal disease. External hemorrhoids originate distal to the dentate line and are lined with modified squamous epithelium. Internal hemorrhoids originate proximal to the dentate line and are covered with mucosa. In some patients the two types coexist.

In Golligher's classification, internal hemorrhoids are subdivided into a further four grades according to the amount of prolapse. In first-degree hemorrhoids there is bleeding but no prolapse. Second-degree hemorrhoids may prolapse beyond the external sphincter and be visible during evacuation but spontaneously reduce. Third-degree hemorrhoids protrude outside the anal canal and require manual reduction, while fourth-degree hemorrhoids are irreducible and are constantly prolapsed. The problem with this classification is that it gives no indication of the extent of the patient's symptoms and emphasis is on prolapse.

Clinical Evaluation

Symptoms

Most patients present with painless bleeding, but some experience swelling, discomfort, discharge, soiling, or pruritus. Pain on defecation with associated bleeding is more suggestive of a thrombosed external hemorrhoid or an anal fissure. Internal hemorrhoids usually become symptomatic only when they prolapse, become ulcerated, bleed, or thrombose. External hemorrhoids may be asymptomatic or be associated with discomfort or bleeding from ulceration, or acute pain if complicated by thrombosis. Bleeding from hemorrhoids rarely causes anemia, and patients who present with anemia require further investigation of the gastrointestinal tract.[9]

Diagnosis

The diagnosis is usually simple on inspection of the perineum, rectal examination, and proctoscopy. This differentiates hemorrhoids from other anorectal pathology, such as skin tags, anal warts, fissures, fistulas, tumors, polyps, and prolapse. Large external hemorrhoids are easily seen on inspection and proctoscopy allows internal hemorrhoids to be visualized in the classical positions.

Patients over the age of 40 who have suspected hemorrhoidal bleeding cannot be assumed to have no other colorectal pathology and should be referred for a specialist opinion. Most will then require additional evaluation by flexible sigmoidoscopy, colonoscopy, CT colonography, or barium enema. Indications for formal colorectal investigation are as follows:

- Iron-deficiency anemia
- Positive fecal occult blood test

Age 50 years or older, with no complete colon evaluation within 10 years
Age 40 years or older, with positive family history for a single first-degree relative with adenoma or colorectal cancer diagnosed at age over 60 years and no complete examination within 10 years
Age 40 years or older, with positive family history for two or more first-degree relatives with adenoma or colorectal cancer diagnosed at age over 60 years and no complete examination within 3 to 5 years
Any history or physical finding indicating malignancy or inflammatory bowel disease

Many colorectal units in the United Kingdom now use protocols that allow direct access to investigation based on standardized proformas completed by general practitioners.

Patients with hemorrhoids and associated soiling or incontinence may require anorectal physiology studies and endoanal ultrasound as these patients have a higher risk of developing incontinence after surgery. These investigations are often instructive in tailoring treatment and in cases where surgery is being considered.

Treatment

Conservative treatment

Dietary fiber supplementation improves symptoms and is generally recommended to all patients.[10] The evidence for other lifestyle modifications, such as improving anal hygiene, taking sitz baths, increasing fluid intake, relieving constipation, and avoiding straining, is scarce, but these measures are routinely employed in the treatment and prevention of hemorrhoids.

Well-designed studies have found no evidence to support the use of any of the myriad of over-the-counter topical preparations that contain low-dose local anesthetics, corticosteroids, keratolytics, protectants, or antiseptics. The use of these agents is widespread for symptomatic relief but the long-term use of these products, particularly steroid preparations, may be detrimental and should be discouraged.

Venotonics, such as flavonoids, have been used as dietary supplements in the treatment of hemorrhoids. The mechanism of action of these drugs remains unclear. They are claimed to improve venous tone, reduce hyperpermeability, and to have anti-inflammatory effects. Meta-analysis of currently available studies does not support the use of these agents, despite their popularity in some parts of the world.[11] The Food and Drug Administration does not currently approve the use of flavonoids in the United States.[12]

Outpatient treatments

A range of interventions are available in the outpatient management of hemorrhoidal disease. These include sclerotherapy, rubber-band ligation, infrared coagulation, hemorrhoidal artery ligation, bipolar diathermy, and cryotherapy.

Sclerotherapy Injection sclerotherapy was first described 2 centuries ago and has been performed with a variety of agents but most commonly with 5% phenol. A proctoscope passed through the anal canal into the rectum is then withdrawn until the hemorrhoidal tissue prolapses into view. The submucosa at the base of the hemorrhoid is then injected with 5 mL of 5% phenol oil. The sclerosant produces an inflammatory reaction with intravascular thrombosis and submucosal fibrosis, which minimizes the extent of the mucosal prolapse and reduces the hemorrhoidal tissue.

Patients undergoing multiple injections can experience pain and discomfort. Injudicious injection of sclerosant must be avoided because it can cause chest and upper abdominal pain if injected directly into the hemorrhoidal vein[13] or cause erectile dysfunction if parasympathetic nerves are damaged.[14] Rare cases of hepatic complications after sclerotherapy for hemorrhoidal disease have been described[15] and local infection and abscess formation are uncommon, but may occur. Antibiotic prophylaxis is indicated for patients with valvular disease or immunodeficiency as transient bacteremia is not unusual after sclerotherapy.[16]

Sclerotherapy is recommended for patients with symptomatic nonprolapsing grades I to II hemorrhoids. It is not suitable for external hemorrhoids. Its popularity has diminished, perhaps as a consequence of evidence indicating that rubber-band ligation produces superior results[17,18] and that conservative treatment with fiber supplementation may be as effective.[19]

Rubber-band ligation The technique of applying rubber bands to hemorrhoids was first described over 40 years ago. Ligation of the hemorrhoidal tissue with a rubber band causes ischemic necrosis and ulceration, which results in reduction of the prolapsed hemorrhoidal tissue and in fixation of the connective tissue to the rectal wall. Band ligation at three sites can be performed at a single clinic visit and improved banding devices allow the procedure to be performed without assistance.

The rubber bands are deployed at the base of the internal hemorrhoid proximal to the dentate line, as banding at or below the dentate can cause severe pain. Common complications include discomfort for several days after the procedure, which can be minimized by sitz baths, mild analgesics, and stool softeners. Injection of a local anesthetic does not reduce the discomfort associated with multiple banding.[20] Other complications include late hemorrhage (1 to 2 weeks after the procedure), slippage of the band, urinary retention, and, rarely, pelvic or perineal sepsis.[21–23] Rubber-band ligation is contraindicated in patients taking anticoagulants because of the risk of delayed hemorrhage.

Meta-analysis of available studies suggests band ligation is the most effective outpatient procedure for hemorrhoids,[21] providing a cure in 79% of patients with grade I to grade III hemorrhoids. Almost 20% of patients have a relapse requiring repeat banding and roughly 2% fail to respond.[24] Dietary fiber supplementation increases the long-term cure rate after banding.[25]

Endoscopic band ligation There is now increasing enthusiasm for endoscopic banding using a flexible scope,[26] as opposed to the conventional method, which employs a rigid proctoscope. Banding is performed in a manner similar to that for banding of esophageal varices. The retroflexed endoscope allows unparalleled views and photographic documentation. Multiple bands can be applied in one session, and further bands can be applied at subsequent sessions. Endoscopic hemorrhoidal ligation appears to be simple, safe, and effective. Results are good for hemorrhoids and mucosal prolapse, and the long-term recurrence rate is low (3.3%–9%).[27] The technique is at least as effective as conventional banding and may require fewer treatment sessions.[28] It has some clear advantages, apart from cost. Indications for use are the same as for conventional banding.

Infrared coagulation This technique employs infrared light, which penetrates the tissue and converts to heat with resultant coagulation and fixation of hemorrhoidal tissue. The infrared probe is applied to the apex of each internal hemorrhoid and repeated three times on each hemorrhoid. Its main limitation is that it can only be used to treat grade I and small grade II hemorrhoids.[18] If an external component is to be treated with infrared coagulation, anesthesia is needed. The main advantages are that it is painless and complications are rare. In a meta-analysis of randomized controlled trials, infrared coagulation was found to be significantly less painful than rubber-band ligation, but required more sessions to relieve symptoms, had a higher recurrence rate, and was more expensive.[21]

Doppler-guided hemorrhoidal artery ligation Doppler-guided hemorrhoidal artery ligation (DGHAL) was first described by Morinaga and colleagues[29] in 1995. This technique uses a Doppler transducer to identify hemorrhoidal arteries, allowing their selective ligation with sutures placed above the dentate line. The insertion of a ring of sutures results in a reduction of hemorrhoidal prolapse while interrupting the feeding vessels. DGHAL, which can be performed as an outpatient procedure with local anesthesia and sedation or as a day case, is successful in the treatment of grade III hemorrhoids. It appears to have none of the drawbacks of formal hemorrhoidectomy, such as pain, incontinence, or stenosis.[29–33] DGHAL does not appear to have a role in the management of grade VI hemorrhoids, but early results are promising[34] and the technique is gaining popularity. Further studies should determine its place in the management hemorrhoidal disease.

Other techniques

Electrocoagulation Bipolar diathermy and direct-current electrotherapy cause coagulation and fibrosis after local application of heat. The success rates of these methods in treating grade I and II hemorrhoids are similar to those of infrared coagulation, with relatively low complication rates.[35]

Cryotherapy Cryotherapy uses cold coagulation (nitrous oxide or liquid nitrogen) to destroy hemorrhoid tissue.[36] The procedure results in profuse, foul-smelling discharge and pain due to necrosis. Recovery is prolonged and cryotherapy is no longer recommended for the treatment of hemorrhoids.

Surgery

Surgery, in the form of formal hemorrhoidectomy, is associated with pain and the risk of uncommon but serious complications of incontinence and anal stenosis. Indicated in less than 10% of patients referred for specialist treatment, it is generally reserved for (1) grade III hemorrhoids not responding to banding, (2) grade IV hemorrhoids (prolapse), (3) large external hemorrhoids or combined internal and external components, and (4) concomitant anorectal pathology requiring surgery.

Surgical hemorrhoidectomy is a very effective treatment with high cure and low recurrence rates. These procedures are now performed in a day-surgery setting in many centers.

Hemorrhoidectomy Excisional hemorrhoidectomy can be performed as an open or closed procedure. In the United Kingdom, the Milligan-Morgan hemorrhoidectomy is the most commonly performed. The hemorrhoid is dissected off the anal sphincter, its vascular pedicle ligated, and the wounds left open to heal by secondary intention with skin and mucosal bridges. The Ferguson hemorrhoidectomy is favored in the United States. The hemorrhoid is exposed in the anoscope, then excised and ligated, and the wounds closed.[37]

Four randomized trials have compared open versus closed hemorrhoidectomy.[38–41] Both techniques are safe and effective, with no consistent difference in postoperative pain, analgesic use, hospital stay, or complication rates. Wound healing showed mixed results, as dehiscence of primarily closed wounds prolonged healing times beyond that of the open technique.

The Harmonic Scalpel and LigaSure have been employed in excisional hemorrhoidectomy. These instruments allow the procedure to be performed more rapidly and provide a dry operating field, but do not appear to offer any other specific advantages and randomized controlled trials show no improvement in postoperative pain.[42–45] These methods have the obvious disadvantage of increased costs.

The complications of hemorrhoidectomy include urinary retention (2%–36%); bleeding (0.03%–6%); infection (0.5%–5.5%); anal stenosis (0%–6%), usually as a result of inadequate mucosal bridges; and incontinence (2%–12%).[21] Sphincter defects associated with incontinence have been documented by endoanal ultrasound and manometry in up to 12% of patients after hemorrhoidectomy.[46–49]

Postoperative pain remains a significant problem and most patients do not return to work for 2 to 4 weeks after surgery.[46] Local anesthesia, glyceryl trinitrate (GTN) paste, and simultaneous lateral internal sphincterotomy have been attempted to reduce postoperative pain without convincing benefit.[50–54] Sphinterotomy should not be performed as it exacerbates continence impairment.[55] Postoperative analgesics, laxatives, and prophylactic metronidazole appear to reduce pain and convalescence after day surgery.[56]

Stapled hemorrhoidopexy Longo developed the stapled hemorrhoidectomy or hemorrhoidopexy in the mid-90s and since then it has gained popularity, particularly in the Far East. The procedure is also known as the procedure for prolapsed hemorrhoids and stapled anopexy. The technique employs a circular stapler, which performs a circumferential resection of mucosa and submucosa above the hemorrhoids, stapling the defect closed with a single firing of the staple gun. The prolapsing hemorrhoidal tissue is resuspended back into the anal canal and the arterial inflow is interrupted in a manner similar to that for DGHAL. The hemorrhoids are not removed, but rather returned to their normal anatomic position.

There are no wounds, less incontinence, less pain, and a shorter recovery period compared with excisional hemorrhoidectomy.[57] Recurrence rates are higher and, although complication rates are no higher than those for conventional hemorrhoidectomy, a number of serious complications were documented following the introduction of the stapled hemorrhoidopexy.[58] These included bleeding, rectal perforation, rectovaginal fistulas, occlusion of the rectum, and perineal and severe pelvic sepsis.[59] Similar complications have been described for most treatments for hemorrhoidal disease. A recent Cochrane systematic review[60] concluded that the procedure was as safe as conventional hemorrhoidectomy but that its main drawback was recurrence. Consequently, with the procedure for prolapsed hemorrhoids, the need for further subsequent procedures is comparable to that for excisional hemorrhoidectomy.

The main role for the procedure for prolapsed hemorrhoids appears to be in the treatment of grade II and III hemorrhoids that have failed outpatient treatment. It may have a role in treating grade IV hemorrhoids that are reducible under anesthesia, but recurrence in this situation appears to be a problem.

Acutely thrombosed hemorrhoids The management of hemorrhoids in an elective setting has been emphasized in this review but patients occasionally present with acutely thrombosed prolapsed hemorrhoids as an emergency. This is a very painful condition that most surgeons would manage, at least initially, with a conservative approach. Ice packs, stool softeners, local anesthetic cream, metronidazole, and ditiazem can be helpful. Emergency surgery is occasionally required for those patients who do not settle, but can be associated with significant morbidity.[61,62]

The management of hemorrhoids in certain special situations in summarized in **Fig. 1**.

Summary

Hemorrhoids remain a common problem and comprise a significant percentage of a colorectal surgeon's workload. A wide and still expanding range of procedures to

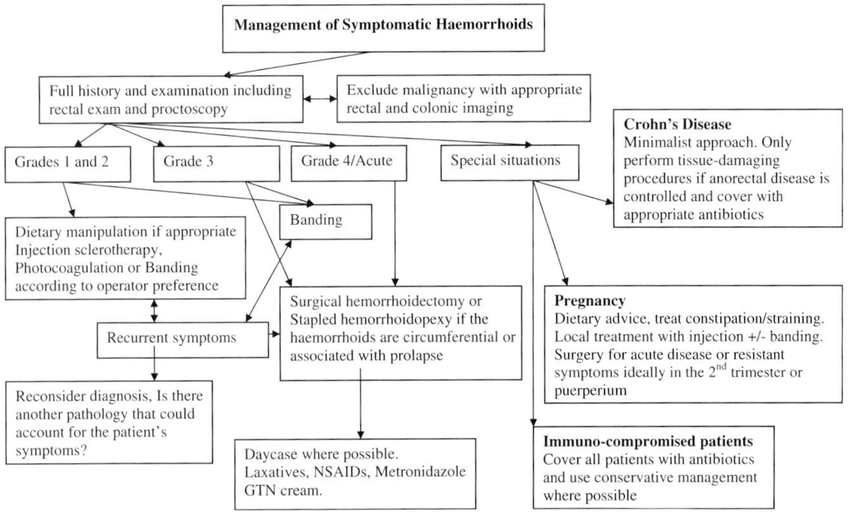

Fig. 1. Management of anal fissure. (*From* Steele SR, Madoff RD. Systematic review: the treatment of anal fissure. Alimentary Pharmacology & Therapeutics 2006;24(2):247–57; with permission.)

treat the condition have been developed and the data generated from studies comparing one technique to another is overwhelming (**Table 1**).

It is safe to say that no one treatment is a panacea. Hemorrhoidal disease is a heterogeneous condition that requires the surgeon to select the most appropriate treatment for the problem that the patient presents. The treatment of hemorrhoidal disease should therefore be tailored to the individual.

FISSURE IN ANO

An anal fissure is a painful tear or split in the distal anal canal. Patients typically complain of severe anal pain during and after defecation, lasting minutes to hours. Bleeding, in the form of bright red blood, is commonly seen either on the toilet tissue or streaking the stool surface.

Table 1
Treatment options for hemorrhoidal disease

Treatment	Indications	Evidence Grading
Sclerotherapy	Grades I and II	Level 1
Rubber-band ligation	Grades I, II, and III	Level 1
Endoscopic banding	Grades I, II, and III	Level 2
DGHAL	Grades II and III	Level 2
Electrocoagulation	Grades I and II	Level 2
Cryotherapy	No current role	
Hemorrhoidectomy	Grades II–IV, external	Level 1
Stapled hemorrhoidopexy	Grades II–III	Level 1

Anal fissures may be classified as acute or chronic according to length of symptoms and typical morphologic appearances. The majority of acute fissures heal spontaneously, but a proportion become chronic and this is usually defined as a persistence of symptoms beyond 6 weeks or by the presence of visible transverse internal anal sphincter (IAS) fibers at the base of a fissure. Associated features include indurated edges, a sentinel pile, and a hypertrophied anal papilla. The medical community should establish clear classifications for fissures. It is likely that the absence of accepted definitions for chronic fissures has led to widely differing healing rates with various interventions reported in the literature. Lindsey and colleagues[63] have described a chronic anal fissure as "the presence of visible transverse internal anal sphincter fibers at the base of an anal fissure of duration not less than 6 weeks."

Anal fissures are most commonly seen in the posterior midline, although 10% to 20% in women and 1% to 10% in men are located in the anterior midline. Fissures located off the midline suggest the presence of underlying pathology, such as Crohn disease, syphilis, or anal cancer, and generally require further evaluation with an examination under anesthesia and biopsy to establish a diagnosis.[64]

Chronic fissures are associated with IAS spasm and ischemia, the relief of which is central to achieving healing whether a surgical or medical approach is taken.[65]

Pathogenesis

The exact mechanism surrounding the pathophysiology of anal fissures has not been clearly established. The current hypotheses are centered on anal sphincter tonicity and blood flow.

It is thought that the initiating factor is trauma to the anal canal, possibly due to the passage of hard stool, but constipation is not always reported and some patients describe repeated episodes of diarrhea. Constipation, by repeated aggravation of the anal canal, is likely to play a role in perpetuating an anal fissure. Increased resting pressures within the IAS in patients with fissures[66–70] has been described as another perpetuating factor and anorectal manometry has consistently demonstrated that IAS tone as measured by the resting pressure is elevated in fissure patients versus controls.[71,72] Maximal voluntary contraction of the external anal sphincter remains similar between the two groups and the IAS alone seems to be responsible for the hypertonicity.[73] There is relative ischemia in posterior midline of the anal canal[74] and this is exacerbated by increased tone, a key factor in preventing fissures from healing.

Internal Anal Sphincter Physiology

The understanding of the physiology of the IAS has improved significantly in recent years and this provides the rationale for current nonsurgical treatment.

The resting tone of the IAS depends on intracellular calcium concentration, and contraction of the smooth muscle cells within the IAS is mediated by influx of calcium through calcium channels and by stimulation of α1-adrenoreceptors at the smooth muscle cells.

Activation of α2-adrenoreceptors in the myenteric inhibitory neurons presynaptically inhibit nonadrenergic, noncholinergic (NANC) relaxation. Relaxation of these cells is mediated through directly decreasing intracellular calcium concentration as well as increasing cyclic guanosine monophosphate and cyclic adenosine monophosphate. Potassium influx hyperpolarizes the cell membrane and decreases calcium entry. In addition, inhibitory neurotransmitters, such as nitric oxide and vasoactive intestinal peptide, mediate NANC relaxation. Nitric oxide is the major neurotransmitter mediating NANC relaxation of the IAS.[75,76] L-arginine, a precursor of nitric oxide, has been found to relax IAS smooth muscle perhaps by increasing substrate for nitric oxide synthase, the enzyme involved in nitric oxide synthesis.[77] A preliminary study has shown reduced nitric oxide synthase in the IAS of patients with anal fissures compared with controls.[78] The reduced production of nitric oxide provides a possible explanation for the high IAS pressures seen in most fissure patients and also why pressures return to pretreatment values in patients whose fissures have healed with medical treatment. The "chemical" sphincteromy lasts only as long as the treatment is continued.[79]

Treatment

Conservative management

The aim of treatment of an acute fissure is to break the cycle of a hard stool, pain, and spasm. This can be accomplished by adequate fluid, fiber, and, if necessary, stool softeners. Up to 90% of patients diagnosed with acute fissures heal with these measures alone, but chronic fissures usually require medical or surgical therapy.

Medical therapy

Increased understanding of anal sphincter physiology, coupled with concerns regarding long-term impaired continence as a consequence of surgery, has driven enthusiasm for pharmacologic treatments for chronic anal fissure. These agents have been developed with the aim of creating a reversible reduction in the abnormally high resting sphincter pressure until the fissure has healed.

Glyceryl trinitrate GTN was the first pharmacologic treatment used in creating a "chemical sphinterotomy." Nitrates are metabolized by smooth muscle cells to release nitric oxide, the principle nonadrenergic, noncholinergic neurotransmitter in the IAS. Its release results in IAS relaxation and increased anodermal blood flow. The usual course is 0.2% GTN, applied topically two or three times daily, for 8 weeks.

The first randomized trial involved patients receiving 0.2% GTN (twice daily for 8 weeks) or placebo.[80] Healing rates were significantly higher in the GTN than in the placebo group (68% versus 8%; $P < 0{\cdot}001$). Perhaps unsurprisingly, there followed great enthusiasm for topical GTN. The treatment significantly reduces pain on defecation after 2 weeks, even in patients who don't heal. Repeated applications may be necessary and are safe. Higher dosing does not improve outcome but, interestingly, does not appear to worsen side effects.[81–83] The most common of these are headache (27%) and hypotension (6%).

However, subsequent trials did not replicate the initial positive results and healing rates are lower than expected with one Italian study demonstrating no difference compared with placebo.[84,85] Medium-term relapse is a problem, side effects common, and compliance is uncertain. The overall healing rate in Nelson's recent Cochrane meta-analysis is 48.6% compared with 37% with placebo, but late recurrence is common, in the range of 50% of those initially cured.[86] The high rates of failure mean that the question of how to treat GTN-resistant fissures is significant. Despite this, GTN is safe, readily available, and has a modest but significant effect compared with placebo. It remains first-line treatment in many centers.

Calcium channel blockers Calcium channel blockers prevent influx of calcium into smooth muscle cells, decreasing intracellular calcium and preventing smooth muscle contraction with a consequent reduction in resting IAS pressure.[87–90] Oral agents appear to have poorer healing rates and higher rates of side effects than topical preparations. Topical calcium channel blockers (diltiazem 2%, nifedipine 0.3%) achieve fissure healing to a degree similar to that reported for topical nitrates, but with fewer side effects and better compliance.[91] Recurrence rates after long-term follow-up appear to be no better than treatment with GTN.

Botulinum A toxin injection Derived from exotoxin produced by the bacterium *Clostridium botulinum*, botulinum A toxin is a potent neurotoxin. Its effects on smooth muscle are well documented and, when injected into the IAS,[92,93] it produces a chemical denervation of motor end plates with a subsequent decrease in resting anal pressure and improved perfusion. The treatment is more invasive than the topical ointments but does not have the same problems with compliance and can be performed in an outpatient setting. It provides a reversible chemical sphincterotomy and represents a novel nonoperative treatment in the management of chronic anal fissure. Side effects, such as temporary minor incontinence and urgency, appear to be infrequent and reversible. Its major disadvantage is its cost, but this has to be set against the cost of surgery.

In one prospective randomized trial that compared injection of 20 U of botulinum toxin with 0.2% GTN twice daily, the botulinum toxin group was associated with significantly improved healing rates (96% versus 60%, $P = .005$).[94] Similar prospective studies, while not achieving such successful rates of healing, have found approximately 80% of patients with initial healing at 6 months.[95,96]

The issue of recurrence after botulin toxin injection remains to be determined and there is still debate regarding the ideal location of injection (into the IAS, external anal sphincter, or the intersphincteric groove) and optimal dose. A number of studies use 20 U divided in one to four injections but there is evidence that higher doses can give better results. In combined analyses botulin toxin was found to be no better or worse than topical nitrates,[97] but botulin toxin is effective in healing 50% to 70% of patients with fissures resistant to topical nitrates,[98] and it may have a role in the treatment of refractory fissures either alone or in combination with topical nitrates.[99]

A Cochrane review of nonsurgical therapy for anal fissure has concluded that medical therapy for nonhealing fissures may be applied with a chance of cure that is marginally but significantly better than that for placebo, but far less effective than surgery and a high recurrence rate.[97] Nonetheless, the risk of using such therapies is not great, without apparent long-term adverse effect, and treatment can be repeated. Medical treatment can therefore be used in individuals wanting to avoid surgery, with surgery being reserved for treatment failures.

Other nonsurgical treatment

A variety of other agents have been used in the treatment of anal fissures. These include the nitrous oxide precursor L-arginine,[100] alpha-1 receptor antagonists,[101] angiotensin-converting enzyme inhibitors,[102] and hyperbaric oxygen.[103] None has demonstrated advantages over currently available therapy and data is limited at present.

Surgery

Surgery represents traditional management of chronic anal fissure. Manual dilatation and internal sphincterotomy have been employed to create a permanent reduction in resting anal pressure.

Manual dilatation of the anus Manual dilatation was once first-line treatment for chronic anal fissure. The aim was to reduce sphincter tone by controlled manual stretching of the internal sphincter. A variable number of fingers are inserted into the anal canal and lateral distraction exerted on the sphincter and sustained for a period. This procedure frequently produced an uncontrolled tearing of the sphincter muscles resulting in incontinence, with characteristic findings on anal endosonography.[104–106]

Speakman and colleagues[104] evaluated 12 men with fecal incontinence after manual dilatation and found that 11 had gross internal sphincter disruption and

3 had associated external sphincter damage. Both prospective[105–109] and retrospective[110–112] studies have documented the risk of incontinence after manual dilatation. Incontinence to flatus is of the order of 0% to 27%. Anal stretch, in its classical form, carries a higher risk of fissure persistence or recurrence and of impaired continence compared with internal sphincterotomy.[113] There is no role for its continued use in the modern management of anal fissure.

However, the concept of anal stretch has been revisited more recently using controlled balloon dilatation with a standardized protocol that overcomes the problem of reproducibility. Limited available data suggest results comparable to those for lateral internal sphincterotomy.[114] Further studies are required to evaluate this technique.

Lateral internal sphincterotomy Internal sphincterotomy was first described by Eisenhammer in 1951.[115] The original method of dividing internal anal sphincter muscle in the posterior midline fissure bed often led to a "keyhole" or "gutter" deformity with associated impaired continence. Lateral internal sphincterotomy (LIS) was then developed by Notaras.[116] The procedure remains the surgical treatment of choice for management of anal fissures refractory to nonsurgical therapy and may be offered without a trial of pharmacologic treatment.[116,117]

The procedure involves division of the internal anal sphincter laterally as an open procedure under direct vision or blindly through a stab incision.[118–120] The length of IAS divided varies, with some surgeons dividing muscle from the distal end of the fissure to the dentate line and others taking muscle equal in length to the fissure,[121] an approach that attempts to diminish the risk of impaired continence. The fissure itself does not require excision or fissurectomy as this encourages deformity. LIS may be done with the patient under local, regional, or general anesthesia, and can be combined with other procedures for concomitant anorectal pathology.[122]

LIS is effective in healing anal fissures with rates of 90% to 100% and low recurrence (1%–3%), but this comes with a price of risk of incontinence, the incidence of which has been variably reported from 0% to 50%.[123] However, incontinence sufficient to cause any measurable impairment in quality of life is uncommon, in the range of 3% to 5%,[124,125] but, unlike continence impairment on medical therapy, it may be permanent. Outcome data on these patients is surprisingly absent and no study has compared incontinence after LIS with other groups with continence impairment.

It is unclear why some series report such high incontinence rates after LIS. The procedure appears to be well controlled with careful division of muscle under vision but it seems that standardization and reproducibility are problems, just as they are with manual dilatation. Sultan and colleagues[126] evaluated the extent of sphincterotomy with the use of anal ultrasonography and showed a high incidence of inadvertent full-length division of the IAS, a problem that appears to be more common in women as a result of overestimation of the length of the shorter female IAS. Farouk and colleagues[127] investigated patients with persistent fissures after LIS by anal ultrasonography and revealed that over 70% had no internal sphincter defect, whereas several had incurred an external sphincter defect. It seems reasonable to conclude that the wide range of continence impairment after LIS may be a function of disparate surgical techniques among units and individual surgeons. Patient selection likely plays a role because others have documented on anorectal physiology and ultrasound unexpected obstetric injuries after LIS.[128]

Patients with preoperative incontinence problems should not undergo LIS and relative contraindications include those with irritable bowel syndrome or diabetes and elderly or postpartum women. Women with a prior obstetric injury and a nonhealing fissure present a difficult problem and it is inadvisable to proceed with LIS in such patients without satisfactory preoperative anal manometry and endoanal ultrasound.

There is no rationale for LIS in patients with a fissure and normal or subnormal IAS tone as hypertonicity is not an issue in this subgroup.[129] Patients with low-pressure fissures and those with significant birth injuries are probably better served with an anal advancement flap.[130,131]

Summary

The choice of treatment remains difficult. Surgery is very effective but high healing rates come with the risk of continence impairment. Publications on treatment and outcome for incontinence after sphincterotomy for fissure are absent and so the duration and magnitude of this problem are uncertain. Medical therapy with GTN is safe and represents a good first line of treatment. The 30% to 50% of patients with chronic fissures resistant to GTN can subsequently be offered second-line treatment with topical diltiazem or botulinum toxin injection and, in some cases, lateral internal sphincterotomy. Patients at high risk of continence disturbance should be identified and evaluated by anorectal manometry and ultrasound before surgery is offered. All patients considered for surgery should be fully cognizant of the potential risks and benefits before giving informed consent as some may wish to persist with an alternative medical therapy.

REFERENCES

1. Gazet JC, Redding W, Rickett JW. The prevalence of haemorrhoids. A preliminary survey. Proc R Soc Med 1970;63(Suppl):78–80.
2. Johanson JF, Sonnenberg A. The prevalence of hemorrhoids and chronic constipation. An epidemiologic study. Gastroenterology 1990;98:380–6.
3. Acheson AG, Scholefield JH. Management of haemorrhoids. BMJ 2008; 336(7640):380–3.
4. Deutsch AA, Moshkovitz M, Nudelman I, et al. Anal pressure measurements in the study of hemorrhoid etiology and their relation to treatment. Dis Colon Rectum 1987;30:855–7.
5. Gaj F, Trecca A. Hemorrhoids and rectal internal mucosal prolapse: one or two conditions? A national survey. Tech Coloproctol 2005;9:163–5.
6. Hulme-Moir M, Bartolo DC. Hemorrhoids. Gastroenterol Clin North Am 2001;30: 183–97.
7. Loder PB, Kamm MA, Nicholls RJ, et al. Haemorrhoids: pathology, pathophysiology and aetiology. Br J Surg 1994;81:946–54.
8. Johannsson HO, Graf W, Pahlman L. Bowel habits in hemorrhoid patients and normal subjects. Am J Gastroenterol 2005;100:401–6.
9. Brill AI, Fleshman JW, Ramshaw BJ, et al. Minimally invasive procedures: what family physicians need to know. J Fam Pract 2005;54(Suppl 1):S1–24.
10. Moesgaard F, Nielsen ML, Hansen JB, et al. High-fiber diet reduces bleeding and pain in patients with hemorrhoids: a double-blind trial of Vi-Siblin. Dis Colon Rectum 1982;25:454–6.
11. Alonso-Coello P, Zhou Q, Martinez-Zapata MJ, et al. Meta-analysis of flavonoids for the treatment of haemorrhoids. Br J Surg 2006;93:909–20.
12. Madoff RD, Fleshman JW. Clinical Practice Committee and American Gastroenterological Association, American Gastroenterological Association technical

review on the diagnosis and treatment of hemorrhoids. Gastroenterology 2004; 126:1463–73.
13. Mann CV, Motson R, Clifton M. The immediate response to injection therapy for first-degree haemorrhoids. J R Soc Med 1988;81:146–8.
14. Pilkington SA, Bateman AC, Wombwell S, et al. Anatomical basis for impotence following haemorrhoid sclerotherapy. Ann R Coll Surg Engl 2000;82:303–6.
15. Suppiah A, Perry EP. Jaundice as a presentation of phenol induced hepatotoxocity following injection sclerotherapy for haemorrhoids. Surgeon 2005;3:43–4.
16. Adami B, Eckardt VF, Suermann RB, et al. Bacteremia after proctoscopy and hemorrhoidal injection sclerotherapy. Dis Colon Rectum 1981;24:373–4.
17. MacRae HM, McLeod RS. Comparison of hemorrhoidal treatment modalities. A meta-analysis. Dis Colon Rectum 1995;38:687–94.
18. Johanson JF, Rimm A. Optimal nonsurgical treatment of hemorrhoids: a comparative analysis of infrared coagulation, rubber band ligation, and injection sclerotherapy. Am J Gastroenterol 1992;87:1600–6.
19. Senapati A, Nicholls RJ. A randomised trial to compare the results of injection sclerotherapy with a bulk laxative alone in the treatment of bleeding haemorrhoids. Int J Colorectal Dis 1988;3:124–6.
20. Law WL, Chu KW. Triple rubber band ligation for hemorrhoids: prospective, randomized trial of use of local anesthetic injection. Dis Colon Rectum 1999;42:363–6.
21. MacRae HM, McLeod RS. Comparison of hemorrhoidal treatments: a meta-analysis. Can J Surg 1997;40:14–7.
22. Scarpa FJ, Hillis W, Sabetta RJ. Pelvic cellulitis: a life-threatening complication of hemorrhoidal banding. Surgery 1988;103:383–5.
23. Clay LD 3rd, White JJ Jr, Davidson JT, et al. Early recognition and successful management of pelvic cellulitis following hemorrhoidal banding. Dis Colon Rectum 1986;29:579–81.
24. Bayer I, Myslovaty B, Picovsky BM. Rubber band ligation of hemorrhoids. Convenient and economic treatment. J Clin Gastroenterol 1996;23:50–2.
25. Jensen SL, Harling H, Tange G, et al. Maintenance bran therapy for prevention of symptoms after rubber band ligation of third-degree haemorrhoids. Acta Chir Scand 1988;154:395–8.
26. Nivatvongs S, Goldberg S. An improved technique of rubber band ligation of hemorrhoids. Am J Surg 1982;144(3):379–80.
27. Su C, Chiu C, Wu Y, et al. Endoscopic hemorrhoidal ligation of symptomatic internal hemorrhoids. Gastrointest Endosc 2001;58(6):871–4.
28. Wehrmann T, Riphaus A, Feinstein J, et al. Hemorrhoidal elastic band ligation with flexible videoendoscopes: a prospective, randomized comparison with the conventional technique that uses rigid proctoscopes. Gastrointest Endosc 2004;60(2):191–5.
29. Morinaga K, Hasuda K, Ikeda T. A novel therapy for internal hemorrhoids: ligation of the hemorrhoidal artery with a newly devised instrument (Moricorn) in conjunction with a Doppler flowmeter. Am J Gastroenterol 1995;90:610–3.
30. Sohn N, Aronoff JS, Cohen FS, et al. Transanal hemorrhoidal dearterialization is an alternative to operative hemorrhoidectomy. Am J Surg 2001;182:515–9.
31. Ramirez JM, Aguilella V, Elia M, et al. Doppler-guided hemorrhoidal artery ligation in the management of symptomatic hemorrhoids. Rev Esp Enferm Dig 2005; 97:97–103.
32. Felice G, Privitera A, Ellul E, et al. Doppler-guided hemorrhoidal artery ligation: an alternative to hemorrhoidectomy. Dis Colon Rectum 2005;48:2090–3.

33. Greenberg R, Karin E, Avital S, et al. First 100 cases with Doppler-guided hemorrhoidal artery ligation. Dis Colon Rectum 2006;49:485–9.
34. Bursics A, Morvay K, Kupcsulik P, et al. Comparison of early and 1 year follow-up results of conventional hemorrhoidectomy and hemorrhoid artery ligation: a randomized study. Int J Colorectal Dis 2004;19:176–80.
35. Dennison A, Whiston RJ, Rooney S, et al. A randomized comparison of infrared photocoagulation with bipolar diathermy for the outpatient treatment of hemorrhoids. Dis Colon Rectum 1990;33:32–4.
36. Smith LE, Goodreau JJ, Fouty WJ. Operative hemorrhoidectomy versus cryodestruction. Dis Colon Rectum 1979;22:10–6.
37. Ferguson JA, Heaton JR. Closed hemorrhoidectomy. Dis Colon Rectum 1959;2:176–9.
38. Ho YH, Seow-Choen F, Tan M, et al. Randomized controlled trial of open and closed haemorrhoidectomy. Br J Surg 1997;84:1729–30.
39. Carapeti EA, Kamm MA, McDonald PJ, et al. Randomized trial of open versus closed day-case haemorrhoidectomy. Br J Surg 1999;86:612–3.
40. Arbman G, Krook H, Haapaniemi S. Closed vs. open hemorroidectomy—Is there any difference? Dis Colon Rectum 2000;43:31–4.
41. Gecosmanoglu R, Sad O, Koc D, et al. Hemorrhoidectomy: open or closed technique? A prospective, randomized clinical trial. Dis Colon Rectum 2002;45:70–5.
42. Khan S, Pawlak SE, Eggenberger JC, et al. Surgical treatment of hemorrhoids: prospective, randomized trial comparing closed excisional hemorrhoidectomy and the Harmonic Scalpel technique of excisional hemorrhoidectomy. Dis Colon Rectum 2001;44:845–9.
43. Tan JJ, Seow-Choen F. Prospective, randomized trial comparing diathermy and Harmonic Scalpel hemorrhoidectomy: a prospective evaluation. Dis Colon Rectum 2001;44:677–9.
44. Armstrong DN, Ambroze WL, Schertzer ME, et al. Harmonic Scalpel vs. electrocautery hemorrhoidectomy: a prospective evaluation. Dis Colon Rectum 2001;44:558–64.
45. Chung CC, Ha JP, Tai YP, et al. Double-blind, randomized trial comparing Harmonic Scalpel hemorrhoidectomy, bipolar scissors hemorrhoidectomy, and scissors excision: ligation technique. Dis Colon Rectum 2002;45:789–94.
46. Ho YH, Tan M. Ambulatory anorectal manometric findings in patients before and after haemorrhoidectomy. Int J Colorectal Dis 1997;12:296–7.
47. Ho YH, Seow-Choen F, Goh HS. Haemorrhoidectomy and disordered rectal and anal physiology in patients with prolapsed hemorrhoids. Br J Surg 1995;82:596–8.
48. Felt-Bersma RJ, van Baren R, Koorevaar M, et al. Unsuspected sphincter defects shown by anal endosonography after anorectal surery. A prospective study. Dis Colon Rectum 1995;38:249–51.
49. Abbasakoor F, Nelson M, Beynon J, et al. Anal endosonography in patients with anorectal symptoms after haemorrhoidectomy. Br J Surg 1998;85:1522–4.
50. Mathai V, Ong BC, Ho YH. Randomized controlled trial of lateral internal sphincterotomy with haemorrhoidectomy. Br J Surg 1996;83(3):380–2.
51. Hussein MK, Taha AM, Haddad FF, et al. Bupivacaine local injection in anorectal surgery. Int Surg 1998;83(1):56–7.
52. Pryn SJ, Crosse MM, Murison MS, et al. Postoperative analgesia for haemorrhoidectomy. A comparison between caudal and local infiltration. Anaesthesia 1989;44(12):964–6.

53. Chester JF, Stanford BJ, Gazet JC. Analgesic benefit of locally injected bupivacaine after hemorrhoidectomy. Dis Colon Rectum 1990;33(6):487–9.
54. Wasvary HJ, Hain J, Mosed-Vogel M, et al. Randomized, prospective, double-blind, placebocontrolled trial of effect of nitroglycerin ointment on pain after hemorrhoidectomy. Dis Colon Rectum 2001;44(8):1069–73.
55. Khubchandani IT. Internal sphincterotomy with hemorrhoidectomy does not relieve pain: a prospective, randomized study. Dis Colon Rectum 2002;45:1452–7.
56. Carapeti EA, Kamm MA, McDonald PJ, et al. Doubleblind randomised controlled trial of effect of metronidazole on pain after day-case haemorrhoidectomy. Lancet 1998;351(9097):169–72.
57. Mehigan BJ, Monson JR, Hartley JE. Stapling procedure for haemorrhoids versus Milligan-Morgan haemorrhoidectomy: randomized controlled trial. Lancet 2000;355:782–5.
58. Nisar PJ, Acheson AG, Neal KR, et al. Stapled hemorrhoidopexy compared with conventional hemorrhoidectomy, a systematic review of randomized controlled trials. Dis Colon Rectum 2004;47:1837–45.
59. Guy RJ, Seow-Choen F. Septic complications after treatment of haemorrhoids. Br J Surg 2003;90:147–56.
60. Jayaraman S, Colquhoun PH, Malthaner RA. Stapled versus conventional surgery for hemorrhoids. Cochrane Database Syst Rev 2006;(4):CD005393.
61. Perrotti P, Antropoli C, Molino D, et al. Conservative treatment of acute thrombosed external hemorrhoids with topical nifedipine. Dis Colon Rectum 2001;44:405–9.
62. Greenspon J, Williams SB, Young HA, et al. Thrombosed external hemorrhoids: outcome after conservative or surgical management. Dis Colon Rectum 2004;47:1493–8.
63. Lindsey I, Jones OM, Cunningham C, et al. Chronic anal fissure. Br J Surg 2004;91(3):270–9.
64. Notaras MJ. Anal fissure and stenosis. Surg Clin North Am 1988;68:1427–40.
65. Lund JN, Scholefield JH. Aetiology and treatment of anal fissure. Br J Surg 1996;83:1335–44.
66. Nothmann BJ, Schuster MM. Internal anal sphincter derangement with anal fissures. Gastroenterology 1974;67:216–20.
67. Abcarian H, Lakshmanan S, Read DR, et al. The role of internal sphincter in chronic anal fissures. Dis Colon Rectum 1982;25:525–8.
68. Chowcat NL, Araujo JGC, Boulos PB. Internal sphincterotomy for chronic anal fissure: long-term effects on anal pressure. Br J Surg 1986;73:915–6.
69. Xynos E, Tzortzinis A, Chrysos E, et al. Anal manometry in patients with fissure-in-ano before and after internal sphincterotomy. Int J Colorectal Dis 1993;8:125–8.
70. Farouk R, Duthie GS, MacGregor AB, et al. Sustained internal sphincter hypertonia in patients with chronic anal fissure. Dis Colon Rectum 1994;37:424–9.
71. Hancock BD. The internal sphincter and anal fissure. Br J Surg 1977;64:92–5.
72. Lin JK. Anal manometric studies in hemorrhoids and anal fissures. Dis Colon Rectum 1989;32:839–42.
73. Gibbons CP, Read NW. Anal hypertonia in fissures: cause or effect? Br J Surg 1986;73:443–5.
74. Klosterhalfen B, Vogel P, Rixen H, et al. Topography of the inferior rectal artery: a possible cause of chronic, primary anal fissure. Dis Colon Rectum 1989;32:43–52.

75. Rattan S. The internal anal sphincter: regulation of smooth muscle tone and relaxation. Neurogastroenterol Motil 2005;17(Suppl 1):50–9.
76. Rattan S, Regan RF, Patel CA, et al. Nitric oxide not carbon monoxide mediates nonadrenergic noncholinergic relaxation in the murine internal anal sphincter. Gastroenterology 2005;129:1954–66.
77. Griffin N, Zimmerman DD, Briel JW, et al. Topical L-arginine gel lowers resting anal pressure: possible treatment for anal fissure. Dis Colon Rectum 2002;45: 1332–6.
78. Lund JN. Nitric oxide deficiency in the internal anal sphincter of patients with chronic anal fissure. Int J Colorectal Dis 2006;21:673–5.
79. Lund JN, Scholefield JH. Internal sphincter spasm in anal fissure. Br J Surg 1997;84:1723–4.
80. Lund JN, Scholefield JH. A randomised, prospective, double-blind, placebo-controlled trial of glyceryl trinitrate ointment in the treatment of anal fissure. Lancet 1997;349:11–4.
81. Carapeti EA, Kamm MA, McDonald PJ, et al. Randomised controlled trial shows that glyceryl trinitrate heals anal fissures, higher doses are not more effective, and there is a high recurrence rate. Gut 1999;44:727–30.
82. Bailey HR, Beck DE, Billingham RP, et al. A study to determine the nitroglycerin ointment dose and dosing interval that best promote the healing of chronic anal fissures. Dis Colon Rectum 2002;45:1192–9.
83. Scholefield JH, Bock JU, Marla B, et al. A dose finding study with 0.1%, 0.2%, and 0.4% glyceryl trinitrate ointment in patients with chronic anal fissures. Gut 2003;52:264–9.
84. Kennedy ML, Sowter S, Nguyen H, et al. Glyceryl trinitrate ointment for the treatment of chronic anal fissure: results of a placebo-controlled trial and long-term follow-up. Dis Colon Rectum 1999;42:1000–6.
85. Altomare DF, Rinaldi M, Milito G, et al. Glyceryl trinitrate for chronic anal fissure—healing or headache? Results of a multicenter, randomized, placebo-controlled, double-blind trial. Dis Colon Rectum 2000;43:174–9.
86. Nelson R. Nonsurgical therapy for anal fissure. Cochrane Database Syst Rev 2006;(4):CD003431.
87. Jonas M, Neal KR, Abercrombie JF, et al. A randomized trial of oral vs. topical diltiazem for chronic anal fissures. Dis Colon Rectum 2001;44:1074–8.
88. Kocher HM, Steward M, Leather AJ, et al. Randomized clinical trial assessing the side-effects of glyceryl trinitrate and diltiazem hydrochloride in the treatment of chronic anal fissure. Br J Surg 2002;89:413–7.
89. Perrotti P, Bove A, Antropoli C, et al. Topical nifedipine with lidocaine ointment vs. active control for treatment of chronic anal fissure: results of a prospective, randomized, double-blind study. Dis Colon Rectum 2002;45:1468–75.
90. Cook TA, Humphreys MM, Mortensen NJ. Oral nifedipine reduces resting anal pressure and heals chronic anal fissure. Br J Surg 1999;86:1269–73.
91. Nash GF, Kapoor K, Saed-Parsy K, et al. The long-term results of diltiazem treatment for anal fissure. Int J Clin Pract 2006;60:1411–3.
92. Maria G, Cassetta E, Gui D, et al. A comparison of botulinum toxin and saline for the treatment of chronic anal fissure. N Engl J Med 1998;338:217–20.
93. Minguez M, Melo F, Espi A, et al. Therapeutic effects of different doses of botulinum toxin in chronic anal fissure. Dis Colon Rectum 1999;42:1016–21.
94. Brisinda G, Maria G, Bentivoglio AR, et al. A comparison of injections of botulinum toxin and topical nitroglycerin ointment for the treatment of chronic anal fissure. N Engl J Med 1999;341:65–9.

95. Jost WH, Schimrigk K. Botulinum toxin in therapy of anal fissure. Lancet 1995; 345:188–9.
96. Minguez M, Herreros B, Espi A, et al. Long-term follow-up (42 months) of chronic anal fissure after healing with botulinum toxin. Gastroenterology 2002;123: 112–7.
97. Nelson R. Nonsurgical therapy for anal fissure. The Cochrane Library, issue 1. Chichester (UK): John Wiley and Sons; 2004.
98. Madalinski MH, Slawek J, Zbytek B, et al. Topical nitrates and the higher doses of botulinum toxin for chronic anal fissure. Hepatogastroenterology 2001;48: 977–9.
99. Lysy J, Israelit-Yatzkan Y, Sestiery-Ittah M, et al. Topical nitrates potentiate the effect of botulinum toxin in the treatment of patients with refractory anal fissure. Gut 2001;48:221–4.
100. Gosselink MP, Darby M, Zimmerman DD, et al. Treatment of chronic anal fissure by application of L-arginine gel: a phase II study in 15 patients. Dis Colon Rectum 2005;48:832–7.
101. Yamato S, Rattan S. Role of alpha adrenoceptors in opossum internal anal sphincter. J Clin Invest 1990;86:424–9.
102. De Godoy MA, Rattan S. Autocrine regulation of internal anal sphincter tone by renin-angiotensin system: comparison with phasic smooth muscle. Am J Physiol Gastrointest Liver Physiol 2005;289:G1164–75.
103. Cundall JD, Gardiner A, Laden G, et al. Use of hyperbaric oxygen to treat chronic anal fissure. Br J Surg 2003;90:452–3.
104. Speakman CT, Burnett SJ, Kamm MA, et al. Sphincter injury after anal dilatation demonstrated by endosonography. Br J Surg 1991;78:1429–30.
105. Nielsen MB, Rasmussen OØ, Pedersen JF, et al. Risk of sphincter damage and anal incontinence after anal dilatation for fissure-in-ano. An endosonographic study. Dis Colon Rectum 1993;36:677–80.
106. Saad AM, Omer A. Surgical treatment of chronic fissure-in-ano: a prospective randomised study. East Afr Med J 1992;69:613–5.
107. Olsen J, Mortensen PE, Krogh-Petersen I, et al. Anal sphincter function after treatment of fissure-in-ano by lateral subcutaneous sphincterotomy versus anal dilatation. A randomized study. Int J Colorectal Dis 1987;2:155–7.
108. Jensen SL, Lund F, Nielsen OV, et al. Lateral subcutaneous sphincterotomy versus anal dilatation in the treatment of fissure in ano in outpatients: a prospective randomised study. BMJ 1984;289:528–30.
109. Fischer M, Thermann M, Trobisch M, et al. Die behandlung der primar-chronischen analfissur durch dehnung des analkanales oder sphincterotomie. Langenbecks Arch Chir 1976;343:35–44.
110. Giebel GD, Horch R. Treatment of anal fissure: a comparison of three different forms of therapy. Nippon Geka Hokan 1989;58:126–33.
111. Collopy B, Ryan P. Comparison of lateral subcutaneous sphincterotomy with anal dilatation in the treatment of fissure in ano. Med J Aust 1979;2: 461–2.
112. Hawley P. The treatment of chronic fissure in ano. A trial of methods. Br J Surg 1969;56:915–8.
113. Nelson R. Operative procedures for fissure in ano. Cochrane Database Syst Rev 2005;(2):CD002199.
114. Renzi A, Brusciano L, Pescatori M, et al. Pneumatic balloon dilatation for chronic anal fissure: a prospective, clinical, endosonographic, and manometric study. Dis Colon Rectum 2005;48:121–6.

115. Eisenhammer S. The surgical correction of chronic internal anal (sphincteric) contracture. S Afr Med J 1951;25:486–9.
116. Notaras MJ. Lateral subcutaneous sphincterotomy for anal fissure—a new technique. Proc R Soc Med 1969;62:713–5.
117. Orsay C, Rakinic J, Perry B, et al. Practice parameters for the management of anal fissures. [revised]. Dis Colon Rectum 2004;47:2003–7.
118. Lewis TH, Corman ML, Prager ED, et al. Longterm results of open and closed sphincterotomy for anal fissure. Dis Colon Rectum 1988;31(5):368–71.
119. Kortbeek JB, Langevin JM, Khoo RE, et al. Chronic fissure-in-ano: a randomized study comparing open and subcutaneous lateral internal sphincterotomy. Dis Colon Rectum 1992;35:835–7.
120. Nelson RL. Meta-analysis of operative techniques for fissure-in-ano. Dis Colon Rectum 1999;42:1424–8.
121. Littlejohn DR, Newstead GL. Tailored lateral sphincterotomy for anal fissure. Dis Colon Rectum 1997;40(12):1439–42.
122. Abcarian H. Surgical correction of chronic anal fissure: results of lateral anal internal sphincterotomy vs. fissurectomy—mid-line sphincterotomy. Dis Colon Rectum 1980;23:31–6.
123. Dykes SL, Madoff RD, et al. The ASCRS textbook of colon and rectal surgery. In: Wolff BG, Fleshner JW, Beck DE, editors. New York: Spinger Science+Business Media; 2007. p. 178–91.
124. Hyman N. Incontinence after lateral internal sphincterotomy: a retrospective study and quality of life assessment. Dis Colon Rectum 2004;47:35–8.
125. Mentes BB, Tezcaner T, Yilmaz U, et al. Results of lateral internal sphincterotomy for chronic anal fissure with particular reference to quality of life. Dis Colon Rectum 2006;49:1045–51.
126. Sultan AH, Kamm MA, Nicholls RJ, et al. Prospective study of the extent of internal anal sphincter division during lateral sphincterotomy. Dis Colon Rectum 1994;37:1031–3.
127. Farouk R, Monson JRT, Duthie GS. Technical failure of lateral sphincterotomy for the treatment of chronic anal fissure: a study using anal ultrasonography. Br J Surg 1997;84:84–5.
128. Bove A, Balzano A, Perrotti P, et al. Different anal pressures profiles in patients with anal fissures. Tech Coloproctol 2004;8:151–6.
129. Leong AF, Seow-Choen F. Lateral sphincterotomy compared with anal advancement flap for chronic anal fissure. Dis Colon Rectum 1995;38:69–71.
130. Nyam DC, Wilson RG, Stewart KJ, et al. Island advancement flaps in the management of anal fissures. Br J Surg 1995;82:326–8.
131. Morin N. 2008 Core Subjects. Hemorrhoids & Fissure-in-Ano. Available at: www.fascrs.org/physicians/education/core_subjects.

responsible for postoperative incontinence,[22] but this was not confirmed in two other studies.[21,23]

Colonic transit time has been shown to be prolonged before surgery.[24] Furthermore, patients with rectal prolapse have an abnormal motility associated with reduced high-amplitude propagated contractions. Colonic transit time performed before and after a Ripstein rectopexy showed a delayed transit postoperatively.[25,26]

Treatment

Correction of rectal prolapse is surgical, but how this should be done is reflected in the following remark of Charles Wells in 1959: "I have traced in the literature between 30 and 50 operations for prolapse in the rectum and would like to add still one more".[27] The traditional treatment for complete rectal prolapse consists of either transabdominal or perineal approaches. The parameters used to assess the success of surgery are the improvement of incontinence and constipation, and a low recurrence rate. Until recently, abdominal rectopexy, with or without high anterior resection, has been advocated as the treatment of choice for complete rectal prolapse.[7,28,29] Because most patients are elderly and are not always fit to undergo an abdominal procedure, various perineal approaches, such as Delorme's procedure or perineal proctosigmoidectomy, have been recommended in the past. Two developments have changed this attitude in the last few years: the introduction of the laparoscopic approach;[30] and the need to consider, because of the frequent association of an enterocele or genital prolapse with the rectal prolapse,[31] some form of obliteration of the Douglas space or colpopexy along with the rectopexy.[32] In a recent meta-analysis that compared the open with the laparoscopic rectopexy both were equally efficacious with regards to the recurrence, morbidity, and length of stay.[33] The laparoscopic approach by minimizing the operative trauma has almost superceded the open approach and can be considered suitable for the elderly population. In many it can be combined with other procedures, such as colpopexy and eventually anterior resection. In this way, perineal operations are only indicated in high-risk groups of patients.

Surgical Technique

Abdominal rectopexy

All classical abdominal procedures, such as the Ripstein-Wells operation, imply different grades of rectal mobilization, with or without anterior resection of the rectum followed by fixation of the rectum to the promontory (rectopexy). Nowadays, laparoscopic approach is the choice for most surgeons for this abdominal fixation, even though it is unclear which procedure is ideal: the posterior rectopexy or the laparoscopic ventral recto(colpo)pexy.

Patients are prepared by giving mechanical bowel preparation and prophylactic antibiotics. The bladder should be emptied before the start of the operation by introducing a catheter.

Modified ripstein procedure by laparoscopic approach

The patient is placed in the supine position on a short "bean bag" with the legs held in leg rests, to facilitate the inspection and digital examination during surgery. The patient is placed in a steep Trendelenburg's position. A four-port technique, placed in the lower abdomen, is used. The 30-degree laparoscope is introduced under the umbilicus, a 12-mm port at the right lower quadrant, another 5-mm port right lateral of the umbilicus, and finally another 5-mm port in the left lower quadrant. If present, the uterus is fixed to the ventral abdominal wall using a temporary suture (**Fig. 2**A). The rectum is subsequently mobilized taking care to identify the left ureter and the

Rectal Prolapse, Rectal Intussusception, Rectocele, Solitary Rectal Ulcer Syndrome, and Enterocele

Richelle J.F. Felt-Bersma, MD, PhD[a,*], M. Tiersma E. Stella, MD, PhD[b], Miguel A. Cuesta, MD, PhD[c]

KEYWORDS

• Rectopexy • Rectocele • Intussusception • SRUS • Enterocele

Rectal prolapse, intussusception (occult rectal prolapse), solitary rectal ulcer syndrome (SRUS), and rectocele are common pelvic floor disorders that share many clinical features and have a common pathogenesis. Chronic constipation, especially an evacuation disorder, is often an underlying problem that leads to these abnormalities. For example, chronic straining may cause intussusception of the rectal mucosa, which subsequently can develop into a full-thickness rectal prolapse. A prolapse may cause excessive stretching of the rectal mucosa that can lead to mucosal injury and cause a rectal ulcer. Furthermore, chronic straining and difficulty with evacuation may induce a rectocele. Because these problems are interrelated, an integrated multidisciplinary approach is required for their management.

RECTAL PROLAPSE

Definition, Etiology, and Pathogenesis

A complete rectal prolapse is defined as the protrusion of all layers of the rectal wall through the anal canal. If the rectal wall prolapses but does not protrude through the anus it is called an "occult rectal prolapse" or a "rectal intussusception." A rectal prolapse should be distinguished from a mucosal prolapse; in the latter there is only

[a] Department of Gastroenterology, University Hospital "Vrije Universiteit," PO Box 7057, 1007 MB Amsterdam, The Netherlands
[b] Department of Gynaecology, University Hospital "Vrije Universiteit," PO Box 7057, 1007 MB Amsterdam, The Netherlands
[c] Department of Surgery, University Hospital "Vrije Universiteit," PO Box 7057, 1007 MB Amsterdam, The Netherlands
* Corresponding author.
E-mail address: rjf.felt@vumc.nl (R.J.F. Felt-Bersma).

Gastroenterol Clin N Am 37 (2008) 645–668
doi:10.1016/j.gtc.2008.06.001 gastro.theclinics.com

protrusion of the rectal or anal mucosa. The incidence of rectal prolapse is approximately 2.5 per 100,000 inhabitants,[1] with a highest incidence among elderly women. In adolescents, the gender ratio is equal.[2]

In the elderly patient with a rectal prolapse both a weak pelvic floor and a mobile rectum are present. Straining over many years (caused by longstanding constipation) is believed gradually to weaken the pelvic floor causing pudendal nerve damage, and this in turn may lead to weakness of the internal and external anal sphincters.[3] These pathophysiologic changes facilitate protrusion of the rectal wall through the anus. Furthermore, pudendal neuropathy caused by either aging or obstetric injury may play a role.[4]

There are two theories regarding the development of rectal prolapse. In 1912, Moschcovitz proposed that a deep pouch of Douglas may allow the small bowel to protrude into the lower anterior rectal wall.[5] This protrusion together with a mobile mesorectum and mesosigmoid may allow the development of a rectal prolapse. In 1968, Broden and Snellman[6] used cinematography and suggested that intussusception from the rectosigmoid region was the main cause.

Symptomatology

The most common complaint is a protrusion of the rectum through the anus, usually no greater than 15 cm (**Fig. 1**). The rectum is often edematous with a fragile mucosa and small ulcerations. It is always possible to push back the prolapse, unless there is strangulation. Passage of mucus and blood is common. Fecal incontinence is associated with rectal prolapse in 20% to 100% of patients, depending on the patient's age.[7] These patients have a very weak pelvic floor with low external anal sphincter pressures.[7–9] Constipation is common and is found in up to 70% of patients with rectal prolapse.[1,7] Pre-existing dysmotility, dyssynergic defecation, or intussusception are also possible predisposing factors.[10,11]

Diagnosis

The diagnosis is made by inspecting the perineum while asking the patient to strain as if to defecate. If the prolapse cannot be evoked on the examination table, the patient is asked to strain in the lavatory. The upright position and privacy are often helpful. Although additional tests are available, they play little role in the patient's management, but provide insights into the pathophysiology and are useful for research purposes.

Imaging Investigations

Defecography can demonstrate prolapse through the anus, but is not necessary for demonstrating a full-thickness rectal prolapse. The anorectal angle is often obtuse in patients with a rectal prolapse, especially in those with coexisting fecal incontinence.[12,13] In addition many other features seen with obstructed defecation, such as rectocele, sigmoidocele, or enterocele, may coexist.[10,11]

Anal endosonography may show asymmetry and thickening of the internal anal sphincter and submucosa. Demonstration of a sphincter defect can be useful if a sphincter reconstruction is being considered.

Anorectal Function Tests

Anal manometry shows low resting pressure and patients with coexisting fecal incontinence have low squeeze pressures.[8,14] After surgery, either there is no change[15] or improvement of the resting pressure and sometimes the sphincter length.[8,16,17] Squeeze pressure may also improve.[16,17] The rectoanal inhibitory reflex may also

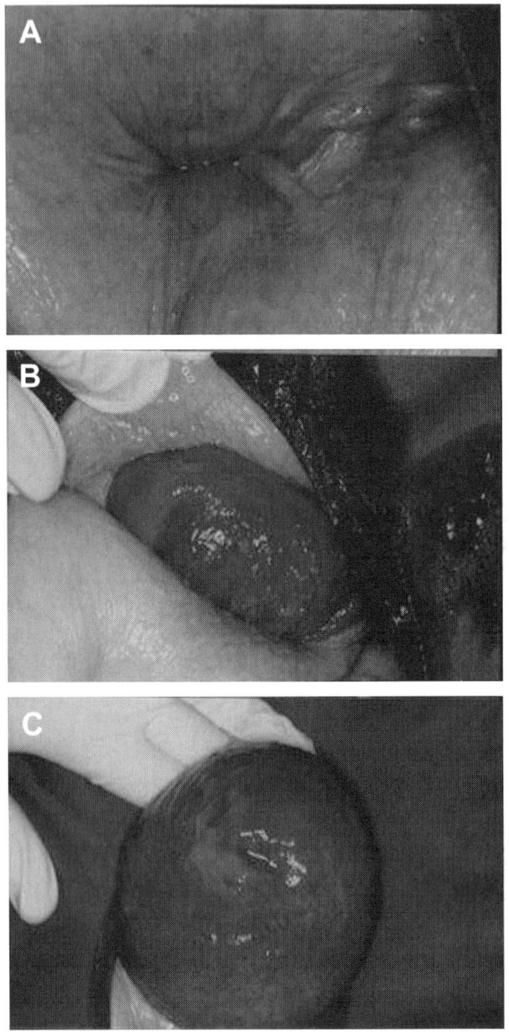

Fig. 1. Rectal prolapse. Before (*A*), during (*B*), and after (*C*) straining.

improve after rectopexy.[8,18] These changes may be caused by cessation of consta dilatation of the internal sphincter by the prolapsed rectum.

Rectal sensitivity and compliance measurements have demonstrated a nor maximal tolerable volume and pressure. After rectopexy, the rectal pressure at m imal tolerable volume increased significantly and the compliance decreased.[19] Bic chanics and visceroperception show diminished rectal sensitivity and complian Anal sensitivity is also diminished in patients with rectal prolapse and remains tered after surgery.[20]

Electromyography has provided insights into the pathogenesis of fecal inconti but has no place in clinical work-up and hardly any in research. Abnormalities found in patients with a rectal prolapse, but these results do not predict con after rectopexy.[21] Another study found that injury to the pudendal nerve

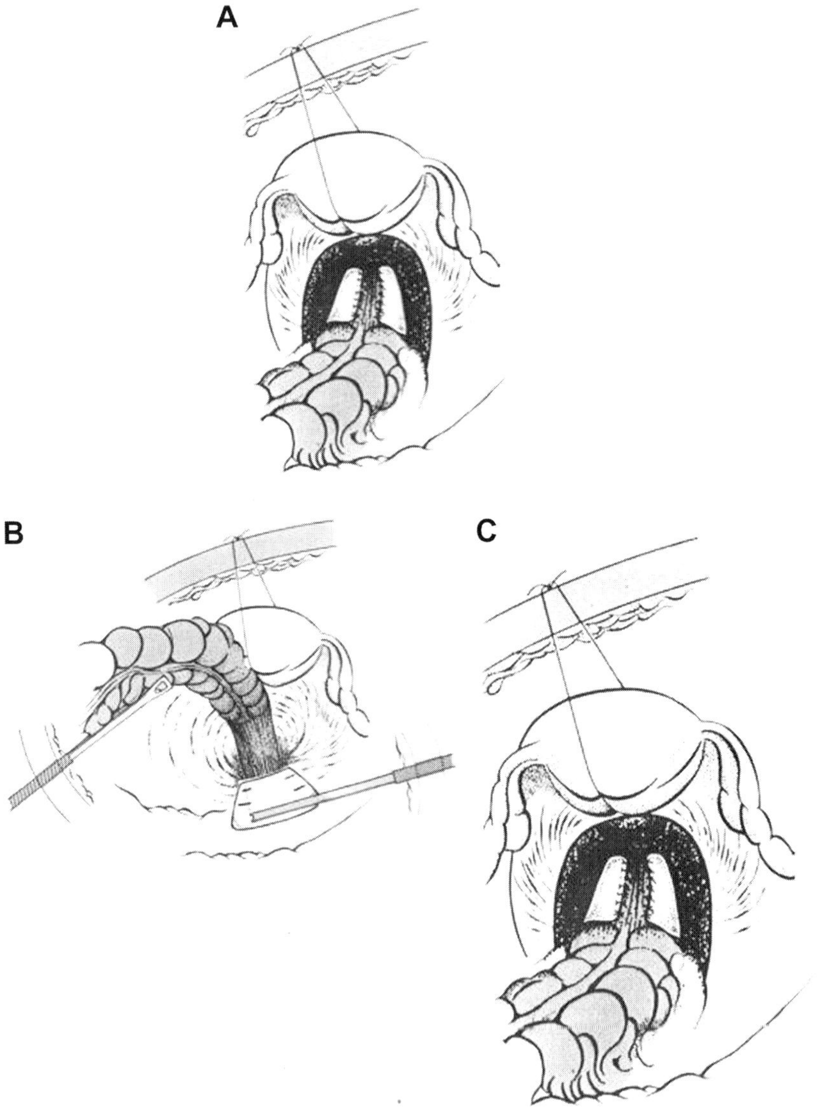

Fig. 2. Laparoscopic modified Ripstein procedure. (*A*) Anterior dissection of the rectum. (*B*) After posterior dissection of the rectum. Fixation of the mesh to the promontory. (*C*) Mesh is attached to the rectum leaving one third of the anterior wall free.

hypogastric nerves. Anteriorly, the rectum is mobilized up to the upper limit of the vagina; posteriorly, the presacral space is entered and dissected up to the level of the coccyx. The lateral ligaments and nervi erigentes are left intact (**Fig. 2**B).

The fixation can be achieved by sutures or by mesh and the fixation can be combined, if indicated, with a high anterior resection. If mesh is used, this is tightly rolled and introduced into the abdomen and attached at the promontory to the presacral fascia using an endoscopic hernia stapler device or nonreabsorbable sutures. Subsequently, the rectum is held without tension, (paying attention that the prolapse is completely reduced) and fixed to the mesh by means of nonabsorbable sutures to the anterolateral wall of the rectum on each side, so that one third of the anterior rectal circumference is left free (**Fig. 2**C).

Laparoscopic ventral(colpo)pexy for rectal prolapse and enterocele

D'Hoore and Penninckx[32] described the technique as follows.

Step 1: dissection After retraction of the rectosigmoid a left peritoneal incision is made over the sacral promontory and extended along the rectum up to the deepest point of Douglas and to the left. Lateral ligaments and right hypogastric nerve are left intact. Rectovaginal septum is broadly opened down to the pelvic floor after probing the vagina to facilitate this maneuver (**Fig. 3**A). Lateral and posterior dissection is avoided, leaving lateral ligaments intact. If the pouch of Douglas is redundant, as in enterocele, the peritoneum is resected. Care is taken to avoid perforation of the rectum during the dissection.

Step 2: mesh fixation A strip of Marlex trimmed to 3 × 17 cm is introduced in the abdomen. The mesh is sutured by means of nonabsorbable sutures to the ventral aspect and both sides of the lateral border of the distal rectum. The mesh is fixed to the sacral promontory using either sutures or an endofascia stapler (Endopath EMS, Johnson and Johnson; C.R. Bard, Inc., Billerica, Massachusetts) (**Fig. 3**B). The prolapse is reduced at the time of mesh fixation.

Step 3: vaginal fornix fixation Posterior vaginal fornix is elevated and sutured to the same strip of mesh. If no enterocele is present, two sutures on the lateral aspect are sufficient. In other cases more sutures are placed. In this way a vaginal vault prolapse (middle pelvic compartment) and the enterocele are corrected (**Fig. 3**C).

Step 4: Neo-Douglas formation Next, the lateral borders of the incised peritoneum are closed over the mesh using nonabsorbable sutures. This elevates the neo-Douglas over the colpopexy. The mesh should be covered with peritoneum to avoid fixation (or fistula formation) of the small bowel (**Fig. 3**D).

Perineal procedures

The two most commonly used perineal procedures are the perineal proctosigmoidectomy according to Altemeier[34] and the Delorme[35] procedure.

In the proctosigmoidectomy (Altmeier), the prolapsed rectum is held under gentle traction and is resected from below, taking care that at least 1 cm of rectum is left proximal to the dentate line to perform a coloanal anastomosis. The intervention procedure may be facilitated by the use of mechanical stapling devices.

In the Delorme procedure, the mucosa is removed from the prolapsed rectum after submucosal injection of epinephrine 1 per 200,000 to avoid unnecessary bleeding. The mucosal stripping is performed by using a circumferential incision, up to 1 cm proximal to the dentate line. After removal of the mucosa from the prolapsed rectum, multiple longitudinal sutures are placed over the exposed muscularis, shortening the rectum and producing an accordion-like effect like a thick muscular ring. Afterward, the remaining mucosal ends are anastomosed with interrupted stitches of absorbable material (**Fig. 4**).

Results

Elderly patients and a longer duration of follow-up are associated with less favorable outcome and a higher recurrence rate.[36] Recurrence rates for different rectopexy techniques are low (0%–8%),[37] although all of these procedures increase risk of

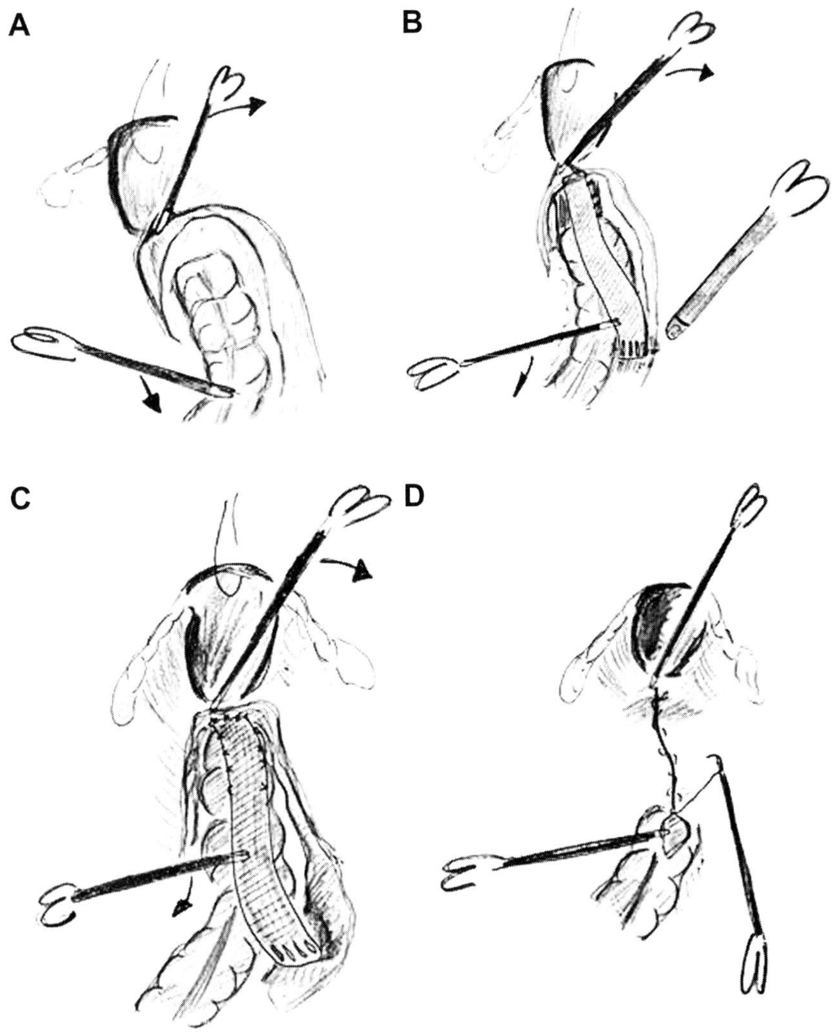

Fig. 3. Laparoscopic ventral (colpo)pexy for rectal prolapse and enterocele. (*A*) Rectovaginal septum is opened after probing the vagina. (*B*) Mesh is fixed on the sacral promontory. (*C*) Posterior vaginal fornix is elevated and sutured to the mesh. (*D*) Lateral borders of the peritoneum are closed.

constipation (up to 50%).[38] The combination of resection with any form of rectopexy decreases constipation in almost 75% of patients.[7,39] Perineal procedures have recurrence rates varying from 5% to 21% with no difference in incidence of constipation.[23,35]

Recently, laparoscopic rectopexy has been developed as an alternative to the previously mentioned approaches, and many surgeons regard this as the standard approach for patients with rectal prolapse. This method combines the good functional outcome of abdominal procedures with the low postoperative morbidity of the minimally invasive surgery.[8,30,32,40,41]

In 28 consecutive laparoscopic operations in the authors' center using a modified Ripstein procedure, only two partial recurrences were seen (7%). Continence

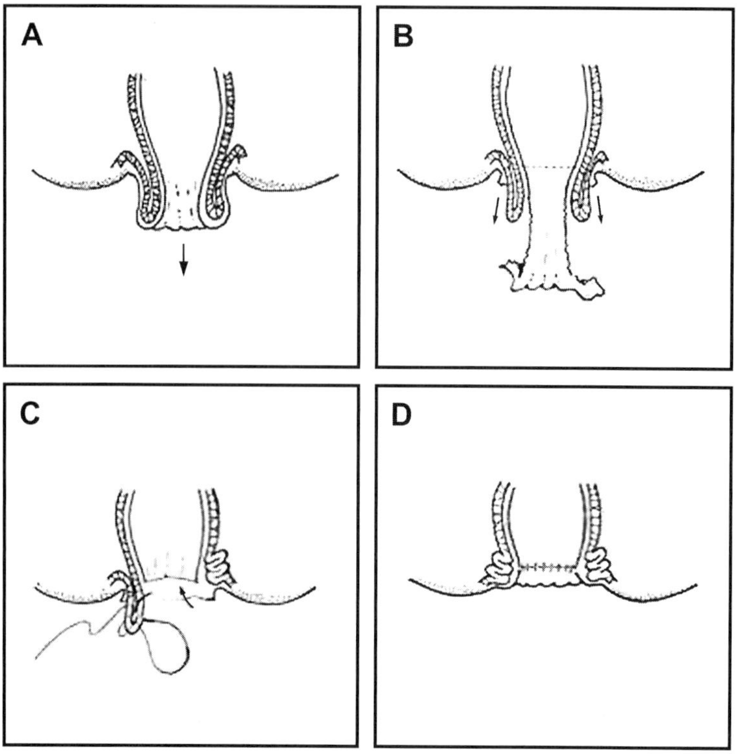

Fig. 4. Delorme's transanal resection. (*A*) Rectal prolapse. (*B*) Dissection of the prolapsed mucosa. (*C*) After extirpation of the prolapsed mucosa the muscular layer is plicated. (*D*) After plication of the muscular layer the anastomosis is made.

improved significantly in 76%; 14% developed mild constipation postoperatively and responded to a high-fiber diet and bulk agents.[8]

After an abdominal rectopexy,[7,36,37,39] most patients (50%–88%) show improvement in fecal incontinence, but after the perineal procedure incontinence rates are higher.[23,35] In the authors' series and others, the return of continence was associated with a small but significant increase in basal sphincter pressure, recovery of the rectoanal inhibitory reflex,[18,30] and normalization of the internal anal sphincter thickness.[30] This suggests that restoration of internal anal sphincter function plays an important role, and this improvement may be caused by cessation of rectoanal inhibition, previously induced by the prolapsed bowel,[18] or improved anal canal sensation.

A major drawback of abdominal rectopexy is constipation. Interestingly, both an improvement of constipation in 76% of patients[39] and an increase in up to 56% of patients has been reported.[36] Colonic denervation resulting in dysmotility and rectal denervation caused by dissection or division of the lateral ligaments and posterior dissection may in part be responsible.[28] Preservation of lateral ligaments was associated with improvement of continence and reduction of constipation.[6] This is reaffirmed by the finding that the rectal sensitivity, which has been proved to be impaired after lateral ligament division, was not changed significantly in patients after the operation.[8] The addition of anterior resection to rectopexy is a common surgical treatment for rectal prolapse in a patient with constipation, but this approach is controversial.[42–44]

Important development is the anterior fixation of the rectum in the ventral recto(colpo)-pexy.[26,32] Rectal prolapse is associated with an enterocele in 40% of patients,[31] but also with different grades of prolapse. Simultaneous obliteration of the deep Douglas space may help prevent symptoms of obstructed defecation. Furthermore, anterior position of the mesh allows colpopexy or vaginal vault fixation and provides permanent support for the neo-Douglas and middle pelvic compartment, and avoids any posterolateral dissection of the rectum and ligaments, improving continence and preventing constipation. The low morbidity (7%), reduced recurrence of 3% to 6%, improved continence in 90%, and resolution of constipation in 84% makes this the preferred operation for these patients.[26,32]

Predicting the outcome of surgery

The results of preoperative manometry do not predict the functional outcome regarding continence, although patients with very low sphincter pressures have a poor prognosis.[26,45] Also, electromyogram abnormalities[21] and prolonged pudendal nerve latency did not predict the risk of postoperative incontinence[21,23] except in one study.[22]

There is a weak correlation between postoperative increased transit time and postoperative emptying difficulties.[35] Division of the lateral ligaments may be related to postoperative constipation.[38]

Postoperative Biofeedback

Postoperative biofeedback can improve external anal sphincter function. In these groups, however, the most important predictor of fecal incontinence was a low internal anal sphincter pressure, an abnormality that cannot be corrected with biofeedback.[46]

Summary

Laparoscopic rectopexy, together with some form of fixation of the middle compartment, offers the best functional results in patients with rectal prolapse and vaginal vault prolapse.

RECTAL INTUSSUSCEPTION

Definition, Etiology, and Pathogenesis

Rectal intussusception, occult rectal prolapse, or internal procidentia is an intussusception of the rectal wall that does not protrude through the anus and can be classified into high-grade (intrarectal) and low-grade (intra-anal) intussusception based on the level of mucosa protruding.[47] Although it is associated with solitary rectal ulcer, rectal prolapse, or perineal descent, the finding per se is not pathologic. In 50% to 60% of healthy volunteers a rectal intussusception can be demonstrated.[23] The rectal intussusception in patients with evacuatory dysfunction is more advanced morpholically, however, than that seen in asymptomatic controls.[48] An intussusception seldom leads to total rectal prolapse.[49] Today, many regard this condition as a consequence of dyssynergic defecation rather than a cause of the problem.

Symptomatology

Patients with high intussusception report feelings of obstructed defecation and incomplete evacuation, although many are asymptomatic. Depending on concurrent problems, such as rectocele, SRUS, pudendal neuropathy, or sphincter damage, additional symptoms, such as soiling, blood loss, or fecal incontinence, may occur.[50] Studies have shown that the presence of an intussusception does not correlate with rectal emptying.[51] Care must be taken when associating symptoms with rectal intussusception.

Diagnosis

Defecography remains the standard for establishing this diagnosis (**Fig. 5**A, B).[11] Sometimes the diagnosis can be made by rectal examination, but in one study an intussusception was palpable in only one third of patients.[52] Even with defecography it can be difficult to distinguish rectal intussusception from normal rectal mucosal folds.[31] Newer techniques, such as dynamic three-dimensional CT[53] and (three-dimensional dynamic) anorectal ultrasonography,[54,55] can also be of value. Dynamic MRI can also demonstrate an enterocele, although the lying position and costs are limitations.[56]

Treatment

Conservative treatment aimed at restoring normal defecation is the first line of treatment. A fiber-enriched diet with additional fiber supplementation and sometimes laxatives may be useful. The next step is biofeedback to restore a normal defecation

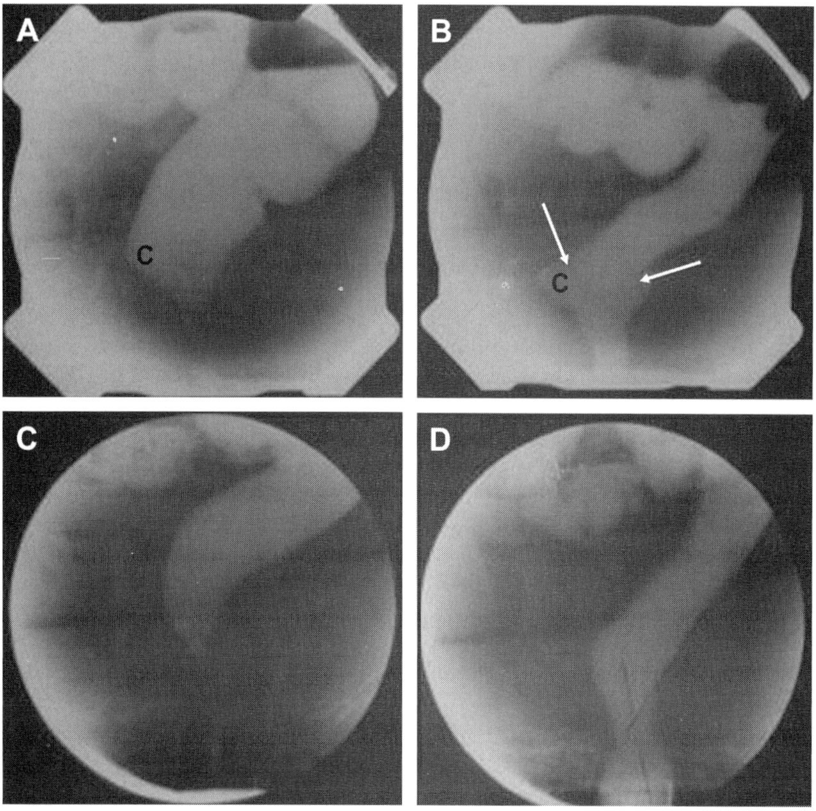

Fig. 5. Defecography in a 65-year-old woman with an intussusception. At rest (*A*) and during straining (*B*). Anteriorly, a rectocele (C) is visible. There is an indentation of the rectal wall both anterior and posterior forming an intussusception (*arrows*). After rectopexy in rest (*C*) and after rectopexy during straining (*D*). The contour of the rectum is sharp without indentation.

pattern; this has favorable results.[49,57] In a study of 34 patients, 52% had complete resolution or improvement of symptoms. Concomitant fecal incontinence also improved.[57] Long-term complaints of more than 9 years had a poor prognosis.

The role of surgical treatment for rectal intussusception is controversial. A Ripstein rectopexy has been performed and incontinence may improve[58] but constipation generally worsens.[59,60] Unlike patients with a rectal prolapse, there was no improvement in anal pressures.[38] Preoperative diarrhea, fecal incontinence, and descending perineum syndrome and proximal intussusception are associated with a poor prognosis.[61] Only a few patients with obstructive defecation improve, although the intussusception has disappeared (**Fig. 5**C, D), indicating that rectal invagination is a consequence of obstructed defecation.[15] Hence, surgery should be avoided. Some patients develop additional complaints of tenesmus and increased defecation frequency or increased straining. Delorme's transrectal excision is an alternative procedure[61,62] and (laparoscopic) resection rectopexy[63,64] is a new procedure that claims better results, but many failures occur. Hence, an intussusception should be considered an epiphenomena and treated conservatively. Surgery should be restricted to highly selected cases with a large intussusception; concomitant resection of part of the rectum (sigmoid) seems the best option.

SOLITARY RECTAL ULCER SYNDROME

Definition, Etiology, and Pathogenesis

SRUS was first described in 1830 by Cruveilhier, but was recognized as a clinical entity in 1969 by Madigan and Morson.[65] The estimated annual incidence is 1 to 3.6 per 100,000.[66] About 80% of patients are less than 50 years. Gender distribution is either equal or there is a slight female preponderance.[66] The mean age of presentation is 49 years, and about 25% present after 60 years.[67] The condition is associated with an evacuation disorder. Defecography has shown that an intussusception is often present and evacuation is delayed.[68,69] Ulceration is thought to occur during forceful straining against an immobile or a nonrelaxing pelvic floor (anismus).[68]

Symptomatology

The classical symptoms of SRUS are rectal bleeding, passage of mucus, rectal pain, excessive straining, and tenesmus. Constipation is present in about 55% of patients.[67] Many patients need digital assistance to defecate but do not admit this. Diarrhea is seen in 20% to 40% of patients.[67] About 25% of patients have no complaints. The median time between presentation and diagnosis varies between 3 months to 30 years. Retrospective analysis has demonstrated that 26% of patients with SRUS are misdiagnosed initially and treated for inflammatory bowel disease. Rarely, massive hemorrhage can occur. In some patients, an underlying psychologic disorder, such as obsessive-compulsive disorder, may be present.[67]

Diagnosis

Sigmoidoscopy with rectal biopsy is diagnostic. The macroscopic appearance of the typical SRUS ulcer is a small, shallow lesion with a white slough or a hyperemic mucosal wall, usually on the anterior wall of the rectum (**Fig. 6**A). Ulceration is present in about 57%. Polypoid lesions are found in about 25%.[66,67,69] Patches of hyperemic mucosa are found in 18%. Lesions are multiple in 30%.[65] SRUS is usually found on the anterior or anterolateral wall of the rectum, centered on a rectal fold. The distance from the anus is about 5 to 10 cm.

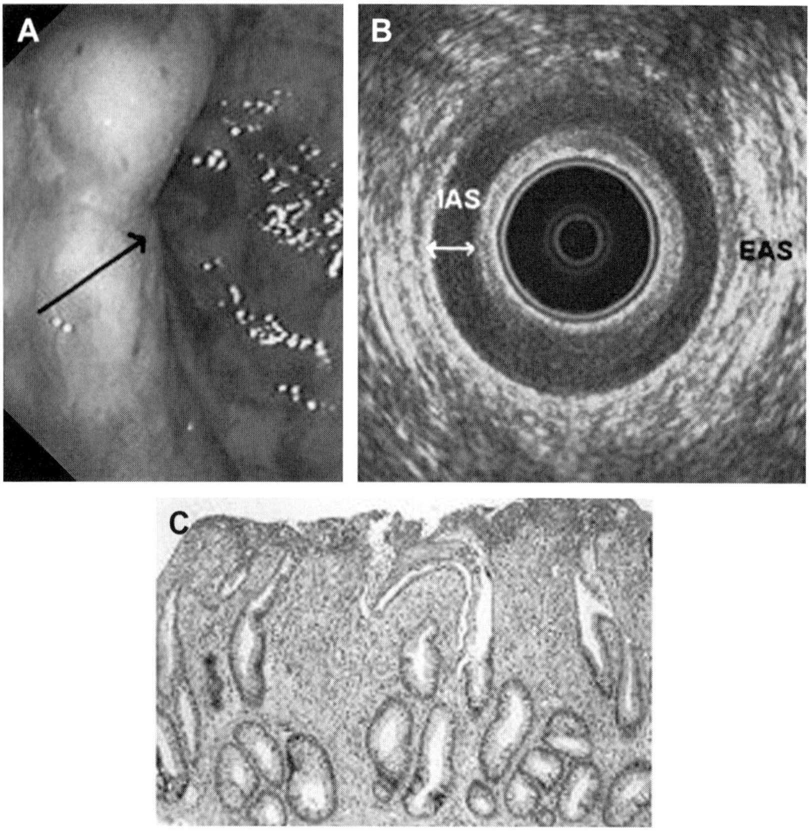

Fig. 6. Solitary rectal ulcer syndrome in a 40-year-old woman. (*A*) Endoscopy. The rectal wall is edematous. A small scar is visible (*arrow*). (*B*) Anal endosonography. The internal anal sphincter (IAS) is thickened 0.5 mm, normal 1.8 ± 0.8 mm. SM, submucosa; EAS, external anal sphincter. (*C*) Histology (hematoxiline-eosine, magnification 400×). Rectal mucosa in solitary ulcer syndrome. The lamina propria shows fibromuscular proliferation. A moderate chronic inflammatory infiltrate is present. The surface is eroded and covered with fibrin and debris. Re-epithelialization is apparent. The crypts are distorted and elongated and the epithelium of the crypts shows depletion of goblet cells. (*Courtesy of* E. Bloemena, MD, PhD, Amsterdam, The Netherlands.)

The histologic appearance of SRUS has been well established (**Fig. 6**C).[65,70] The mucosa is elongated with distorted glands, especially at the base. When the glands are displaced to the submucosa, superficial bleeding can occur. The lamina propria is edematous and contains proliferation of fibroblasts. It is also thickened, particularly the inner circular muscular layer, with less prominent thickening (edema) of the submucosa. Sometimes there are unique features, such as decussation of the two muscular layers, nodular induration of inner layer, and grouping of outer longitudinal layer into bundles.[70]

Histologic proof is necessary to differentiate SRUS from ulcers caused by nonsteroidal anti-inflammatory drugs, malignant conditions, or possibly from malignant transformation.[71] Also, rectal endometriosis should be considered in the differential diagnosis.[72]

Radiologic Investigations

Defecography can provide insights regarding its pathophysiology, but has a limited role in establishing diagnosis. Abnormalities are found in about 75% of patients with SRUS, intussusception being most frequently seen in about 45% to 80%. Prolonged preoperative evacuation time may predict poor outcome after rectopexy.[69,73]

Barium enema may reveal nodularity of the rectal mucosa, thickening of the rectal folds, stricture formation, polypoid lesions, or ulceration. It is an unreliable method of diagnosis because it cannot differentiate SRUS from more sinister conditions.[69]

Ultrasonography can show marked thickening of the internal anal sphincter, submucosa, and external anal sphincter. The rectal wall and the muscularis propria may also be thickened.[74]

Anorectal Function Tests

Anorectal function tests do not help in establishing the diagnosis or predicting therapeutic response. Either no differences in anal pressure or lower pressures have been found.[67,75] The rectum is hypersensitive, the maximum tolerable rectal volume is reduced [44] and a high incidence of dyssynergic defecation can be found,[68,75] and balloon expulsion time may be prolonged.

Treatment and Prognosis

Therapy should be aimed at restoring a normal pattern of defecation. The patient should be instructed to avoid excessive straining and to regulate their defecation habits, in collaboration with a therapist for pelvic floor exercises or behavioral retraining. The diet should contain enough fiber and sufficient fluid intake. Modest use of laxatives should be considered. Psychologic factors should be addressed whenever appropriate. If these measures do not resolve the problem, surgery may be considered.

Conservative treatment

Diet and fiber A high-fiber diet can help but by itself is insufficient to obtain healing. Response rates vary between 19% and 70%.[67] Avoiding excessive straining can improve symptoms in about 67%[76] of patients and sigmoidoscopic improvement of the ulcer may occur in about 30%.

Local treatment Topical steroids and sulphasalazine enemas are not effective.[77] Sucralfate enemas have shown some improvement in six patients.[78] Local application of human fibrin sealant has been tried with some improvement in six patients.[79]

Physiotherapy and biofeedback training This is the most useful approach. Three studies have described favorable results of biofeedback. In one study, biofeedback therapy before and after surgery showed a lower recurrence rate.[76] No prognostic factors were identified.[80] Recently, two studies have emerged demonstrating the effect of biofeedback as first-line treatment in patients with SRUS.

In one study, 16 patients with SRUS and 26 healthy controls were studied. Laser Doppler mucosal flowmetry was performed before and after biofeedback treatment. Twelve (75%) of 16 patients reported symptomatic improvement after treatment. Five (31%) of the 16 patients had sigmoidoscopic ulcer resolution. Biofeedback resulted in a significant improvement in rectal mucosal blood flow in subjects who felt subjectively better after biofeedback.[81] Another study of 11 patients with refractory SRUS underwent biofeedback treatment. Nine (82%) patients exhibited dyssynergia. After biofeedback, straining effort and stool frequency decreased. All five patients discontinued digital maneuvers and bleeding stopped in 56%. There was complete healing in four (36%) patients; more than 50% healing in two (18%) patients; and less than 50% healing in four (36%) patients.[82]

Surgery

The strong association between chronic straining and SRUS suggests that surgery should be reserved for selected cases, especially because surgery can induce constipation, which is an underlying mechanism for the problem. Generally, a rectopexy is performed, although anterior resection with rectopexy and Delorme's procedure has also been used. Some short-term favorable results have been reported.[83,84] Surgical procedures are disappointing, with persistence of symptoms, postoperative bleeding, and sexual dysfunction.[83,84]

RECTOCELE

Definition, Etiology, and Pathogenesis

A rectocele is a protrusion of the anterior rectal wall usually toward the vagina. Weakness of the pelvic floor leads to a deficiency in the rectovaginal septum (the fascia of Denonvilliers, which is continuous with the perineal body) (**Fig. 7**). Deficiency in the upper half of the septum produces a high rectocele, and that of the lower half a low rectocele. A rectocele can be classified as low, midvaginal, or high according to the new standardized terminology.[85]

Obstetric injury is the major cause of rectocele. Most patients are multiparous but the condition also occurs in nullipara.[86] During childbirth direct damage to the rectovaginal septum, pelvic floor musculature, and pudendal nerve may lower the pelvic floor and enlarge the vaginal outlet (ie, it assumes a more vertical position, and lacks support from below). In this position, the vaginal opening is unable to close during straining, creating a pressure gradient between the rectum, which is subjected to high pelvic pressure and the vagina, which is at atmospheric pressure. Loose ligamentous structures attached to the uterus and upper vagina complete the scenario for a rectocele. Postmenopausal status is a predisposing factor, especially in nulliparous women. Hysterectomy is also associated with a rectocele. There is also an association

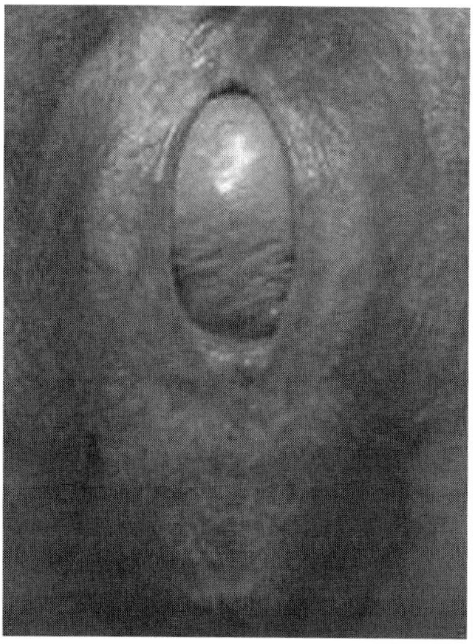

Fig. 7. Physical examination of a rectocele during straining.

between anismus and rectocele. A rectocele can be a cause or a consequence of chronic constipation and is often seen with dyssynergic defecation and intussusception.[87]

Symptomatology

Most symptoms are associated with pelvic floor weakness and rectocele. Few, however, are specific. Pelvic pain, feeling of prolapse, dragging, constant pressure, and backache can occur. Constipation and especially difficulty with evacuation of feces is often reported. Digitally supporting the posterior vaginal wall may promote defecation. Sometimes patients assist defecation anally. Fecal soiling and urologic complaints and dyspareunia may occur. Many women with uterovaginal prolapse, however, frequently have symptoms related to bowel function, but this is not associated with the severity of prolapse.[88]

Diagnosis

The diagnosis is made on inspection and digital examination. The patient is asked to strain in the left lateral or in dorsal lithotomy position. Bulging of the posterior vaginal wall may become obvious. Additional rectal palpation may help with the diagnosis. The vagina may be best examined with a single blade of a speculum with separate blades placed to push the posterior compartment away from the anterior compartment and then vice versa. Physical examination detects most rectoceles and cystoceles. In contrast, enteroceles and sigmoidoceles are difficult to palpate.[89] An enterocele can be confirmed versus a high rectocele with the patient straining, with the index finger in the rectum and the thumb (or index finger of the other hand) in the vagina.[90]

Pelvic Organ Prolapse Quantification

Traditionally, pelvic organ prolapse is graded with the Baden and Walker grading system.[91] Since 1996, a more detailed pelvic organ prolapse quantification system devised by the International Continence Society is being used.[85] Pelvic organ prolapse quantification uses six measurements to describe the distance from the cervix (or vaginal vault after hysterectomy) and defined points of the anterior and posterior vaginal walls to the hymen during maximum straining. Measurements of the height of the perineal body, the vaginal orifice, and the total vaginal length are also included in the pelvic organ prolapse quantification. These measurements result in four stages of genital prolapse and can be used to draw a schematic picture of the genital prolapse.

Radiologic Investigation

Defecography can demonstrate the presence and size of a rectocele (**Fig. 6**B) and other rectal wall aberrations and an enterocele. Also it can assess the magnitude of the rectocele and identify concomitant retention. Its use in clinical work-up is, however, limited.[92]

The amount of barium trapped in the rectocele, the evacuation time, and the effect of digital evacuation can be investigated. The finding of a rectocele is not necessarily abnormal, because small rectoceles are found in 80% of asymptomatic controls.[23] Rectoceles are associated with poor rectal emptying, especially those over 2 cm,[93] but with poor correlation with symptoms.[94] Surgical reduction of the rectocele size improves rectal emptying but not necessarily symptoms.[95] This underlines the importance of caution in interpreting radiologic findings. Only rectoceles greater than 3 cm or with significant contrast retention may clinically be relevant. Vaginal opacification during defecography can demonstrate displacement of the vagina; cephalad displacement is suggestive of an enterocele or a rectocele.[96] Defecography cannot predict the outcome of rectocele repair.[92] MRI can also provide good visualization of a rectocele and pelvic floor movements.[97]

Anorectal Function Tests

There are no physiologic findings that are specific for a rectocele. Basal and squeeze pressures, rectoanal inhibitory reflex, rectal sensation, and rectal compliance are significantly unchanged, although pelvic floor descent is increased and rectal sensitivity decreased. Anal manometry can show dyssynergia in some patients.[98,99] Surgery does not affect anal or rectal sensation.[98]

Treatment

Conservative treatment

The underlying defecation disorder should be treated first. A fiber-enriched diet, bulk-forming agents, and laxatives should be tried. If dyssynergic defecation is present, biofeedback should be tried first before considering surgical repair.[99]

Surgery

When there is a large rectocele with complaints of a bulge into the vagina or a feeling of prolapse, surgery should be considered. The success rate of surgery is approximately 75%.[100] According to a recent Cochrane review, vaginal approach is associated with a lower rate of recurrent rectocele or enterocele than transanal approach.[101] Complications, such as constipation and sexual dysfunction, however, are common[100] and care must be taken when advising surgery.

Posterior colporrhaphy This is the most commonly performed surgical procedure. The patient is positioned in dorsal lithotomy position. A longitudinal incision is made in the midline of the posterior vagina wall up to a point above the rectocele, and as far as the fornix when a high rectocele or enterocele are present. Next, the epithelium is mobilized laterally from the underlying fascia and anterior rectal wall by a combination of blunt and sharp dissection, with countertraction on the rectum. Repair includes correction of the rectal defect with one or more layers of fine separate or running sutures from proximal to distal. Next, the posterior vaginal wall is sutured, once the excess lateral edges of the vaginal epithelium have been trimmed to preserve a proper vaginal caliber. In addition, correction of the perineum may be performed (perineorrhaphy).[102]

In sexually active patients the perineal correction should be limited and performed with special care to prevent dyspareunia. Sutures running through the puborectalis portions of the levator ani to support the perineum should be omitted and be replaced by sutures running through only the bulbocavernosus.

Vaginal protrusion surgery may benefit from the use of vaginal meshes, because they may reduce the risk of recurrent protrusion. Meshes have been associated with erosion, shrinkage, and dyspareunia. Recent studies applying newly developed meshes (eg, polypropylene, monofilamentous, pore size >75 μm) report reduced risks of these complications compared with earlier studies with previously developed meshes.[103] Various meshes and push-through techniques to position the meshes to both the anterior and the posterior vaginal wall (if required) have recently been developed. The basic steps are as follows. The vaginal epithelium is resected together with the rectovaginal fascia. Needle-like guides with cannula's are placed through the obturatum membranes and the sacrospinous ligaments from the outside in, on both sides. The guides are removed and retrieval devices are passed through the cannulas on both sides. The meshes are positioned against the anterior rectal wall and the straps of the meshes are pulled back with the retrieval devices until the wings of the meshes exit the skin. The meshes are tension-free fixated by sutures. The parts of the straps exiting the skin are cut and sutures close the vaginal epithelium.[103] Although, new meshes are promising, long-term results are awaited. To date, the application of these meshes is mainly reserved for recurrent prolapses in elderly women.[104]

Transrectal approach The transanal approach is ideal for a rectocele associated with dyssynergic defecation. After placing the patient in a jackknife position and gently introducing the anal retractor, the submucosal plane is infiltrated with a solution of epinephrine 1 per 200,000. The anterior mucosa above the dentate line is incised in a transversal direction, and in orad direction a rectangular portion of at least 5 cm is excised depending on the size of the rectocele. The muscular defect in the anterior wall is plicated longitudinally or transversely with absorbable sutures. The mucosa is then closed with a continuous absorbable suture.

It is possible to combine the transvaginal and rectal technique.[92] The disadvantage is the formation of a thick fibrotic septum that often causes dyspareunia. A non-randomized study[105] compared the transvaginal with the transanal techniques and good results were obtained with both in 46% of patients.

Other techniques Other techniques, such as site-specific vaginal rectocele repair [69] or abdominal[106] or laparoscopic rectovaginopexy,[33,107] are described with results comparable with the conventional posterior colporrhaphy.

Prognosis

Although surgery corrects the anatomic defect and symptoms, many side effects may occur. In one study, posterior colporrhaphy corrected the vaginal defect in 76% of women and diminished prolapse-related symptoms in 50%. However, there was a higher incidence of constipation, incomplete bowel emptying, fecal incontinence and sexual dysfunction[107,108]. The correlation between symptoms and anatomic defects is weak, especially below stage 2 pelvic organ prolapse quantification (hymen $\pm$ 1 cm). Bulging is the principle symptom that correlates with prolapse severity.[108] Transanal approach to rectocele repair may compromise anal sphincter pressures.[109] It is important to determine the prognostic factors. Digital or perineal assistance with defecation is either associated with a favorable outcome[95,110] or makes little difference, whereas hysterectomy, a large rectocele, use of enemas, and laxatives are associated with a poor result.[95] Slow transit constipation is also associated with a poor outcome.[111] The effect of dyssynergia on surgical outcome is unclear, with better [112] or similar [92] outcome than those without.

ENTEROCELE

Definition, Cause, Pathogenesis

Enterocele is defined as a peritoneum-lined sac herniating down between the vagina and rectum filled with abdominal content, often the small bowel.[113] It was first reported in 1932 and considered a rare clinical entity, until in 1973 after a larger series was presented[114] the phenomena became more known in the gynecologic literature. With the increasing interest in dyssynergic defecation gastroenterologists and colorectal surgeons have focused more on pelvic floor abnormalities.[115] The frequency is unknown. Women are more affected and there is a high correlation between pelvic surgery (hysterectomy) and enterocele formation. In a series of 912 defecographies, 104 (11%)

enteroceles were seen and 92% were women. In 76% of patients concomitant findings, such as rectocele, perineal descent, and rectal intussusception, were seen.[115]

Symptoms

Characteristic symptoms are pelvic pain or heaviness especially when standing, difficulty with evacuation, and feeling of incomplete emptying can be present.[115] The pain and heaviness may disappear when lying down, because of repositioning of the bowel.

Diagnosis

Enterocele may be diagnosed with physical examination, but it is best made during defecography (**Fig. 8**).[11,116] It is important to opacify the small bowel with contrast. Typically, oral contrast is given 1 hour before the test. Newer techniques, such as dynamic three-dimensional CT [53] and (three-dimensional dynamic) anorectal ultrasonography[54,55] and dynamic MRI,[56] may prove useful. Frequently, an enterocele is found during posterior colporrhaphy.

Treatment

Because an enterocele lacks specific symptoms, conservative treatment by regulating defecation and biofeedback should be tried first. Patients with persistent pelvic pain and constant urge to defecate may require surgical repair. In a study of 25 isolated enteroceles,[115] five underwent surgery and only one had complete relief of symptoms; the other four had improvement in straining sensation but defecatory difficulties persisted.

The choice of surgical procedure is unclear.[115] Various procedures have been reported to obliterate the deep Douglas' pouch. The abdominal procedures include approximation of the uterosacral ligaments, transverse obliteration of the enterocele sac, or circumferential obliteration of the pelvic inlet with Mersilene mesh. The transvaginal approach includes repair of vaginal enterocele. Recently, laparoscopic treatment has been introduced.[117]

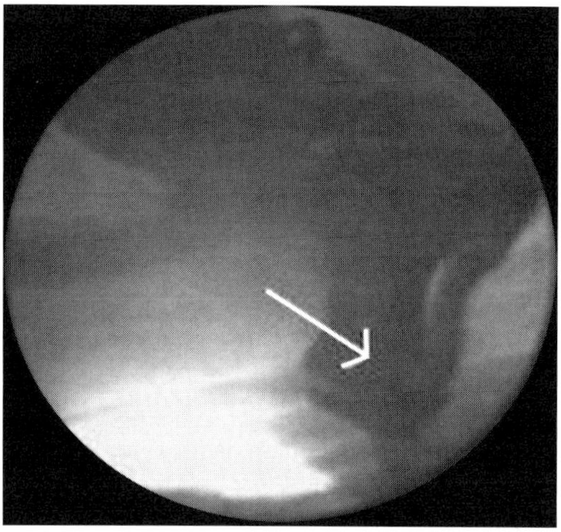

Fig. 8. Enterocele (*arrow*) reducing the rectum to a concave structure.

REFERENCES

1. Kairaluoma MV, Kellokumpu IH. Epidemiologic aspects of complete rectal prolapse. Scand J Surg 2005;94:207–10.
2. Nicholls J. Rectal prolase and the solitary ulcer syndrome. Petersfield (UK): Wrightson Biomedical Publishing Ltd; 1994. p. 289.
3. Neill ME, Parks AG, Swash M. Physiological studies of the anal sphincter musculature in faecal incontinence and rectal prolapse. Br J Surg 1981;68:531–6.
4. Snooks SJ, Swash M, Henry MM, et al. Risk factors in childbirth causing damage to the pelvic floor innervation. Int J Colorectal Dis 1986;1:20–4.
5. Moschvowitz AV. The pathogenesis, anatomy and cure of prolapseof the rectum. Surg Gynecol Obstet 1912;15:7.
6. Broden B, Snellman B. Procidentia of the rectum studied with cineradiography: a contribution to the discussion of causative mechanism. Dis Colon Rectum 1968;11:330–47.
7. Madoff RD, Mellgren A. One hundred years of rectal prolapse surgery. Dis Colon Rectum 1999;42:441–50.
8. Poen AC, de BM, Felt-Bersma RJ, et al. Laparoscopic rectopexy for complete rectal prolapse: clinical outcome and anorectal function tests. Surg Endosc 1996;10:904–8.
9. Felt-Bersma RJ, Janssen JJ, Klinkenberg-Knol EC, et al. Soiling: anorectal function and results of treatment. Int J Colorectal Dis 1989;4:37–40.
10. Pescatori M, Spyrou M, Pulvirenti dUA. A prospective evaluation of occult disorders in obstructed defecation using the iceberg diagram. Colorectal Dis 2006;8: 785–9.
11. Renzi A, Izzo D, Di SG, et al. Cinedefecographic findings in patients with obstructed defecation syndrome: a study in 420 cases. Minerva Chir 2006;61: 493–9.
12. Felt-Bersma RJ, Luth WJ, Janssen JJ, et al. Defecography in patients with anorectal disorders. Which findings are clinically relevant? Dis Colon Rectum 1990; 33:277–84.
13. Agachan F, Pfeifer J, Wexner SD. Defecography and proctography: results of 744 patients. Dis Colon Rectum 1996;39:899–905.
14. Dvorkin LS, Chan CL, Knowles CH, et al. Anal sphincter morphology in patients with full-thickness rectal prolapse. Dis Colon Rectum 2004;47:198–203.
15. Boccasanta P, Rosati R, Venturi M, et al. Comparison of laparoscopic rectopexy with open technique in the treatment of complete rectal prolapse: clinical and functional results. Surg Laparosc Endosc 1998;8:460–5.
16. Zittel TT, Manncke K, Haug S, et al. Functional results after laparoscopic rectopexy for rectal prolapse. J Gambl Stud 2000;4:632–41.
17. Kohler A, Athanasiadis S. The value of posterior levator repair in the treatment of anorectal incontinence due to rectal prolapse: a clinical and manometric study. Langenbecks Arch Surg 2001;386:188–92.
18. Farouk R, Duthie GS, MacGregor AB, et al. Rectoanal inhibition and incontinence in patients with rectal prolapse. Br J Surg 1994;81:743–6.
19. Felt-Bersma RJ, Sloots CE, Poen AC, et al. Rectal compliance as a routine measurement: extreme volumes have direct clinical impact and normal volumes exclude rectum as a problem. Dis Colon Rectum 2000;43:1732–8.
20. Felt-Bersma RJ, Poen AC, Cuesta MA, et al. Anal sensitivity test: what does it measure and do we need it? Cause or derivative of anorectal complaints. Dis Colon Rectum 1997;40:811–6.

21. Schultz I, Mellgren A, Nilsson BY, et al. Preoperative electrophysiologic assessment cannot predict continence after rectopexy. Dis Colon Rectum 1998;41: 1392–8.
22. Birnbaum EH, Stamm L, Rafferty JF, et al. Pudendal nerve terminal motor latency influences surgical outcome in treatment of rectal prolapse. Dis Colon Rectum 1996;39:1215–21.
23. Shorvon PJ, McHugh S, Diamant NE, et al. Defecography in normal volunteers: results and implications. Gut 1989;30:1737–49.
24. Brown AJ, Horgan AF, Anderson JH, et al. Colonic motility is abnormal before surgery for rectal prolapse. Br J Surg 1999;86:263–6.
25. Mollen RM, Kuijpers JH, van HF. Effects of rectal mobilization and lateral ligaments division on colonic and anorectal function. Dis Colon Rectum 2000;43: 1283–7.
26. Schultz I, Mellgren A, Oberg M, et al. Whole gut transit is prolonged after Ripstein rectopexy. Eur J Surg 1999;165:242–7.
27. Wells C. New operation for rectal prolapse. Proc R Soc Med 1959;52:602–3.
28. Ripstein CB. Surgical treatment of rectal prolapse. Pac Med Surg 1967;75: 329–32.
29. Duthie GS, Bartolo DC. Abdominal rectopexy for rectal prolapse: a comparison of techniques. Br J Surg 1992;79:107–13.
30. Cuesta MA, Borgstein PJ, de JD, et al. Laparoscopic rectopexy. Surg Laparosc Endosc 1993;3:456–8.
31. Mellgren A, Bremmer S, Johansson C, et al. Results of investigations in 2,816 patients. Dis Colon Rectum 1994;37:1133–41.
32. D'Hoore A, Penninckx F. Laparoscopic ventral recto(colpo)pexy for rectal prolapse: surgical technique and outcome for 109 patients. Surg Endosc 2006; 20:1919–23.
33. Slawik S, Soulsby R, Carter H, et al. Laparoscopic ventral rectopexy, posterior colporrhaphy and vaginal sacrocolpopexy for the treatment of recto-genital prolapse and mechanical outlet obstruction. Colorectal Dis 2008;10:138–43.
34. Kimmins MH, Evetts BK, Isler J, et al. The Altemeier repair: outpatient treatment of rectal prolapse. Dis Colon Rectum 2001;44:565–70.
35. Lechaux JP, Lechaux D, Perez M. Results of Delorme's procedure for rectal prolapse: advantages of a modified technique. Dis Colon Rectum 1995;38:301–7.
36. Aitola PT, Hiltunen KM, Matikainen MJ. Functional results of operative treatment of rectal prolapse over an 11-year period: emphasis on transabdominal approach. Dis Colon Rectum 1999;42:655–60.
37. Madden MV, Kamm MA, Nicholls RJ, et al. Abdominal rectopexy for complete prolapse: prospective study evaluating changes in symptoms and anorectal function. Dis Colon Rectum 1992;35:48–55.
38. Scaglia M, Fasth S, Hallgren T, et al. Abdominal rectopexy for rectal prolapse: influence of surgical technique on functional outcome. Dis Colon Rectum 1994;37:805–13.
39. Bruch HP, Herold A, Schiedeck T, et al. Laparoscopic surgery for rectal prolapse and outlet obstruction. Dis Colon Rectum 1999;42:1189–94.
40. Raftopoulos Y, Senagore AJ, Di GG, et al. Recurrence rates after abdominal surgery for complete rectal prolapse: a multicenter pooled analysis of 643 individual patient data. Dis Colon Rectum 2005;48:1200–6.
41. Purkayastha S, Tekkis P, Athanasiou T, et al. A comparison of open vs. laparoscopic abdominal rectopexy for full-thickness rectal prolapse: a meta-analysis. Dis Colon Rectum 2005;48:1930–40.

42. Hsu A, Brand MI, Saclarides TJ. Laparoscopic rectopexy without resection: a worthwhile treatment for rectal prolapse in patients without prior constipation. Am Surg 2007;73:858–61.
43. Johnson E, Stangeland A, Johannessen HO, et al. Resection rectopexy for external rectal prolapse reduces constipation and anal incontinence. Scand J Surg 2007;96:56–61.
44. Lechaux JP, Atienza P, Goasguen N, et al. Prosthetic rectopexy to the pelvic floor and sigmoidectomy for rectal prolapse. Am J Surg 2001;182:465–9.
45. Yoshioka K, Hyland G, Keighley MR. Anorectal function after abdominal rectopexy: parameters of predictive value in identifying return of continence. Br J Surg 1989;76:64–8.
46. Hamalainen KJ, Raivio P, Antila S, et al. Biofeedback therapy in rectal prolapse patients. Dis Colon Rectum 1996;39:262–5.
47. Shorvon PJ, Marshall MM. Evacuation proctography. London: Springer Verlag; 2005.
48. Dvorkin LS, Gladman MA, Epstein J, et al. Rectal intussusception in symptomatic patients is different from that in asymptomatic volunteers. Br J Surg 2005;92:866–72.
49. Choi SH, Han JK, Kim SH, et al. Intussusception in adults: from stomach to rectum. AJR Am J Roentgenol 2004;183:691–8.
50. Dvorkin LS, Knowles CH, Scott SM, et al. Rectal intussusception: characterization of symptomatology. Dis Colon Rectum 2005;48:824–31.
51. Karlbom U, Pahlman L, Nilsson S, et al. Relationships between defecographic findings, rectal emptying, and colonic transit time in constipated patients. Gut 1995;36:907–12.
52. Ihre T, Seligson U. Intussusception of the rectum-internal procidentia: treatment and results in 90 patients. Dis Colon Rectum 1975;18:391–6.
53. Okamoto N, Maeda K, Kato R, et al. Dynamic pelvic three-dimensional computed tomography for investigation of pelvic abnormalities in patients with rectocele and rectal prolapse. J Gastroenterol 2006;41:802–6.
54. Brusciano L, Limongelli P, Pescatori M, et al. Ultrasonographic patterns in patients with obstructed defaecation. Int J Colorectal Dis 2007;22:969–77.
55. Murad-Regadas SM, Regadas FS, Rodrigues LV, et al. A novel three-dimensional dynamic anorectal ultrasonography technique (echodefecography) to assess obstructed defecation: a comparison with defecography. Surg Endosc 2008;22:974–9.
56. Kaufman HS, Buller JL, Thompson JR, et al. Dynamic pelvic magnetic resonance imaging and cystocolpoproctography alter surgical management of pelvic floor disorders. Dis Colon Rectum 2001;44:1575–83 [discussion: 83-4].
57. Hwang YH, Person B, Choi JS, et al. Biofeedback therapy for rectal intussusception. Tech Coloproctol 2006;10:11–5 [discussion: 5-6].
58. Lazorthes F, Gamagami R, Cabarrot P, et al. Is rectal intussusception a cause of idiopathic incontinence? Dis Colon Rectum 1998;41:602–5.
59. Christiansen J, Hesselfeldt P, Sorensen M. Treatment of internal rectal intussusception in patients with chronic constipation. Scand J Gastroenterol 1995;30:470–2.
60. Graf W, Karlbom U, Pahlman L, et al. Functional results after abdominal suture rectopexy for rectal prolapse or intussusception. Eur J Surg 1996;162:905–11.
61. Sielezneff I, Malouf A, Cesari J, et al. Selection criteria for internal rectal prolapse repair by Delorme's transrectal excision. Dis Colon Rectum 1999;42:367–73.

62. Berman IR, Harris MS, Rabeler MB. Delorme's transrectal excision for internal rectal prolapse: patient selection, technique, and three-year follow-up. Dis Colon Rectum 1990;33:573–80.
63. Tsiaoussis J, Chrysos E, Athanasakis E, et al. Rectoanal intussusception: presentation of the disorder and late results of resection rectopexy. Dis Colon Rectum 2005;48:838–44.
64. von Papen M, Ashari LH, Lumley JW, et al. Functional results of laparoscopic resection rectopexy for symptomatic rectal intussusception. Dis Colon Rectum 2007;50:50–5.
65. Madigan MR, Morson BC. Solitary ulcer of the rectum. Gut 1969;10:871–81.
66. Haray PN, Morris-Stiff GJ, Foster ME. Solitary rectal ulcer syndrome: an underdiagnosed condition. Int J Colorectal Dis 1997;12:313–5.
67. Tjandra JJ, Fazio VW, Church JM, et al. Clinical conundrum of solitary rectal ulcer. Dis Colon Rectum 1992;35:227–34.
68. Womack NR, Williams NS, Mist JH, et al. Anorectal function in the solitary rectal ulcer syndrome. Dis Colon Rectum 1987;30:319–23.
69. Mahieu PH. Barium enema and defaecography in the diagnosis and evaluation of the solitary rectal ulcer syndrome. Int J Colorectal Dis 1986;1:85–90.
70. Kang YS, Kamm MA, Engel AF, et al. Pathology of the rectal wall in solitary rectal ulcer syndrome and complete rectal prolapse. Gut 1996;38:587–90.
71. Tsuchida K, Okayama N, Miyata M, et al. Solitary rectal ulcer syndrome accompanied by submucosal invasive carcinoma. Am J Gastroenterol 1998;93:2235–8.
72. Daya D, O'Connell G, DeNardi F. Rectal endometriosis mimicking solitary rectal ulcer syndrome. Mod Pathol 1995;8:599–602.
73. Halligan S, Nicholls RJ, Bartram CI. Evacuation proctography in patients with solitary rectal ulcer syndrome: anatomic abnormalities and frequency of impaired emptying and prolapse. AJR Am J Roentgenol 1995;164:91–5.
74. Van Outryve MJ, Pelckmans PA, Fierens H, et al. Transrectal ultrasound study of the pathogenesis of solitary rectal ulcer syndrome. Gut 1993;34:1422–6.
75. Keighley MR, Shouler P. Clinical and manometric features of the solitary rectal ulcer syndrome. Dis Colon Rectum 1984;27:507–12.
76. Ho YH, Ho JM, Parry BR, et al. Solitary rectal ulcer syndrome: the clinical entity and anorectal physiological findings in Singapore. Aust N Z J Surg 1995;65:93–7.
77. Kennedy DK, Hughes ES, Masterton JP. The natural history of benign ulcer of the rectum. Surg Gynecol Obstet 1977;144:718–20.
78. Zargar SA, Khuroo MS, Mahajan R. Sucralfate retention enemas in solitary rectal ulcer. Dis Colon Rectum 1991;34:455–7.
79. Ederle A, Bulighin G, Orlandi PG, et al. Endoscopic application of human fibrin sealant in the treatment of solitary rectal ulcer syndrome. Endoscopy 1992;24:736–7.
80. Vaizey CJ, Roy AJ, Kamm MA. Prospective evaluation of the treatment of solitary rectal ulcer syndrome with biofeedback. Gut 1997;41:817–20.
81. Jarrett ME, Emmanuel AV, Vaizey CJ, et al. Behavioural therapy (biofeedback) for solitary rectal ulcer syndrome improves symptoms and mucosal blood flow. Gut 2004;53:368–70.
82. Rao SS, Ozturk R, De Ocampo S, et al. Pathophysiology and role of biofeedback therapy in solitary rectal ulcer syndrome. Am J Gastroenterol 2006;101:613–8.
83. Sitzler PJ, Kamm MA, Nicholls RJ, et al. Long-term clinical outcome of surgery for solitary rectal ulcer syndrome. Br J Surg 1998;85:1246–50.

84. Torres C, Khaikin M, Bracho J, et al. Solitary rectal ulcer syndrome: clinical findings, surgical treatment, and outcomes. Int J Colorectal Dis 2007;22: 1389–93.
85. Bump RC, Mattiasson A, Bo K, et al. The standardization of terminology of female pelvic organ prolapse and pelvic floor dysfunction. Am J Obstet Gynecol 1996;175:10–7.
86. Beevors MA, Lubowski DZ, King DW, et al. Pudendal nerve function in women with symptomatic utero-vaginal prolapse. Int J Colorectal Dis 1991;6:24–8.
87. Rieger NA, Wattchow DA, Sarre RG, et al. Prospective study of biofeedback for treatment of constipation. Dis Colon Rectum 1997;40:1143–8.
88. Weber AM, Walters MD, Ballard LA, et al. Posterior vaginal prolapse and bowel function. Am J Obstet Gynecol 1998;179:1446–9.
89. Kelvin FM, Hale DS, Maglinte DD, et al. Female pelvic organ prolapse: diagnostic contribution of dynamic cystoproctography and comparison with physical examination. AJR Am J Roentgenol 1999;173:31–7.
90. Stanton SL, Zimmern S. Investigations. In: Stanton SL, Zimmern S, editors. Female Pelvic Reconstructive Surgery. London: Springer-Verlag; 2003. p. 227–30.
91. Baden W. Surgical repair of vaginal defects. In: Book surgical repair of vaginal defects. Philadelphia: Lippincott; 1992.
92. van Dam JH, Ginai AZ, Gosselink MJ, et al. Role of defecography in predicting clinical outcome of rectocele repair. Dis Colon Rectum 1997;40:201–7.
93. Karlbom U, Nilsson S, Pahlman L, et al. Defecographic study of rectal evacuation in constipated patients and control subjects. Radiology 1999;210:103–8.
94. Kenton K, Shott S, Brubaker L. The anatomic and functional variability of rectoceles in women. Int Urogynecol J Pelvic Floor Dysfunct 1999;10:96–9.
95. Karlbom U, Graf W, Nilsson S, et al. Does surgical repair of a rectocele improve rectal emptying? Dis Colon Rectum 1996;39:1296–302.
96. Low VH, Ho LM, Freed KS. Vaginal opacification during defecography: direction of vaginal migration aids in diagnosis of pelvic floor pathology. Abdom Imaging 1999;24:565–8.
97. Comiter CV, Vasavada SP, Barbaric ZL, et al. Grading pelvic prolapse and pelvic floor relaxation using dynamic magnetic resonance imaging. Urology 1999;54: 454–7.
98. van Dam JH, Schouten WR, Ginai AZ, et al. The impact of anismus on the clinical outcome of rectocele repair. Int J Colorectal Dis 1996;11:238–42.
99. Mellgren A, Lopez A, Schultz I, et al. Rectocele is associated with paradoxical anal sphincter reaction. Int J Colorectal Dis 1998;13:13–6.
100. Kahn MA, Stanton SL. Posterior colporrhaphy: its effects on bowel and sexual function. Br J Obstet Gynaecol 1997;104:82–6.
101. Maher C, Baessler K. Surgical management of posterior vaginal wall prolapse: an evidence-based literature review. Int Urogynecol J Pelvic Floor Dysfunct 2006;17:84–8.
102. Bachoo P, Brazzelli M, Grant A. Surgery for complete rectal prolapse in adults. Cochrane Database Syst Rev 2000: CD001758.
103. Fatton B, Amblard J, Debodinance P, et al. Transvaginal repair of genital prolapse: preliminary results of a new tension-free vaginal mesh (Prolift technique). A case series multicentric study. Int Urogynecol J Pelvic Floor Dysfunct 2007;18: 743–52.
104. Huebner M, Hsu Y, Fenner DE. The use of graft materials in vaginal pelvic floor surgery. Int J Gynaecol Obstet 2006;92:279–88.

105. Porter WE, Steele A, Walsh P, et al. The anatomic and functional outcomes of defect-specific rectocele repairs. Am J Obstet Gynecol 1999;181:1353–8.
106. Nygaard IE, McCreery R, Brubaker L, et al. Abdominal sacrocolpopexy: a comprehensive review. Obstet Gynecol 2004;104:805–23.
107. Silvis R, Gooszen HG, van EA, et al. Abdominal rectovaginopexy: modified technique to treat constipation. DisColon Rectum 1999;42:82–8.
108. Ghetti C, Gregory WT, Edwards SR, et al. Pelvic organ descent and symptoms of pelvic floor disorders. Am J Obstet Gynecol 2005;193:53–7.
109. Ho YH, Ang M, Nyam D, et al. Transanal approach to rectocele repair may compromise anal sphincter pressures. DisColon Rectum 1998;41:354–8.
110. Watson SJ, Loder PB, Halligan S, et al. Transperineal repair of symptomatic rectocele with Marlex mesh: a clinical, physiological and radiologic assessment of treatment. J Am Coll Surg 1996;183:257–61.
111. Mellgren A, Anzen B, Nilsson BY, et al. Results of rectocele repair: a prospective study. DisColon Rectum 1995;38:7–13.
112. Tjandra JJ, Ooi BS, Tang CL, et al. Transanal repair of rectocele corrects obstructed defecation if it is not associated with anismus. DisColon Rectum 1999;42:1544–50.
113. Aigner F, Zbar AP, Ludwikowski B, et al. The rectogenital septum: morphology, function, and clinical relevance. DisColon Rectum 2004;47:131–40.
114. Kinzel GE. Enterocele: a study of 265 cases. Am J Obstet Gynecol 1961;81: 1166–74.
115. Takahashi T, Yamana T, Sahara R, et al. Enterocele: what is the clinical implication? DisColon Rectum 2006;49:S75–81.
116. Bremmer S, Mellgren A, Holmstrom B, et al. Peritoneocele and enterocele: formation and transformation during rectal evacuation as studied by means of defaeco-peritoneography. Acta Radiol 1998;39:167–75.
117. Cook JR, Seman EI, O'Shea RT. Laparoscopic treatment of enterocele: a 3-year evaluation. Aust N Z J Obstet Gynaecol 2004;44:107–10.

Ileal Pouch Dysfunction: Diagnosis and Management

Paris P. Tekkis, MD, FRCS[a,b,c,*], R. John Nicholls, MD, FRCS[b,c]

KEYWORDS

- Restorative proctocolectomy • Pouch dysfunction
- Pouchitis • Pouch salvage

Restorative proctocolectomy (RPC) is the elective surgical procedure of choice for most patients who have ulcerative colitis or familial adenomatous polyposis. RPC involves removal of the colon and rectum, construction of a reservoir or pouch from the last 30 to 40 cm of ileum, followed by an ileoanal anastomosis. Today, most surgeons use a J pouch or two-loop pouch configuration, owing to the ease of construction, although other designs such as the W pouch or four-loop pouch may result in lower frequency of defecation. It is, however, technically more difficult to construct. In forming the ileoanal anastomosis, the surgeon either can staple or hand-sew the pouch to the anal canal. This is an important difference, because stapling leaves a 1 to 2 cm cuff of residual rectum in situ, which may become symptomatic and is at risk of dysplasia. The hand sewn technique includes a mucosectomy to remove virtually all anorectal mucosa and places the anastomosis just above the dentate line, but it may be associated with a higher incidence of minor anal leakage.[1] When an ileostomy is performed, it is closed at about 8 weeks, provided the anastomosis has healed as judged by digital examination and a contrast enema.

RPC results in good functional outcomes and quality of life in most patients but fails in between 3.5% and 17% per cent, necessitating excision of the pouch or indefinite fecal diversion. The failure rate increases with the duration of follow-up and may occur early, within the first postoperative year, or at any time thereafter. The overall

[a] Department of Academic Surgery, Chelsea and Westminster Hospital, Division of Surgery, Oncology, Reproductive Biology, and Anaesthetics, Imperial College, Fulham Road, London, SW10 9NH, UK
[b] Department of Surgery, St. Mark's Hospital, Division of Surgery, Oncology, Reproductive Biology and Anaesthetics, Imperial College, Harrow, HA1 3UJ, UK
[c] Department of Biosurgery and Surgical Technology, St. Mary's Hospital, Division of Surgery, Oncology, Reproductive Biology and Anaesthetics, Imperial College, Praed Street, London, W2 1NY, UK
* Corresponding author. Department of Academic Surgery, 3rd Floor, Chelsea and Westminster Hospital, 369 Fulham Road, London, SW10 9NH, UK.
E-mail address: p.tekkis@imperial.ac.uk (P.P. Tekkis).

Gastroenterol Clin N Am 37 (2008) 669–683
doi:10.1016/j.gtc.2008.07.003 gastro.theclinics.com

cumulative failure taking all patients irrespective of diagnosis is approximately 5% at 5 years, 10% at 10 years and 15% at 15 years.[2]

Reports of long-term function over 10 to 20 years have demonstrated a median stool frequency per 24 hours of four to eight, with about half of patients needing to evacuate at night. This is stable over 25 years. Urgency is uncommon (5%), although there is some evidence that it increases with time.[3,4] Fecal leakage during the day occurs in less than 4% of patients and is stable over 25 years. At night, these rates are 4% at 10 years, rising to 9% at 25 years. Seepage during the day and at night occurs in 7% and 9% of patients, rising to 11% and 18% of patients, respectively, at 25 years. Antidiarrheal medication is required in about a third of patients at 10 years and in 45% of patients at 25 years.[5]

For patients in whom failure is threatened, revisional or redo surgery may be indicated. There are four causes of ileal pouch failure: (1) acute and chronic sepsis, (2) poor function for mechanical or functional reasons, (3) mucosal inflammation (pouchitis), and (4) neoplastic transformation. Of these, sepsis is the most common, being responsible for over 50% of all failures.[2] Poor function accounts for about a third of failures and pouchitis for 10%.[6] Neoplastic transformation is uncommon,[6] and in these patients excision of the pouch is indicated. For the larger group of patients without neoplastic transformation in whom failure is threatened, various factors need to be considered when advising revisional pouch surgery. These include the feasibility of success, the magnitude of the proposed operation, the overall duration of treatment, and the patient's wishes. The potential morbidity of excision of the reservoir resulting in a permanent ileostomy also should be discussed, including the possibility of a high-output ileostomy, pelvic nerve damage, and an unhealed perineal wound. These complications occur in 50% or more of patients undergoing excision of the pouch.[7]

SEPSIS

Pelvic sepsis after restorative proctocolectomy occurs in 3% to 25% of cases and its incidence appears to decrease as surgical experience increases.[8] Pelvic sepsis may present in the early postoperative period, or it may be delayed, manifesting as abscess formation (usually presacral) or fistulation (in females usually into the vagina), often with a history of an anastomotic complication.

Early Sepsis

Patients who develop sepsis in the early postoperative period have a cumulative incidence of subsequent failure five times that of the whole population of patients undergoing restorative proctocolectomy. Symptoms of early pelvic sepsis include fever, anal pain, tenesmus, and discharge of pus or secondary hemorrhage through the anus. The diagnosis is established by digital examination (under anesthesia if necessary), combined with imaging, including contrast pouchography, CT, and MRI.

Management

In a proportion of patients the condition resolves spontaneously. Others need operative endoanal, or imaging-guided percutaneous, drainage. If drainage of the cavity is unsatisfactory, an attempt can be made to deroof the abscess and curette the cavity through the anus, creating a large communication between the abscess and the reservoir. Sometimes several local procedures are needed to eradicate sepsis. Rarely, an abdominal approach is indicated. When sepsis is severe enough to warrant a laparotomy, the functional outcome is poor, often followed by failure.[9]

When anastomotic disruption is the cause of pelvic sepsis, after drainage and curettage, transanal repair of the anastomosis or advancement of the ileum and resuturing of the ileoanal anastomosis have been advocated. In a report of 15 patients who were found to have partial anastomotic disruption between 7 and 90 days after surgery, seven were treated by resuturing of the anastomotic defect and counter drainage, with success in three. Seven others underwent a pouch advancement procedure, with success in five. Thus, over a follow-up of 1 to 22 months, successful salvage was achieved in eight of the 15 patients.[10]

Severe acute pelvic sepsis with extensive anastomotic breakdown occurs in 5% to 15% of patients and results in early failure in around 30% of patients, despite adequate drainage. Attempts at salvage by direct suture may work for some patients. The occurrence of early sepsis renders the patient at increased risk of subsequent failure compared with the total population. In a report by Heuschen and colleagues,[11] only 16.8% of the 131 patients who had sepsis could be managed conservatively, the rest requiring some form of surgical procedure. Patients who had early postoperative sepsis, however, were not distinguished from those in whom sepsis developed during subsequent follow-up, although there was no significant difference in the failure rate when salvage surgery was undertaken within or beyond 6 months of restorative proctocolectomy. As might be expected, failure was related to the magnitude of the procedure, 6.1% per cent after minor intervention (33 patients) compared with 47.3% after major surgery (74 patients).

Delayed Sepsis

Delayed abdominal or pelvic sepsis presents as chronic abscess formation with or without fistulation. MRI using short-tau inversion recovery (STIR) settings may make the diagnosis in some patients in whom clinical examination, contrast radiography, or CT has not been successful. When sepsis is limited, there is a good chance of healing, provided that drainage is adequate. If resolution does not occur, there are two surgical options, including excision of the pouch or an attempt at salvage, usually by means of an abdominal approach.

Management

There is a considerable variation in the reported success of abdominal salvage surgery. Satisfactory success rates were reported in a series of 35 patients who had chronic sepsis, either abscess or fistulation,[12] including 22 who had ulcerative colitis, 10 who had Crohn's disease, one who had indeterminate colitis, and two who had familial adenomatous polyposis. Twenty-nine patients had leakage from the ileoanal anastomosis and four from the upper pouch. Overall a pelvic abscess was present in 25 patients, and 10 had a vaginal and 12 a perineal fistula. All underwent abdominal revision with detachment of the ileoanal anastomosis, curettage of any chronic abscess cavity with drainage or repair of fistula, and reanastomosis. The median interval between the first operation and revision was 24 months. At a median follow-up of 18 (range 6 to 105) months, 30 patients had preserved anal function. Twenty-one of the 22 patients who had ulcerative colitis retained anal function, but the functional outcome was not satisfactory in all cases. The median frequency of defecation per 24 hours was 9.6 times, but the range was considerable, from 4 to 35. Urgency was common and was constantly present in four patients and intermittent in 14. The quality of life was reported as good or excellent by 17 patients and fair or poor by 13. Despite disappointing function in some patients, it is clear that major surgical revision can result in worthwhile salvage in many.

Others, however, have reported poorer results. In a series of 114 patients who underwent abdominal salvage surgery for various reasons after RPC, 29 had procedures for intra-abdominal sepsis.[13] These included drainage of abscess (three patients), diverting ileostomy (18), revision of the pouch (six) and primary closure of fistula (four). Of the 29 patients, 17 still had an ileostomy at the time of assessment, and in 10, the pouch had been removed. Only 10 had satisfactory anal function. The authors showed, importantly, that failure continues with the passage of time; at 2 years, 34 procedures had failed, and at 5 years, the probability of remaining free of pouch excision was 75%.

A similar experience was reported in 131 patients who developed early sepsis out of a total of 706 who had RPC for ulcerative colitis (494) and polyposis (212).[11] The occurrence of early sepsis conferred a higher chance of cumulative failure compared with that in patients who did not develop early sepsis. Furthermore, failure after attempted salvage rose from 20% at 3 years to 40% at 10 years. Of the 131 patients followed for 51 (interquartile range 31 to 96) months, sepsis was caused by fistulation in 76% of cases, anastomotic separation in 15% of cases, and abscess formation alongside the pouch in 10% of cases. The authors classified the site of fistulation into three levels: level 1 (upper pouch) in 19% of cases, level 2 (lower pouch, rectal cuff) in 31% of cases, and level 3 (ileoanal anastomosis) in 50% of cases. Sepsis was treated conservatively in 24 cases (18%), by minor surgery in 33 cases (25%), and by major surgery in 74 cases (56%). As might be expected, the failure rate was higher after major (47%) than after minor (6%) surgery. Overall, failure was related to sepsis at level 3, the presence of a pouch–vaginal fistula (43%), an original diagnosis of ulcerative colitis, and the number of salvage procedures. It was also cumulative with time, even after salvage intervention.

The largest series of abdominal salvage surgery published to date included 112 patients, with the following original pathology: ulcerative colitis (n = 86), indeterminate colitis (n = 11), familial adenomatous polyposis (n = 10), and other conditions (n = 5). At a median follow-up of 46 (range 1 to 147) months, 24 (21%) patients experienced pouch failure, the incidence of which increased with time. The pouch failed in all patients who had Crohn's disease. Successful salvage at 5 years was associated with a nonseptic (85%) rather than a septic (61%) indication (P = .016) as shown in **Fig. 1**. Frequency of nighttime defecation and fecal urgency improved after salvage surgery.[14]

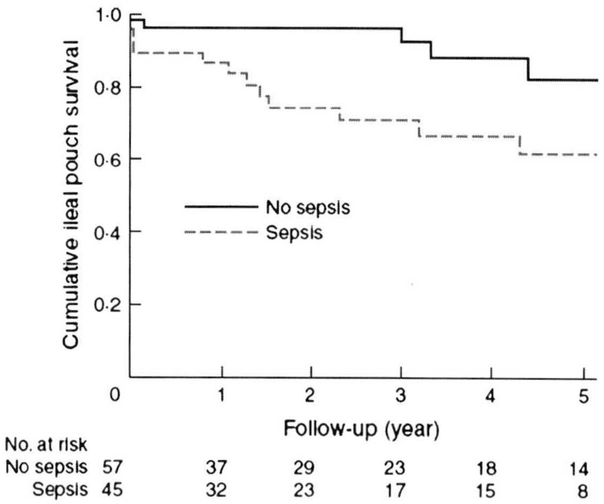

Fig. 1. Cumulative pouch survival after abdominal salvage for patients with and without sepsis. Log rank statistic = 5.78, 1 degrees of freedom, P = .016 (log rank test). (*From* Tekkis PP, Heriot AG, Smith JJ, et al. Long-term results of abdominal salvage surgery following restorative proctocolectomy. Br J Surg 2006;93(2):231–7; with permission.)

POOR FUNCTION

Function varies from day to day, and the patient's own perception is probably the most important factor in the identification of poor function. Most patients with poor function have a stool frequency of 10 evacuations per 24 hours or more, usually associated with the passage of small-volume stool. There also may be urgency, incontinence, and difficulty in evacuation. An assessment of the extent to which these impair quality of life should be made. Pouch function tends to improve with time, and a reasonable period should be allowed to pass before considering any form of salvage surgery. In a prospective study of patients over 12 years, however, there was no change in bowel frequency, although there was an increase in major day continence in 18% and improvement in only 1% of patients. Most patients had stable function over the 12 years.[15]

Differential diagnosis

The diagnosis is made on clinical examination combined with investigations, including pouchoscopy with mucosal biopsy, contrast pouchography, physiologic tests of sphincter function, and estimation of reservoir capacity. Pouchitis often is invoked as the cause of poor function. A degree of acute inflammation in a mucosal biopsy often is seen, however, and this may not be the reason necessarily. Frequently, more than one lesion coexists. For example, stenosis of the ileoanal anastomosis,

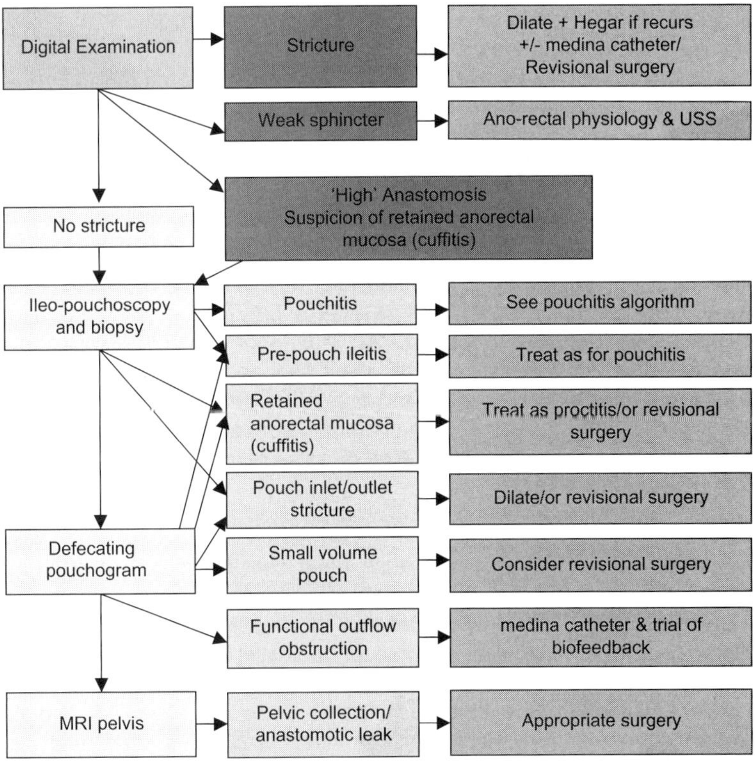

Fig. 2. Algorithm for the investigation of pouch dysfunction. (*From* McLaughlin SD, Clark SK, Tekkis PP, et al. Review article: restorative proctocolectomy, indications, management of complications and follow-up–a guide for gastroenterologists. Aliment Pharmacol Ther 2008;27(10):895–909; with permission.)

chronic abscess, and retained rectum may occur in the same patient. An algorithm is shown in **Fig. 2** for investigating patients who have ileal pouch dysfunction.

Mechanical Outlet Obstruction

The causes of mechanical outlet obstruction include: stricture of the ileoanal anastomosis, retained rectum after ileorectal anastomosis, and long efferent limb of an S-reservoir (no longer relevant).

Examination and contrast radiology may show evidence of narrowing or obstruction either at the level of the ileoanal anastomosis or in the distal part of the reservoir. In some patients, outlet obstruction may not be associated with evidence of mechanical narrowing; it then is presumed to be caused by a functional disorder of unknown etiology. Surgery is not indicated in these patients.

The symptoms of outflow obstruction are typical and almost diagnostic. The patient experiences difficulty in evacuation with the characteristic frequent passage of small volumes of stool. Frequency may be as high as 20 to 30 defecations per 24 hours with the expulsion of no more than a few milliliters of stool on each occasion. Such symptoms are an indication for further investigation.

Long efferent limb

The original ileal reservoir[16] and the isoperistaltic reconstruction[17] both involved the creation of an efferent limb of terminal ileum, which formed the proximal side of the ileoanal anastomosis. Neither reconstruction is performed today. With a limb of up to 8 cm in length in the early years of the reservoir, over 50% of patients were unable to evacuate spontaneously and needed to catheterize the pouch through the anus to do so. Contrast radiological studies showed outflow obstruction that was roughly proportional to the length of the limb. Accordingly, this was shortened to 2 cm, resulting in spontaneous evacuation in around 90% of patients.[18]

Patients usually accepted the need for catheterization as a reasonable price to pay for avoiding an ileostomy, but some were unable to tolerate the situation. Further surgery has some prospect of improving matters for such patients, with restoration of spontaneous evacuation. It may be possible to remove the problematic segment endoanally, but this is technically possible in less than 30% of patients. In most, an abdominoanal salvage procedure is required. The pouch is mobilized and the ileoanal anastomosis detached. The efferent limb is excised, and a new anastomosis is constructed manually between the pouch and anal canal. Of a total of 35 patients, failure occurred in six, and improved function, including conversion from catheterization to spontaneous evacuation occurred in 18 of 26 patients in whom a functional assessment was made.[19–21]

Stricture of the ileoanal anastomosis

Narrowing of the ileoanal anastomosis requiring at least one dilatation under anesthesia has been reported in 4% to 40% of patients.[10,13,22–25] Factors leading to fibrosis include pelvic sepsis and anastomotic tension causing separation, although no statistical difference has been shown in the incidence of stenosis in patients who develop septic complications compared with those who do not. Stenosis may be more common in patients who have ulcerative colitis than in those who have FAP, and also after a stapled anastomosis, particularly when an instrument with a small head has been used.[23] In a series of 266 patients, stenosis occurred in 14.2% and 39.6%, respectively, after manual and stapled anastomosis.[25]

The severity of the stricture is assessed by digital examination to determine the diameter, longitudinal length, and the extent of surrounding induration. Contrast radiology is used to assess the length and the degree of dilatation of the proximal bowel. An apparent stricture may be noted when digital examination is performed for the first time after operation. This is often caused by lateral adhesions across the anastomosis creating a web effect, which is divided easily by gentle passage of the finger. Usually this resolves the problem.

In one study, 35 of 50 patients who had stenosis were treated by dilatation, including 26 with and nine without general anesthesia.[25] Repeated dilatations were necessary in the former group. The stenosis persisted in 37 of the 50 patients, and in only 13 did it resolve. In another study, 42 patients who developed a stricture among 982 undergoing restorative proctocolectomy were followed up for 31 (range 1 to 98) months.[13] All patients underwent dilatation under anesthesia, with recurrence in 25 and failure in seven. In 23 patients who required repeated dilatation, function was satisfactory, and in 11 it was poor. Thus reasonable function was achieved by dilatation in about half the patients.

If symptoms of outflow obstruction persist despite dilatation, surgery may be indicated depending on their severity. In some patients who have a tight but short stricture, a posterior stricturotomy may be successful, although there are no published data on the results. This operation runs the risk of sepsis and hemorrhage, and should be performed under direct vision by means of electrocoagulation. A transanal approach involving excision of the stricture and advancement of the pouch distally has been described in three patients who had stricture, two of whom had a simultaneous vaginal fistula. At follow-up of 3 to 11 months, all had satisfactory function.[15,26]

The endoanal approach is difficult for patients who are unsuitable for this or who do not respond to dilatation. The available options include removal of the reservoir with the establishment of a permanent ileostomy or a major salvage procedure. Removal has been reported to be necessary in 2.5% to 15% of patients who have stricture.[13,17] Abdominal salvage involves mobilization of the reservoir from the pelvis, followed by excision of the stenosis and reanastomosis of the apex of the reservoir to the distal anal canal. It is usually necessary to perform a mucosectomy to achieve this.[27] Technical details of importance include the need to dissect close to the reservoir to avoid damage to pelvic structures, including the autonomic nerves, and removal of as much of the fibrosis in the area of structuring as possible. Any associated chronic abscess cavity should be curetted and the operation covered by a defunctioning ileostomy.

There is little information in the literature on the outcome of major abdominal surgery for stricture. In one study, five patients treated for stricture were followed for a minimum of 6 months.[27] The median frequency of defecation fell from 17 (range 10 to 26) to 6 (range 4 to 24) times per day after operation, with a successful outcome in four. In another study of 23 patients who underwent abdominal salvage for various reasons, the indication was an anastomotic complication in three, all of whom had a successful result.[21]

Retained rectum after ileorectal anastomosis

The aim of restorative proctocolectomy is to remove all disease-prone mucosa. The original technique therefore included a mucosectomy of the upper anal canal with an anastomosis just above the dentate line. With the introduction of stapling techniques,[28] the anastomosis usually came to lie more proximal at, or above, the level of the anorectal junction. Some degree of inflammation in biopsies taken from the anal columnar epithelium is common. This may be severe enough to cause symptoms in 2% to 15% of patients.[29–32] In a series of 217 patients who had a stapled anastomosis, 48 (22.1%) had evidence of persisting inflamed mucosa distal to the anastomosis. Of these, 32 patients were symptomatic, and 28 needed treatment.[30]

The symptoms of retained inflamed mucosa are those of proctitis, including bleeding, burning, and urgency. Disordered evacuation with the frequent passage of small amounts of stool also may occur, and patients are at continuing risk of neoplastic transformation.[33] The diagnosis of retained rectum may be made on digital palpation, which will demonstrate the anastomosis to be above the level of the anorectal junction. This will be confirmed by contrast radiology and endoscopy by taking biopsies from above and below the anastomosis.

Treatment with local steroids may relieve the symptoms in some patients, but in others it may not result in a satisfactory long-term solution. Thus in patients who have unacceptable function despite medical treatment, surgery is indicated. If there is a short longitudinal length of persisting inflamed mucosa, it may be possible to remove it by means of an endoanal approach.[34] In most patients, however, a combined abdominoanal approach is necessary, with removal of the retained rectal stump followed by mucosectomy of the anal stump and a manual ileoanal anastomosis.

In a larger series of 22 patients followed for a median of 22.5 (range 4 to 114) months, failure with excision of the reservoir occurred in five. Seventeen patients had anal function, and in these, the median 24-hour frequency before and after surgery was 12 (range 4 to 20) and 6 (range 3 to 12) months, respectively.[35] Median night-time frequency fell from 4 (range 0 to 8) to 0.5 (range 0 to 4). Fifteen of the 17 patients reported subjective improvement in the quality of life, giving an overall success rate of 15 of 22 patients.

Small-Volume Reservoir

A compliant pouch of good volume appears to be a factor determining function. There is an inverse relationship between the maximum tolerated volume of the reservoir and frequency of defecation.[36,37] Patients with a small-capacity reservoir have high stool frequency, sometimes with urge incontinence. The original straight ileoanal anastomosis reconstruction is an extreme example of this. The diagnosis is made by contrast radiology to give a direct image of the size of the reservoir, and by balloon volumetry, which gives a functional measure of urge and maximum tolerated volume.

If medical treatment fails to reduce unacceptable stool frequency, a reservoir augmentation procedure should be considered using an abdominal approach. It may be possible to add a loop of immediately proximal ileum to the upper part of the reservoir. When this is not technically possible, it is necessary to mobilize the reservoir entirely, including detachment of the ileoanal anastomosis, to allow a complete remodeling. In a report of five patients with functional failure caused by low pouch capacity whose reservoir was converted to a pouch, mean 24-hour and nocturnal stool frequency fell from 13.8 and 3.0 to 5.8 and 0.3 respectively after augmentation.[38]

Sphincter Dysfunction

Some degree of anal discharge occurs in up to 30% of patients, but fecal incontinence caused by poor sphincter function is less common, with a reported frequency of less than 5%. Preoperative assessment of the sphincter may avoid some failures by appropriate patient selection. Previous anal surgery is not, however, necessarily a contraindication to the operation. In patients who have postoperative incontinence clinical examination, anorectal physiologic testing, and anal ultrasonography should determine the nature of the sphincter lesion.[39]

There is little information in the literature on the results of salvage surgery for an incompetent sphincter. One study reported two patients who underwent sphincter repair, both with a satisfactory outcome.[40]

Pouchitis

Some degree of inflammation in the ileal pouch develops in about 50% of cases. The intensity of this fluctuates. Pouchitis is diagnosed when histologically proven acute inflammation is associated with symptoms of frequency, urgency, and liquid stool in the presence of endoscopic evidence of inflammation. It is important to understand that there are various causes of frequency; not all are caused by pouch inflammation. There is a difference between incidence and prevalence. Quoted incidences of pouchitis of up to 50%[41,42] may be misleading, because these are based on cumulative life table analysis methodology. In many cases, the diagnosis has not been confirmed histologically. In clinical practice, prevalence the true marker of patients suffering significantly, is the important consideration. This is much lower, being around 5%.[43,44]

The etiology is unknown but is likely to be related to the vast increase ($\times 10^{6-7}$) in the concentration of bacterial flora within the pouch. Treatment with antibiotics is successful in most patients, although this may need to be repeated. Patients who have chronic unremitting pouchitis may not respond. Only 10% of failures of RPC are caused by pouchitis.[45]

Examination of serial biopsies of the pouch over several years has allowed the division of patients into three groups. Type A includes patients whose biopsies show normal mucosa or mild villous atrophy with no or mild inflammation. In Type B, the mucosa fluctuates between moderate-to-severe villous atrophy and normal. In Type C, there is persistent subtotal or total villous atrophy developing early after closure of the defunctioning ileostomy accompanied by acute and chronic inflammation. Patients with type C changes have pouchitis and are more likely to have primary sclerosing cholangitis.[46,47]

Diagnosis

In clinical practice, the diagnosis of pouchitis requires a triad of compatible symptoms and endoscopic and histologic findings. Scoring systems have been devised to grade pouchitis. These include the Moskowitz score,[48] the pouchitis disease activity index,[49] the Heidelberg system,[50] and the Objective Pouchitis Score (OPS).[51] The PDAI and Heidelberg Pouchitis Activity Score (PAS) give numbers to clinical, endoscopic, and histologic features. These systems, however, contain the fallacy that histologic evidence of acute inflammation is not an essential requisite for the diagnosis.

Management

All patients should have a flexible pouchoscopy and biopsy, as symptoms do not always correlate with the endoscopic and histologic findings.[48–50] Other disorders can present with poor function and may respond to antibiotics temporarily. For patients who have frequent episodes of established pouchitis, it is reasonable to start antibiotics without repeating the pouchoscopy. Many patients have asymptomatic inflammation in the pouch. Some will have inflammation along a suture line; this is a normal variant and not pouchitis. Inflammation may be patchy in distribution, and biopsies therefore may not be representative.

For practical purposes pouchitis can be classified as acute or chronic. Acute pouchitis is defined as less than 4 weeks in duration, responding to a single antibiotic, and occurring less than three times per year. This category includes most patients.

Chronic pouchitis can be divided further into: chronic relapsing, chronic antibiotic-dependent, or chronic refractory. Chronic relapsing pouchitis is defined as three or more episodes per year that respond to antibiotic treatment. Chronic antibiotic-dependent pouchitis is defined as that in which symptoms are controlled when maintained on a single antibiotic, but promptly return when this is withdrawn. Most authors define chronic antibiotic refractory pouchitis as when the patient no longer responds to a single antibiotic.

Treatment

Nonsteroidal anti-inflammatory drugs (NSAIDs) are associated with pouchitis, and withdrawal may induce remission.[52] Ciprofloxacin or metronidazole for 14 days should be used as first-line treatment. Their efficacy is similar, but ciprofloxacin is tolerated better and does not cause peripheral neuropathy.[53] If this fails or early relapse occurs, combined ciprofloxacin and metronidazole for 30 days is usually effective.[54] In patients intolerant to oral metronidazole, good results may be obtained with metronidazole administered per anum. A combination of ciprofloxacin and rifaximin is also effective.[55] Ciprofloxacin combined with tinidazole additionally has been shown to be effective in some patients who do not respond to ciprofloxacin and metronidazole. Co-amoxiclav or clarithromycin may be useful; however there are no published controlled studies.[56]

Treatment with topical or oral budesonide has been shown to be beneficial but only in patients who do not respond to a single antibiotic.[57]

Patients with chronic pouchitis who achieve remission following antibiotic therapy but show a tendency to relapse should be treated with maintenance ciprofloxacin (250 to 500 mg twice daily) given the long-term adverse effects of metronidazole. This appears to be safe and well-tolerated, although there are no published long-term data. It may be possible to reduce the dose to 250 mg daily.

The probiotic VSL#3 has been shown in two randomized–controlled trials (RCTs) to maintain remission in 85% of patients with chronic pouchitis up to 1 year.[58,59] In this study, it should be noted, however, that patients who did not achieve endoscopic and clinical remission were excluded from the study. Furthermore, the trial dose cannot be given in clinical practice, because the commercially available sachets are of a different strength to that used in the original studies. These factors may explain why the results obtained by the authors and others have been disappointing. In the authors' experience, 87% of treated patients relapsed at 2 months. In a further study,[60] 25 (80%) of 31 patients after antibiotic-induced remission rapidly relapsed following treatment with VSL#3. There is no evidence that other drugs, including 5-ASA agents, systemic steroids, or immunosuppressants, are effective. **Fig. 3** demonstrates a suggested algorithm for the treatment of pouchitis.

Prepouch ileitis

A few patients develop inflammation in the ileum immediately proximal to the pouch. This usually is associated with pouchitis, but it may occur in isolation. Symptoms include those of pouchitis and also of intestinal obstruction. Prepouch ileitis occurs in about 3% of patients after RPC[61] Ileo-pouchoscopy or video capsule endoscopy will determine the extent of inflammation. CD should be considered in patients with extensive prepouch ileitis or where skip lesions are evident, particularly in the presence of a normal pouch.

Treatment

Various treatments have been described including oral steroids, 5-ASA drugs, and antibiotics. There are no controlled studies; however treatment with ciprofloxacin and metronidazole is usually effective.

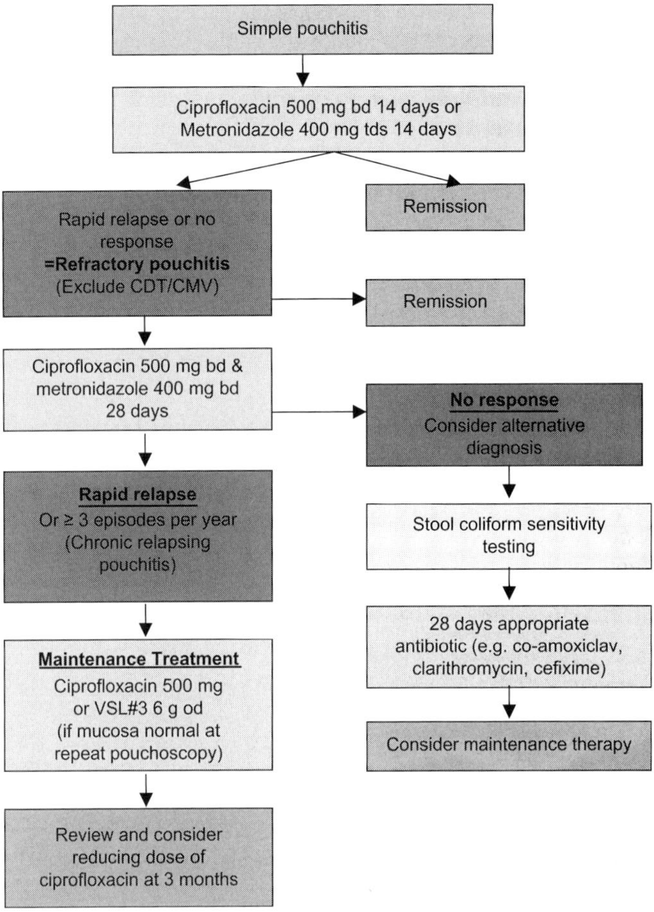

Fig. 3. Algorithm for the treatment of acute and chronic pouchitis. (*From* McLaughlin SD, Clark SK, Tekkis PP, et al. Review article: restorative proctocolectomy, indications, management of complications and follow-up–a guide for gastroenterologists. Aliment Pharmacol Ther 2008;27(10):895–909; with permission.)

Bile salt malabsorption

Bile salt malabsorption has been reported to be associated with pouch dysfunction.[62] The cause is probably multifactorial. Reduced absorption and depletion of bile salts may occur due in some manner to the vast increase of pouch bacteria and the change of mucosal morphology including colonic metaplasia and villous atrophy. There are no published effective treatments (ursodeoxycholic acid is ineffective).

Investigating Pouch Dysfunction

There is considerable overlap of symptoms between the various causes of pouch dysfunction that can make diagnosis difficult. Digital anal examination will reveal a weak sphincter, mechanical obstruction at the anastomosis, and a high rectal anastomosis indicating a retained rectal stump. The initial investigation should include stool culture and antigen testing for clostridium difficile toxin and other pathogens. Celiac antibody screening should be performed in patients presenting with frequency given the high incidence of celiac disease. Flexible pouchoscopy with biopsy is essential to assess the pouch and prepouch ileal mucosa. It is the most useful first-line investigation. A pouchogram may demonstrate a small reservoir. Physiology of the sphincter and pouch balloon volumetry will give an objective assessment of sphincter competence and pouch capacitance.

SUMMARY

RPC has revolutionized the surgical treatment of ulcerative colitis and, in some cases FAP. This major advance has offered an alternative to permanent ileostomy in these patients. Thus far, the good outcomes appear durable, but careful follow-up of patients is required after this type of surgery to describe the long-term results.

REFERENCES

1. Lovegrove RE, Constantinides VA, Heriot AG, et al. Comparison of hand-sewn versus stapled ileal pouch anal anastomosis (IPAA) following proctocolectomy: a meta-analysis of 4183 patients. Ann Surg 2006;244(1):18–26.
2. Tulchinsky H, Hawley PR, Nicholls J. Long-term failure after restorative proctocolectomy for ulcerative colitis. Ann Surg 2003;238(2):229–34.
3. Hahnloser D, Pemberton JH, Wolff BG, et al. Results at up to 20 years after ileal pouch–anal anastomosis for chronic ulcerative colitis. Br J Surg 2007;94(3): 333–40.
4. Bengtsson J, Borjesson L, Lundstam U, et al. Long-term function and manovolumetric characteristics after ileal pouch-anal anastomosis for ulcerative colitis. Br J Surg 2007;94(3):327–32.
5. Tekkis PP, Lovegrove RE, Tilney HS, et al. Restorative proctocolectomy in the United Kingdom: a multicentre study of 2491 patients. Colorectal Dis 2007; 9(Suppl 3):1.
6. Das P, Johnson MW, Tekkis PP, et al. Risk of dysplasia and adenocarcinoma following restorative proctocolectomy for ulcerative colitis. Colorectal Dis 2007; 9(1):15–27.
7. Karoui M, Cohen R, Nicholls J. Results of surgical removal of the pouch after failed restorative proctocolectomy. Dis Colon Rectum 2004;47(6):869–75.
8. Meagher AP, Farouk R, Dozois RR, et al. J ileal pouch–anal anastomosis for chronic ulcerative colitis: complications and long-term outcome in 1310 patients. Br J Surg 1998;85(6):800–3.
9. Scott NA, Dozois RR, Beart RW Jr, et al. Postoperative intra-abdominal and pelvic sepsis complicating ileal pouch-anal anastomosis. Int J Colorectal Dis 1988;3(3): 149–52.
10. Fleshman JW, McLeod RS, Cohen Z, et al. Improved results following use of an advancement technique in the treatment of ileoanal anastomotic complications. Int J Colorectal Dis 1988;3(3):161–5.
11. Heuschen UA, Allemeyer EH, Hinz U, et al. Outcome after septic complications in J pouch procedures. Br J Surg 2002;89(2):194–200.
12. Fazio VW, Wu JS, Lavery IC. Repeat ileal pouch–anal anastomosis to salvage septic complications of pelvic pouches: clinical outcome and quality-of-life assessment. Ann Surg 1998;228(4):588–97.
13. Galandiuk S, Scott NA, Dozois RR, et al. Ileal pouch–anal anastomosis. Reoperation for pouch-related complications. Ann Surg 1990;212(4):446–52.
14. Tekkis PP, Heriot AG, Smith JJ, et al. Long-term results of abdominal salvage surgery following restorative proctocolectomy. Br J Surg 2006;93(2):231–7.

15. Bullard KM, Madoff RD, Gemlo BT. Is ileoanal pouch function stable with time? Results of a prospective audit. Dis Colon Rectum 2002;45(3):299–304.
16. Parks AG, Nicholls RJ. Proctocolectomy without ileostomy for ulcerative colitis. Br Med J 1978;2(6130):85–8.
17. Fonkalsrud EW, Bustorff-Silva J. Reconstruction for chronic dysfunction of ileoanal pouches. Ann Surg 1999;229(2):197–204.
18. Vasilevsky CA, Rothenberger DA, Goldberg SM. The S ileal pouch–anal anastomosis. World J Surg 1987;11(6):742–50.
19. Nicholls RJ, Gilbert JM. Surgical correction of the efferent ileal limb for disordered defaecation following restorative proctocolectomy with the S ileal reservoir. Br xJ Surg 1990;77(2):152–4.
20. Ogunbiyi OA, Korsgen S, Keighley MR. Pouch salvage. Long-term outcome. Dis Colon Rectum 1997;40(5):548–52.
21. Sagar PM, Dozois RR, Wolff BG, et al. Disconnection, pouch revision, and reconnection of the ileal pouch–anal anastomosis. Br J Surg 1996;83(10):1401–5.
22. Marcello PW, Roberts PL, Schoetz DJ Jr, et al. Long-term results of the ileoanal pouch procedure. Arch Surg 1993;128(5):500–3.
23. Lewis WG, Kuzu A, Sagar PM, et al. Stricture at the pouch–anal anastomosis after restorative proctocolectomy. Dis Colon Rectum 1994;37(2):120–5.
24. Metcalf AM, Dozois RR, Kelly KA, et al. J pouch–anal anastomosis. Clinical outcome. Ann Sur 1985;202(6):735–9.
25. Senapati A, Tibbs CJ, Ritchie JK, et al. Stenosis of the pouch anal anastomosis following restorative proctocolectomy. Int J Colorectal Dis 1996;11(2):57–9.
26. Breen EM, Schoetz DJ Jr, Marcello PW, et al. Functional results after perineal complications of ileal pouch–anal anastomosis. Dis Colon Rectum 1998;41(6): 691–5.
27. Herbst F, Sieleznеff I, Nicholls RJ. Salvage surgery for ileal pouch outlet obstruction. Br J Surg 1996;83(3):368–71.
28. Heald RJ, Allen DR. Stapled ileoanal anastomosis: a technique to avoid mucosal proctectomy in the ileal pouch operation. Br J Surg 1986;73(7):571–2.
29. Curran FT, Hill GL. Symptomatic colitis in the anal canal after restorative proctocolectomy. Aust N Z J Surg 1992;62(12):941–3.
30. Lavery IC, Sirimarco MT, Ziv Y, et al. Anal canal inflammation after ileal pouch–anal anastomosis. The need for treatment. Dis Colon Rectum 1995;38(8): 803–6.
31. Schmitt SL, Wexner SD, Lucas FV, et al. Retained mucosa after double-stapled ileal reservoir and ileoanal anastomosis. Dis Colon Rectum 1992;35(11):1051–6.
32. Thompson-Fawcett MW, Mortensen NJ, Warren BF. Cuffitis and inflammatory changes in the columnar cuff, anal transitional zone, and ileal reservoir after stapled pouch—anal anastomosis. Dis Colon Rectum 1999;42(3):348–55.
33. Sequens R. Cancer in the anal canal (transitional zone) after restorative proctocolectomy with stapled ileal pouch–anal anastomosis. Int J Colorectal Dis 1997; 12(4):254–5.
34. Fazio VW, Tjandra JJ. Transanal mucosectomy. Ileal pouch advancement for anorectal dysplasia or inflammation after restorative proctocolectomy. Dis Colon Rectum 1994;37(10):1008–11.
35. Tulchinsky H, McCourtney JS, Rao KV, et al. Salvage abdominal surgery in patients with a retained rectal stump after restorative proctocolectomy and stapled anastomosis. Br J Surg 2001;88(12):1602–6.
36. Oresland T, Fasth S, Nordgren S, et al. Pouch size: the important functional determinant after restorative proctocolectomy. Br J Surg 1990;77(3):265–9.

37. Heppell J, Kelly KA, Phillips SF, et al. Physiologic aspects of continence after colectomy, mucosal proctectomy, and endorectal ileoanal anastomosis. Ann Surg 1982;195(4):435–43.
38. Klas J, Myers GA, Starling JR, et al. Physiologic evaluation and surgical management of failed ileoanal pouch. Dis Colon Rectum 1998;41(7):854–61.
39. Thompson-Fawcett MW, Jewell DP, Mortensen NJ. Ileoanal reservoir dysfunction: a problem-solving approach. Br J Surg 1997;84(10):1351–9.
40. Thompson JS, Quigley EM. Anal sphincteroplasty for incontinence after ileal pouch–anal anastomosis. Report of two cases. Dis Colon Rectum 1995;38(2):215–8.
41. Stahlberg D, Gullberg K, Liljeqvist L, et al. Pouchitis following pelvic pouch operation for ulcerative colitis. Incidence, cumulative risk, and risk factors. Dis Colon Rectum 1996;39(9):1012–8.
42. Romanos J, Samarasekera DN, Stebbing JF, et al. Outcome of 200 restorative proctocolectomy operations: the John Radcliffe hospital experience. Br J Surg 1997;84(6):814–8.
43. Hurst RD, Molinari M, Chung TP, et al. Prospective study of the incidence, timing, and treatment of pouchitis in 104 consecutive patients after restorative proctocolectomy. Arch Surg 1996;131(5):497–500.
44. Lovegrove RE, Tilney HS, Heriot AG, et al. A comparison of adverse events and functional outcomes after restorative proctocolectomy for familial adenomatous polyposis and ulcerative colitis. Dis Colon Rectum 2006;49(9):1293–306.
45. Price AB. Overlap in the spectrum of nonspecific inflammatory bowel disease—colitis indeterminate. J Clin Pathol 1978;31(6):567–77.
46. Veress B, Reinholt FP, Lindquist K, et al. Different types of mucosal adaptation in the ileal reservoir after restorative proctocolectomy. A two-year follow-up study. APMIS 1990;98(9):786–96.
47. Setti Carraro P, Talbot IC, Nicholls RJ. Long-term appraisal of the histological appearances of the ileal reservoir mucosa after restorative proctocolectomy for ulcerative colitis. Gut 1994;35(12):1721–7.
48. Moskowitz RL, Shepherd NA, Nicholls RJ. An assessment of inflammation in the reservoir after restorative proctocolectomy with ileoanal ileal reservoir. Int J Colorectal Dis 1986;1(3):167–74.
49. Sandborn WJ, Tremaine WJ, Batts KP, et al. Pouchitis after ileal pouch–anal anastomosis: a pouchitis disease activity index. Mayo Clin Proc 1994;69(5):409–15.
50. Heuschen UA, Allemeyer EH, Hinz U, et al. Diagnosing pouchitis: comparative validation of two scoring systems in routine follow-up. Dis Colon Rectum 2002;45(6):776–86.
51. Johnson MW, Maestranzi S, Dewar DH, et al. Validation of the new PhiCal faecal calprotectin test as a diagnostic tool for pouchitis. Gut 2006;56(Supp II):A112.
52. Shen B, Fazio VW, Remzi FH, et al. Effect of withdrawal of nonsteroidal anti-inflammatory drug use on ileal pouch disorders. Dig Dis Sci 2007;52:3321–8.
53. Shen B, Achkar JP, Lashner BA, et al. A randomized clinical trial of ciprofloxacin and metronidazole to treat acute pouchitis. Inflamm Bowel Dis 2001;7(4):301–5.
54. Mimura T, Rizzello F, Helwig U, et al. Four-week open-label trial of metronidazole and ciprofloxacin for the treatment of recurrent or refractory pouchitis. Aliment Pharmacol Ther 2002;16(5):909–17.
55. Gionchetti P, Rizzello F, Venturi A, et al. Antibiotic combination therapy in patients with chronic, treatment-resistant pouchitis. Aliment Pharmacol Ther 1999;13(6):713–8.
56. Pardi DS, Sandborn WJ. Systematic review: the management of pouchitis. Aliment Pharmacol Ther 2006;23(8):1087–96.

57. Gionchetti P, Rizzello F, Poggioli G, et al. Oral budesonide in the treatment of chronic refractory pouchitis. Aliment Pharmacol Ther 2007;25(10):1231–6.
58. Gionchetti P, Rizzello F, Venturi A, et al. Oral bacteriotherapy as maintenance treatment in patients with chronic pouchitis: a double-blind, placebo-controlled trial. Gastroenterology 2000;119(2):305–9.
59. Mimura T, Rizzello F, Helwig U, et al. Once-daily high-dose probiotic therapy (vsl#3) for maintaining remission in recurrent or refractory pouchitis. Gut 2004;53(1):108–14.
60. Shen B, Brzezinski A, Fazio VW, et al. Maintenance therapy with a probiotic in antibiotic-dependent pouchitis: experience in clinical practice. Aliment Pharmacol Ther 2005;22(8):721–8.
61. Bell AJ, Price AB, Forbes A, et al. Prepouch ileitis: a disease of the ileum in ulcerative colitis after restorative proctocolectomy. Colorectal Dis 2006;8(5):402–10.
62. Bain IM, Mostafa AB, Harding LK, et al. Bile acid absorption from ileoanal pouches using enema scintigraphy. Br J Surg 1995;82(5):614–7.

Functional and Chronic Anorectal and Pelvic Pain Disorders

Adil E. Bharucha, MBBS, MD[a,*], Emanuel Trabuco, MD[b]

KEYWORDS

- Anorectal pain • Pelvic pain • Levator ani syndrome
- Proctalgia fugax • Interstitial cystitis • Chronic prostatitis

Several organic and functional disorders of the urinary bladder, reproductive tract, anorectum, and the pelvic floor musculature cause pelvic pain. This article describes functional disorders in which chronic pelvic and anorectal pain cannot be explained by a structural or other specified pathology.[1] Currently, these functional disorders are classified into urogynecologic conditions (ie, chronic prostatitis and chronic pelvic pain syndrome [CP-CPPS] or interstitial cystitis and painful bladder syndrome [IC-PBS]); anorectal disorders (ie, proctalgia fugax); and the levator ani syndrome. Although these disorders are defined by predominant pain, they can be associated with functional disturbances (ie, disordered voiding or defecation). Although this nomenclature suggests that these conditions are distinct, there is considerable overlap of their symptoms, which is perhaps inevitable because the urogenital tract and anorectum are in proximity and intimately related to the levator ani, because visceral discomfort is poorly localized, and because pelvic floor dysfunctions can impair urogenital and anorectal functioning. Indeed, these disorders have much in common. Not only is there overlap among urogynecologic symptoms (eg, CP, benign prostatic hypertrophy, and IC)[2] but also between pain in the urinary bladder (eg, in IC) and sacrum, coccyx, and anus.[3]

Cardinal features of chronic functional anorectal and urogynecologic disorders include the following:

- Disorders are diagnosed by symptoms, supplemented by objective findings in IC
- Predominant symptom is discomfort or pain; patients may also have dysfunctional voiding or defecation

This study was supported in part by USPHS National Institutes of Health grant P01 DK068055, and by the Mayo CTSA grant M01-RR00585 from the National Institutes of Health in support of the Physiology Laboratory and Patient Care Cores.
[a] Division of Gastroenterology and Hepatology, College of Medicine, Mayo Clinic, 200 First Street, SW, Rochester, MN 55905, USA
[b] Department of Obstetrics and Gynecology, College of Medicine, Mayo Clinic, 200 First Street, SW, Rochester, MN 55905, USA
* Corresponding author. Clinical Enteric Neuroscience Translational and Epidemiologic Research Program (CENTER), Mayo Clinic, 200 First Street, SW, Rochester, MN 55905.
E-mail address: bharucha.adil@mayo.edu (A.E. Bharucha).

Gastroenterol Clin N Am 37 (2008) 685–696
doi:10.1016/j.gtc.2008.06.002
gastro.theclinics.com

Clinical Features

Among women with chronic pelvic pain, gynecologic conditions (eg, endometriosis, ovarian cysts), painful intercourse, and urinary urgency and frequency were more common than in age-matched controls.[9] In patients presenting for care, chronic pelvic pain is frequently severe and interferes with lifestyle.[9] Indeed, the sickness impact is similar to that for myocardial infarction and Crohn's disease.[72] Compared with age-matched controls, men with CP-CPPS are more likely to have cardiovascular disease, neurologic disease, sinusitis, and anxiety or depression.[73]

Diagnostic Testing

Testing to try and identify specific and it is hoped treatable causes of pelvic pain should be performed. In most men, however, no such cause is identified. In addition to history and physical examination (including digital rectal examination), urinalysis and urine cultures should be performed. A preprostate and postprostate massage urine is as sensitive and specific as the four-glass test for diagnosing chronic bacterial prostatitis.[74] Other tests for consideration, which are detailed elsewhere, include prostatic ultrasound, urethral swab, urodynamic studies, and prostate-specific antigen.

Management

Although the evidence is mixed, a 4- to 6-week course of antibiotics in men with CP-CPPS is frequently prescribed.[68] Repeated courses of antibiotics are not advisable. α_1-Adrenergic antagonists may also be effective when used for at least 3 months or longer. Tricyclic antidepressants (eg, nortriptyline beginning at 10 mg a day and increasing gradually up to a maximum of 75–100 mg daily if necessary) may ameliorate pain by inhibiting neuronal uptake of norepinephrine and serotonin and thereby modulating visceral hypersensitivity. Other agents that have been tried with variable benefit include finasteride and the anti-inflammatory bioflavonoid quercetin.

Pelvic floor physical therapy not only improved overall symptoms but also improved sexual dysfunction.[75] Acupuncture has also been suggested.[76] Prostate-specific therapies, such as microwave thermotherapy or transurethral needle ablation, have limited efficacy.[77]

REFERENCES

1. Clemens JQ. Male and female pelvic pain disorders: is it all in their heads? J Urol 2008;179:813–4.
2. Barry MJ, Link CL, McNaughton-Collins MF, et al. Boston Area Community Health I. Overlap of different urological symptom complexes in a racially and ethnically diverse, community-based population of men and women. BJU Int 2008;101(1): 45–51.
3. Lilius HG, Oravisto KJ, Valtonen EJ. Origin of pain in interstitial cystitis: effect of ultrasound treatment on the concomitant levator ani spasm syndrome. Scand J Urol Nephrol 1973;7(2):150–2.
4. Williams RE, Hartmann KE, Steege JF. Documenting the current definitions of chronic pelvic pain: implications for research. Obstet Gynecol 2004;103(4): 686–91.
5. Thiele GH. Coccygodynia: cause and treatment. Dis Colon Rectum 1963;6: 422–36.
6. Grant SR, Salvati EP, Rubin RJ. Levator syndrome: an analysis of 316 cases. Dis Colon Rectum 1975;18(2):161–3.

7. Drossman DA, Li Z, Andruzzi E, et al. U.S. householder survey of functional gastrointestinal disorders: prevalence, sociodemography, and health impact. Dig Dis Sci 1993;38(9):1569–80.
8. Peters KM, Carrico DJ, Kalinowski SE, et al. Prevalence of pelvic floor dysfunction in patients with interstitial cystitis. Urology 2007;70(1):16–8.
9. Tu FF, Holt JJ, Gonzales J, et al. Physical therapy evaluation of patients with chronic pelvic pain: a controlled study. Am J Obstet Gynecol 2008;198(3): 272.e1–7.
10. Grimaud JC, Bouvier M, Naudy B, et al. Manometric and radiologic investigations and biofeedback treatment of chronic idiopathic anal pain. Dis Colon Rectum 1991;34(8):690–5.
11. Anderson RU, Orenberg EK, Chan CA, et al. Psychometric profiles and hypothalamic-pituitary-adrenal axis function in men with chronic prostatitis/ chronic pelvic pain syndrome. [see comment]. J Urology 2008;179(3):956–60.
12. Bharucha AE, Wald A, Enck P, et al. Functional anorectal disorders. Gastroenterology 2006;130(5):1510–8.
13. Heymen S, Wexner SD, Gulledge AD. MMPI assessment of patients with functional bowel disorders. Dis Colon Rectum 1993;36(6):593–6.
14. Sohn N, Weinstein MA, Robbins RD. The levator syndrome and its treatment with high-voltage electrogalvanic stimulation. Am J Surg 1982;144(5):580–2.
15. Nicosia JF, Abcarian H. Levator syndrome: a treatment that works. Dis Colon Rectum 1985;28(6):406–8.
16. Billingham RP, Isler JT, Friend WG, et al. Treatment of levator syndrome using high-voltage electrogalvanic stimulation. Dis Colon Rectum 1987;30(8):584–7.
17. Ger GC, Wexner SD, Jorge JM, et al. Evaluation and treatment of chronic intractable rectal pain: a frustrating endeavor. Dis Colon Rectum 1993;36(2):139–45.
18. Gilliland R, Heymen JS, Altomare DF, et al. Biofeedback for intractable rectal pain: outcome and predictors of success. Dis Colon Rectum 1997;40(2):190–6.
19. Heah SM, Ho YH, Tan M, et al. Biofeedback is effective treatment for levator ani syndrome. Dis Colon Rectum 1997;40(2):187–9.
20. Thiele GH. Tonic spasm of the levator ani, coccygeus and piriformis muscle: relationship to coccygodynia and pain in the region of the hip and down the leg. Transactions of the American Proctologic Society 1936;37:145–55.
21. Oyama IA, Rejba A, Lukban JC, et al. Modified Thiele massage as therapeutic intervention for female patients with interstitial cystitis and high-tone pelvic floor dysfunction. Urology 2004;64(5):862–5.
22. Dodi G, Bogoni F, Infantino A, et al. Hot or cold in anal pain? A study of the changes in internal anal sphincter pressure profiles. Dis Colon Rectum 1986; 29(4):248–51.
23. Thompson WG. Proctalgia fugax. Dig Dis Sci 1981;26(12):1121–4.
24. Rao SS, Hatfield RA. Paroxysmal anal hyperkinesis: a characteristic feature of proctalgia fugax. Gut 1996;39:609–12.
25. Eckardt VF, Dodt O, Kanzler G, et al. Anorectal function and morphology in patients with sporadic proctalgia fugax. Dis Colon Rectum 2004;39:755–62.
26. Pilling LF, Swenson WM, Hill JR. The psychologic aspects of proctalgia fugax. Dis Colon Rectum 1965;8(5):372–6.
27. Kamm MA, Hoyle CH, Burleigh DE, et al. Hereditary internal anal sphincter myopathy causing proctalgia fugax and constipation: a newly identified condition. Gastroenterology 1991;100(3):805–10.
28. Celik AF, Katsinelos P, Read NW, et al. Hereditary proctalgia fugax and constipation: report of a second family. Gut 1995;36(4):581–4.

69. Pontari MA. Chronic prostatitis/chronic pelvic pain syndrome. Urol Clin N Am 2008;35(1):81–9, vi.
70. Yang CC, Lee JC, Kromm BG, et al. Pain sensitization in male chronic pelvic pain syndrome: why are symptoms so difficult to treat? J Urol 2003;170(3):823–6 [discussion: 6–7].
71. Mehik A, Hellstrom P, Sarpola A, et al. Fears, sexual disturbances and personality features in men with prostatitis: a population-based cross-sectional study in Finland. BJU Int 2001;88(1):35–8.
72. Tripp DA, Curtis Nickel J, Landis JR, et al. Predictors of quality of life and pain in chronic prostatitis/chronic pelvic pain syndrome: findings from the National Institutes of Health Chronic Prostatitis Cohort Study. BJU Int 2004;94(9):1279–82.
73. Wenninger K, Heiman JR, Rothman I, et al. Sickness impact of chronic nonbacterial prostatitis and its correlates. J Urol 1996;155(3):965–8.
74. Pontari MA, McNaughton-Collins M, O'Leary MP, et al. A case-control study of risk factors in men with chronic pelvic pain syndrome. BJU Int 2005;96(4):559–65.
75. Nickel JC, Shoskes D, Wang Y, et al. How does the pre-massage and post-massage 2-glass test compare to the Meares-Stamey 4-glass test in men with chronic prostatitis/chronic pelvic pain syndrome? J Urol 2006;176(1):119–24.
76. Anderson RU, Wise D, Sawyer T, et al. Sexual dysfunction in men with chronic prostatitis/chronic pelvic pain syndrome: improvement after trigger point release and paradoxical relaxation training. J Urol 2006;176(4 Pt 1):1534–8 [discussion: 8–9].
77. Chen R, Nickel JC. Acupuncture ameliorates symptoms in men with chronic prostatitis/chronic pelvic pain syndrome. [see comment]. Urology 2003;61(6):1156–9 [discussion: 9].
78. Zeitlin SI. Heat therapy in the treatment of prostatitis. Urology 2002;60(6 Suppl): 38–40 [discussion: 1].
79. Barry MJ, Fowler FJ Jr, O'Leary MP, et al. The American Urological Association symptom index for benign prostatic hyperplasia. The Measurement Committee of the American Urological Association. J Urol 1992;148(5):1549–57 [discussion: 64].
80. Litwin MS, McNaughton-Collins M, Fowler FJ Jr, et al. The National Institutes of Health chronic prostatitis symptom index: development and validation of a new outcome measure. Chronic Prostatitis Collaborative Research Network. J Urol 1999;162(2):369–75.

Urinary and Fecal Incontinence in Nursing Home Residents

Felix W. Leung, MD[a,b], John F. Schnelle, PhD[c,*]

KEYWORDS

• Fecal incontinence • Constipation • Urinary incontinence

Urinary incontinence (UI) and fecal incontinence (FI) are commonly encountered in nursing home residents, and are associated with significant morbidity and use of health care resources. UI has been estimated to affect between 50% and 65% of nursing home residents, and most of these residents also have FI.[1–3] The fact that so many nursing home residents have both UI and FI suggests a common cause.[3] A recent follow-up study of residents in skilled nursing facilities in Wisconsin[4] confirmed that dementia and advancing age were consistently associated with the development of incontinence, but the strongest associations were impairment of activities of daily living and the use of patient restraints.

PATHOPHYSIOLOGY OF URINARY INCONTINENCE

Numerous physical disorders contribute to the pathogenesis of UI among nursing home residents. Urologic, gynecologic, and neurologic disorders, and functional impairments, particularly dementia and lack of mobility (including bed restraints), are primary factors.[5] Many cross-sectional studies have demonstrated that UI and FI are associated with urinary tract infections, respiratory infections, constipation, and other disorders.[6–9] Recent studies suggest, however, that reducing UI and FI alone does not improve skin health or reduce hospitalizations or decrease urinary tract

Supported in part by VA Clinical Merit Research Funds (FWL) and National Institutes of Health grant 1R02 AG 23,555-01A1 "Interventions to Improve Fecal Incontinence" (JFS).
[a] David Geffen School of Medicine at University of California, Los Angeles, Los Angeles, CA 90024, USA
[b] Sepulveda Ambulatory Care Center, VA Greater Los Angeles Healthcare System, 16111 Plummer Street, North Hills, CA 91343, USA
[c] Center for Quality Aging, Vanderbilt University Medical Center, Department of Medicine, 1161 21st Avenue South, S-1121 Medical Center North, VUMC, Nashville, TN 37232–2400, USA
* Corresponding author.
E-mail address: john.schnelle@vanderbilt.edu (J.F. Schnelle).

Gastroenterol Clin N Am 37 (2008) 697–707
doi:10.1016/j.gtc.2008.06.005 gastro.theclinics.com

infections.[10,11] Multifaceted interventions may be necessary to improve the chronic health problems associated with both forms of incontinence among nursing home residents.[12]

It is important to diagnose and treat the underlying disorders, especially reversible conditions, to reduce the severity and frequency of incontinence episodes. Even when physiologic conditions are improved, however, nursing home residents may continue to have "functional" incontinence for several primary reasons: (1) lack of mental awareness; (2) physical inability to properly toilet themselves; (3) failure of understaffed nursing homes to provide residents with frequent assistance in toileting (prompted voiding); and (4) tendency by staff to rely heavily on special undergarments and absorbent pads. This article reviews the risk factors for the development of UI and FI and addresses how nursing homes can reduce incontinence by providing residents with adequate toileting assistance in the face of staff and funding limitations.

Medical documentation about the daily care delivery may be so erroneous that even the best-intentioned efforts to improve the care received by residents may not be successful.[13] A culture of inaccurate documentation is largely created by a discrepancy between expectations for health care placed on nursing homes by regulatory guidelines and inadequate reimbursement and staffing to fulfill these expectations. Nursing home staff has little incentive to implement the technologies necessary to audit and ensure data quality if accurate documentation reveals that care consistent with regulatory guidelines is not or cannot be provided because of inadequate staff. A survey process that largely focuses on chart documentation to assess quality provides further incentive for care-process documentation as opposed to care-process delivery.

There are two potential solutions to this problem. The first solution is to maximize the efficiency of available staff resources by targeting residents for toileting programs who are most responsive. This at least makes it more feasible for staff to provide adequate toileting assistance to a subset of residents and in so doing increases the probability of accurate documentation. Validated methods to accomplish such targeting are described later in this article. The second solution is to implement quality monitoring programs that collect information for improvement purposes as opposed to for compliance purposes. This information could be stored out of the medical record and hence protected from survey scrutiny, which reduces another source of motivation for inaccurate documentation. Methods to collect accurate data about care and the type of data that are useful for improvement have been described.[14]

URINARY INCONTINENCE AMONG NURSING HOME RESIDENTS

Immobility and dementia are the most critical factors contributing to the development of UI in nursing home residents. In three clinical trials assessing the prevalence of UI,[12,15,16] 60% to 90% of incontinent nursing home residents had significant mobility problems and the average Mini-Mental Status Score for incontinent residents ranged from 8 to 14, indicating severe cognitive impairment. These data support the conclusions of other research identifying immobility and dementia as the primary risk factors for developing UI.[17]

Immobility increases the likelihood of incontinence among nursing home residents by preventing them from getting to the toilet; dementia reduces their motivation to do so. There is also ample evidence of dysfunction in the lower urinary tract among nursing home residents.[5,18,19] Any intervention in the nursing home setting, however, must consider immobility and dementia as first-stage treatment priorities. Treating the bladder abnormalities alone will not alleviate UI especially if the resident lacks consistent access to and motivation to use a toilet.

Constipation, fecal impaction, and overflow FI are common events in nursing home residents. Until recently, in the absence of comprehensive anorectal testing, drug-induced constipation was considered the most likely explanation. The high prevalence of constipation in nursing home residents, however, is only partly caused by adverse drug effects.[35] A recent study reported systematic anorectal testing of nursing home residents with FI. This preliminary report documented for the first time impaired sphincter function (risk factor for FI), decreased rectal sensation, and sphincter dyssynergia (risk factor for constipation and impaction) affecting up to 75% of the assessed residents.[36] The sphincter dyssynergia documented in these nursing home residents with FI[36] has shed new light on the frequent association between constipation and FI in nursing home residents.

TREATMENT OPTIONS FOR FECAL INCONTINENCE AMONG NURSING HOME RESIDENTS

Unlike UI there is a paucity of data derived from randomized controlled trials of treatment regimens of FI in the nursing home setting. A Medline search of publications from 1966 to 2008 performed on May 10, 2008, yielded the following number of citations: FI (n = 6469); nursing home (n = 27343); randomized controlled trial (n = 56019); evidence based (n = 40500); FI and nursing home (n = 126); FI, nursing home, and randomized controlled trial (n = 0); FI, nursing home, and evidence based (n = 0). Much of what follows is a narration of clinical experience repeatedly reviewed in the literature.

When FI is associated with diarrhea, it is important to treat underlying disorders, such as lactose malabsorption (or intolerance), bile salt malabsorption, and inflammatory bowel disease. Antidiarrheal medications, such as loperamide[37] and diphenoxylate,[37] or bile acid binders, such as cholestyramine,[38] may help. Gradually increasing the intake of dietary fiber can relieve constipation for many elderly subjects. Stool softeners, saline laxatives, stimulant laxatives, and single-agent osmotic products are frequently administered as prophylactic treatment against constipation and impaction. In a study of institutionalized elderly patients,[39] the use of a single osmotic agent with a rectal stimulant and weekly enemas to achieve complete rectal emptying reduced the frequency of FI by 35% and the incidence of soiling by 42%. If fecal impaction is not relieved by laxatives and better toileting, a regimen should be implemented using manual disimpaction, tap water enemas two or three times weekly, and possible use of rectal suppositories.[40] In the presence of impaired sphincter function and decreased rectal sensation, however, the fluidity of the stool induced by the use of laxatives and stool softeners administered to prevent constipation and impaction may predispose the nursing home residents to manifest FI. The recent finding of anal sphincter dyssynergia in a high proportion of nursing home residents with FI[36] suggests that a new approach to the management of FI should consist of neuromuscular conditioning to improve the dyssynergic sphincter function. Even though the efficacy of biofeedback therapy has been demonstrated by a randomized controlled trial in ambulatory patients,[41] in nursing home residents dementia and immobility may limit the effectiveness of such treatment. Other novel approaches deserve to be considered.

SKIN CARE IN NURSING HOME RESIDENTS WITH INCONTINENCE

The use of a defined skin care regimen that includes a cleanser and a moisture barrier is associated with a low rate of incontinence-associated dermatitis in these incontinent residents, and use of a polymer skin barrier film three times weekly is effective in preventing incontinence-associated skin breakdown.[42] One uncontrolled trial focused on an innovative adult brief that encouraged skin cleansing during incontinence care. The system was easily and effectively incorporated into the nursing home, and was used and favored by certified nurse assistants whenever available (97% of the time). Patterns of incontinence care differed at follow-up with one-step incontinence system compared with wipes placed at the bedside, with fewer linens used, fewer wipes used, and less certified nurse assistant interruption during care.[43]

SUMMARY

Multiple studies have shown that dementia and health-related or restraint-related immobility contribute to UI and FI. These factors must be considered when developing interventions to improve UI or FI in nursing home residents. Two clinical intervention trials[11,27] that evaluated the effects of prompted voiding on UI and FI have demonstrated that scheduled toileting significantly increased the rates of appropriate urinary and fecal voids and can decrease the frequency of UI. Only the trial that combined prompted voiding with a fluid intake and exercise protocol, however, resulted in a significant decrease in the frequency of FI episodes. Even in this successful trial,[11] the overall rate of bowel movements remained low: during 2 days of hourly checks, 43% of residents had no bowel movements, despite consistent toileting assistance, exercise, and increased fluid intake and exercise. Fifty-six percent of the control subjects who received no intervention also had no bowel movements during the 2 days of hourly checks. The recently described high prevalence of sphincter dyssynergia in nursing home residents with FI[36] may offer the missing link in this enigma.

FUTURE RESEARCH

Longer measurement periods, control for laxatives and medications with constipating side effects, and an intervention to increase both food and fluid intake are necessary. Feeding assistance protocols that significantly improve caloric intake in this population[44] should also be considered. Staff time requirements need to be documented. The addition of simple behavioral modification of advice to refrain from straining, so as not to trigger the development of sphincter dyssynergia, and the use of bulking agents[45–58] combined with scheduled toileting[11,27] should be compared with usual laxative prophylactic management. Finally, the role that inadequate staffing and staff management have in contributing to incontinence in so many residents should continue to be documented until policy-level changes are made in how nursing homes are reimbursed and evaluated. For FI treatment, toileting assistance is logical. The effectiveness and time requirement of a comprehensive program addressing not only immobility and dementia but also other factors including physical activity, medications, disimpaction, and resolution of sphincter dyssynergia remain to be evaluated.

REFERENCES

1. Johanson JF, Irizarry F, Doughty A. Risk factors for fecal incontinence in a nursing home population. J Clin Gastroenterol 1997;24:156–60.
2. Harrington C, Carrillo H, Thollaug SC, et al. Nursing facilities, staffing, residents, and facility deficiencies, 1993 through 1999. San Francisco (CA): Department of Social and Behavioral Sciences, University of California; 2000.
3. Chiang L, Ouslander J, Schnelle JF, et al. Dually incontinent nursing home residents: clinical characteristics and treatment differences. J Am Geriatr Soc 2000;48:673–6.
4. Nelson RL, Furner SE. Risk factors for the development of fecal and urinary incontinence in Wisconsin nursing home residents. Maturitas 2005;52(1):26–31.

5. Ouslander JG, Schnelle JF. Incontinence in the nursing home. Ann Intern Med 1995;122:438–49.
6. Schnelle JF, Adamson GM, Cruise PA, et al. Skin disorders and moisture in incontinent nursing home residents: intervention implications. J Am Geriatr Soc 1997; 45:1182–8.
7. Beck-Sague C, Banerjee S, Jarvis WR. Infectious diseases and mortality among US nursing home residents. Am J Epidemiol 1993;83:1739–42.
8. Murtaugh C, Freiman MP. Nursing home residents at risk of hospitalization and the characteristics of their hospital stays. Gerontologist 1995;35:35–43.
9. Brandeis GH, Ooi WL, Hossain M, et al. A longitudinal study of risk factors associated with the formation of pressure ulcers in nursing homes. J Am Geriatr Soc 1994;42:388–93.
10. Bates-Jensen BM, Alessi CA, Al-Samarrai NR, et al. The effects of an exercise and incontinence intervention on skin health outcomes in nursing home residents. J Am Geriatr Soc 2003;51:348–55.
11. Schnelle JF, Kapur K, Alessi CA, et al. Does an exercise and incontinence intervention save health care costs in a nursing home population. J Am Geriatr Soc 2003;51:161–8.
12. Schnelle JF, MacRae PG, Ouslander JG, et al. Functional incidental training, mobility performance, and incontinence care with nursing home residents. J Am Geriatr Soc 1995;43:1356–62.
13. Schnelle JF, Bates-Jensen BM, Chu L, et al. Accuracy of nursing home medical record information about care-process delivery: implications for staff management and improvement. J Am Geriatr Soc 2004;52(8):1378–83.
14. Schnelle JF. Continuous quality improvement in nursing homes: public relations or a reality? J Am Med Dir Assoc 2007;8(1):S2–5.
15. Schnelle JF, Alessi CA, Simmons SF, et al. Translating clinical research into practice: a randomized controlled trial of exercise and incontinence care with nursing home residents. J Am Geriatr Soc 2002;50:1476–83.
16. Ouslander JG, Schnelle JF, Uman G, et al. Does oxybutynin add to the effectiveness of prompted voiding for urinary incontinence among nursing home residents? J Am Geriatr Soc 1995;43:610–7.
17. Resnick NM, Yalla SV, Laurino E. The pathophysiology of urinary incontinence among institutionalized elderly persons. N Engl J Med 1989;320:1–7.
18. Resnick NM, Yalla SV. Detrusor hyperactivity with impaired contractile function: an unrecognized but common cause of incontinence in elderly patients. J Am Med Assoc 1987;257:3076–81.
19. Schnelle JF. Treatment of urinary incontinence in nursing home patients by prompted voiding. J Am Geriatr Soc 1990;38:356–60.
20. Schnelle JF. Incontinence. In: Bellack AS, Hersen M, editors. Comprehensive clinical psychology. New York: Pergamon; 1998. p. 433–54.
21. Schnelle JF, Ouslander JG, Simmons SF. Predicting nursing home resident responsiveness to a urinary incontinence treatment protocol. Int Urogynecol J 1993;4:89–94.
22. Ouslander JG, Schnelle JF, Uman G, et al. Predictors of successful prompted voiding among incontinent nursing home residents. J Am Med Assoc 1995; 273:1366–70.
23. Schnelle JF, Ouslander JG. Management of incontinence in long term care. Missouri (MO): Mosby Year book Inc.; 1997. p. 405–13.
24. Johnson TM, Ouslander JG, Uman GC, et al. Urinary incontinence treatment preferences in long-term care. J Am Geriatr Soc 2001;49:710–8.

25. Chassagne P, Landrin I, Neveu C, et al. Fecal incontinence in the institutionalized elderly: incidence, risk factors, and prognosis. Am J Med 1999;106:185–90.
26. Borrie MJ, Davidson HA. Incontinence in institutions: costs and contributing factors. CMAJ 1992;147:322–8.
27. Ouslander JG, Simmons S, Schnelle JF, et al. Effects of prompted voiding on fecal continence among nursing home residents. J Am Geriatr Soc 1996;44:424–8.
28. Rao SSC, Leung F. Treatment of fecal incontinence in the elderly. In: Mezey M, editor. The encyclopedia of elder care: the comprehensive resource on geriatric and social care. New York: Springer; 2001. p. 261–4.
29. Leung FW, Karyotakis NC, Rahman HU, et al. Fecal incontinence in a nursing home and an ambulatory population. [abstract]. Gastroenterology 1998;114:A778.
30. Muller-Lissner S. General geriatrics and gastroenterology: constipation and faecal incontinence. Best Pract Res Clin Gastroenterol 2002;16:115–33.
31. De Lillo AR, Rose S. Functional bowel disorders in the geriatric patient: constipation, fecal impaction, and fecal incontinence. Am J Gastroenterol 2000;95:901–5.
32. Madoff RD, Williams JG, Caushaj PF. Fecal incontinence. N Engl J Med 1992;326: 1002–7.
33. Hirsh T, Lembo T. Diagnosis and management of fecal incontinence in elderly patients. Am Fam Physician 1996;54:1559–64.
34. Kinnunen O, Jauhonen P, Salokannel J, et al. Diarrhea and fecal impaction in elderly long-stay patients. Z Gerontol 1989;22:321–3.
35. van Dijk KN, de Vries CS, van den Berg PB, et al. Constipation as an adverse effect of drug use in nursing home patients: an overestimated risk. Br J Clin Pharmacol 1998;46(3):255–61.
36. Leung FW, Beard MH, Grbic V, et al. Dyssynergia: key pathophysiologic mechanism for fecal incontinence (FI) in nursing home residents. Am J Gastroenterol 2007;102(S2):386 [abstract].
37. Harford WV, Krejs GJ, Santa Ana CA, et al. Acute effect of diphenoxylate with atropine (Lomotil) in patients with chronic diarrhea and fecal incontinence. Gastroenterology 1980;78(3):440–3.
38. Remes-Troche JM, Ozturk R, Philips C, et al. Cholestyramine: a useful adjunct for the treatment of patients with fecal incontinence. Int J Colorectal Dis 2008;23(2): 189–94 [Epub 2007 Oct 16].
39. Chassagne P, Jego A, Gloc P, et al. Does treatment of constipation improve faecal incontinence in institutionalized elderly patients? Age Ageing 2000;29: 159–64.
40. Whitehead WE, Wald A, Norton NJ. Treatment options for fecal incontinence. Dis Colon Rectum 2001;44(1):131–42 [discussion: 142–4].
41. Rao SS, Seaton K, Miller M, et al. Randomized controlled trial of biofeedback, sham feedback, and standard therapy for dyssynergic defecation. Clin Gastroenterol Hepatol 2007;5(3):331–8.
42. Bliss DZ, Zehrer C, Savik K, et al. An economic evaluation of four skin damage prevention regimens in nursing home residents with incontinence: economics of skin damage prevention. J Wound Ostomy Continence Nurs 2007;34(2): 143–52.
43. Al-Samarrai NR, Uman GC, Al-Samarrai T, et al. Introducing a new incontinence management system for nursing home residents. J Am Med Dir Assoc 2007;8(4): 253–61.
44. Simmons S, Osterweil D, Schnelle JF. Improving food intake in nursing home residents with feeding assistance: a staffing analysis. J Gerontol A Biol Sci Med Sci 2001;56A:M790–4.

45. Karam SE, Nies DM. Student/staff collaboration: a pilot bowel management program. J Gerontol Nurs 1994;20(3):32–40.
46. Khaja M, Thakur CS, Bharathan T, et al. Fiber 7 supplement as an alternative to laxatives in a nursing home. Gerodontology 2005;22(2):106–8.
47. Simmons SF, Schnelle JF. Strategies to measure nursing home residents' satisfaction and preferences related to incontinence and mobility care: implications for evaluating intervention effects. Gerontologist 1999;39:345–55.
48. Bowers B, Becker M. Nurse's aides in nursing homes: the relationship between organization and quality. Gerontologist 1992;32:360–6.
49. Bowers BJ, Esmond S, Jacobson N. The relationship between staffing and quality in long-term care facilities: exploring the view of nurse aides. J Nurs Care Qual 2000;14:55–64.
50. Lekan-Rutledge D, Palmer MH, Belyea M. In their own words: nursing assistants' perceptions of barriers to implementation of prompted voiding in long-term care. Gerontologist 1998;38:370–8.
51. Schnelle JF, Cretin S, Saliba D, et al. Minimum nurse aide staffing required to implement best practice care in nursing homes. Report to Congress: appropriateness of minimum nurse staffing ratios in nursing homes, vol. II. Health Care Financing Administration; 2000 [chapter 14].
52. Schnelle JF, Simmons SF, Cretin S. Minimum nurse aide staffing required to implement best practice care in nursing homes. Report to Congress: phase II final. Appropriateness of minimum nurse staffing ratios in nursing homes, vol. I. Health Care Financing Administration; 2001 [chapter 3].
53. Feuerberg M. Report to Congress (executive summary). Appropriateness of minimum nurse staffing ratios in nursing homes, vol. I. Health Care Financing Administration; 2000 [chapter 1].
54. Schnelle JF, Newman DR, Fogarty TE. Management of patient continence in long-term care nursing facilities. Gerontologist 1990;30:373–6.
55. Schnelle JF, Newman D, White M, et al. Maintaining continence in nursing home residents through the application of industrial quality control. Gerontologist 1993;33:114–21.
56. Schnelle JF, McNees P, Crooks V, et al. The use of a computer-based model to disseminate an incontinence management program. Gerontologist 1995;35:656–65.
57. Levy-Storms L, Schnelle JF, Simmons SF. What do family members notice following an intervention to improve mobility and incontinence care for nursing home residents? An analysis of open-ended comments. Gerontologist 2007;47(1):14–20.
58. Schnelle JF, Cadogan MP, Yoshii J, et al. The minimum data set urinary incontinence quality indicators: do they reflect differences in care processes related to incontinence. Med Care 2003;41:909–22.

Pediatric Anorectal Disorders

Paola Masi, MD, Erasmo Miele, MD, Annamaria Staiano, MD*

KEYWORDS

- Functional constipation • Organic constipation • Therapy
- Fecal incontinence

Anorectal disorders include a diverse group of functional and pathologic conditions that cause significant patient discomfort and disability. They are common in children and are usually mild and short-lived if the child receives prompt and adequate attention during the early phase of the disorder. Frequently, however, the child presents long after the appearance of initial symptoms, when the symptoms may have become more difficult to treat. Altered stool frequency and altered behavior with defecation are common presenting symptoms in children who have anorectal disorders. These alterations may be affected by several factors such as diet, social habit, convenience, parents' cultural beliefs, interrelationships within the family, and daily timing of activities. In addition, all of the previously described factors may vary in relation to the age and the degree of psychophysical development of the child.[1] It has been estimated that 10% of children are brought to medical attention because of an anorectal disorder, and constipation is the chief reason for these visits to pediatricians.[2]

This article reports the clinical, physiopathologic, diagnostic, and therapeutic aspects of the most common anorectal disorders in children. In particular, it focuses on the differential diagnosis between organic and functional constipation. In addition, the authors separately examine some of the clinical conditions such as atopy, neurologic diseases, and anorectal malformations, in which chronic constipation may be an important clinical manifestation.

CONSTIPATION

Constipation is a symptom rather than a disease and often constitutes a major problem for the child and his or her family. Unfortunately, there is no universally accepted definition of chronic constipation.[3] Recently, a group of pediatric gastroenterologists and pediatricians with an interest in gastrointestinal (GI) motility reached agreement on defining childhood functional defecation disorders.[4] Based on this consensus,

Department of Pediatrics, University of Naples Federico II, Via Pansini, 5, 80131 Naples, Italy
* Corresponding author.
E-mail address: staiano@unina.it (A. Staiano).

Gastroenterol Clin N Am 37 (2008) 709–730
doi:10.1016/j.gtc.2008.07.002

constipation was defined as the occurrence of two or more of the following six characteristics during the previous 8 weeks:

Two or less bowel movements in the toilet per week
One or more episodes of fecal incontinence per week
History of retentive posturing and withholding behavior
History of painful defecation
Presence of large stools in the rectum or palpable on abdominal examination
History of large diameter stools that may obstruct the toilet

The group also adopted the term fecal incontinence to replace the terms encopresis and soiling.[4] With 84% of constipated children suffering from this disorder, the involuntary passing of fecal material in the underwear is one of the major features of childhood constipation.[5–7] Hence, it is important to distinguish between constipation with fecal incontinence and functional nonretentive fecal incontinence (FNRFI), because different pathophysiological mechanisms are involved. Both entities can result in fecal incontinence, but in children who have FNRFI, there are no signs of constipation. In many studies, constipated children who have fecal incontinence and children who have FNRFI are grouped into one study population, because both groups have fecal incontinence. Nevertheless, about 80% of children who have fecal incontinence experience chronic constipation.[6–9]

The normal frequency of bowel movements at different ages has been well-characterized (**Table 1**).[10]

Infants have a mean of 4 stools per day during the first week of life. This frequency gradually declines to a mean average of 1.7 stools per day at 2 years of age and 1.2 stools per day at 4 years of age. Some normal breast-fed babies do not have stools for several days or longer. After 4 years, the frequency of bowel movements remains unchanged.[2,11,12]

A normal pattern of stool evacuation is thought to be a sign of good health in children of all ages. Often, during the first months of life, parents pay close attention to the frequency and characteristics of their child's defecation. Any deviation from what is thought by a family member to be the norm for the child may trigger a call to the nurse or a visit to the pediatrician. In fact, chronic constipation is a source of anxiety for parents who worry that it may be a symptom of serious disease.[12]

Table 1
Normal frequency of bowel movements in children[10]

Age	Bowel Movements Per Week[a]	Bowel Movements Per Day[b]
0–3 months		
Breast-fed	5–40	2.9
Formula-fed	5–28	2
6–12 months	5–28	1.8
1–3 years	4–21	1.4
More than 3 years	3–14	1.0

[a] Approximately mean ± 2SD.
[b] Mean.

Data from Baker S, Di Lorenzo C, Liptak G, et al. Evaluation and the treatment of constipation in infants and children: recommendation of the North American Society for Pediatric Gastroenterology, Hepatology and Nutrition. J Pediatr Gastroenterol Nutr 2006;43:e1–13.

EPIDEMIOLOGY

Constipation is the main complaint in 3% of pediatric outpatient visits.[13]

This percentage increases to 25% to 45% in specific pediatric–GI motility clinics. To date, the worldwide prevalence of constipation in children varies widely and is estimated to range between 0.6% and 29.6%.[14–16] This wide range could be caused by differences in survey methods, age distribution, or definition.[17]

Organic causes actually affect less than 10% of children presenting with constipation. In children who have cerebral palsy or autism, constipation is reported in 26.5% to 74% of subsets.[18,19]

In very low birth weight infants (<750 g), constipation is very common (32%). When evaluated between 10 and 14 years of age, these children continue to experience higher rates of toileting problems such as encopresis and withholding behavior, and neuro-developmental impairment when compared with age-matched children of higher birth weight.[20]

Some children may be genetically predisposed to developing constipation. A family history of constipation has been found in 28% to 50% of cases, and there is a higher incidence in monozygotic twins when compared with dizygotic twins. It has been reported that in some children constipation is associated with specific dermatoglyphic pattern.[21,22] Constipation usually is reported to be more common in boys than in girls, with a 2:1 ratio, although some describe an equal prevalence between the sexes.[23]

PHYSIOLOGY OF DEFECATION

A brief review of the physiology of defecation indicates that there are several motor patterns normally responsible for the movement of colonic contents:

- Segmental, nonpropagated, phasic contractions mixing luminal contents
- Powerful high-amplitude propagated contractions (HAPCs) that propel stools aborally
- Changes in colonic tone[24–26]

An increase in colonic motility and tone after a meal, also known as the gastrocolonic response, moves the stools from the more proximal colon to the rectosigmoid region. The HAPCs are the most powerful contractions found in the large bowel and are the manometric equivalent of the mass movements described in the radiologic literature. The descending fecal bolus distends the empty rectum, stimulating sensory receptors in the bowel wall and pelvic floor. Ascending sensory fibers allow conscious awareness of rectal distension. There is a transient contraction of the voluntary striated muscles, the external anal sphincter (EAS), and the puborectalis sling, the so-called inflation reflex. Transmission of the nerve impulse distally by the myenteric plexus of the lower rectal wall produces a reflex inhibition of the involuntary internal anal sphincter (IAS), the recto–anal inhibitory reflex (RAIR), and of the EAS involving reflex pathways. Several studies in term and preterm infants have shown that the RAIR is present in infants older than 26 weeks gestation.[23] Relaxation of the puborectalis muscle allows widening of the anorectal angle (from resting 60° to 105° to 140°), resulting in an unobstructed anal canal. The increased abdominal pressure and rectal peristalsis result in expulsion of feces and emptying of the entire rectum. Before the acquisition of voluntary control, rectal distension results in EAS loss of electrical activity and tone (inhibition reflex). By 24 to 30 months of age, the maturation of myenteric ganglion cells is associated with persistence of EAS tonic activity mediated by a spinal reflex and augmented by supraspinal cortical centers, allowing the normal inflation reflex and conscious control of defecation.

The sensitive lining of the anoderm perceives the stool, and a conscious decision is made whether to expel it or to postpone defecation by contracting the external anal sphincter and the puborectalis muscle. If defecation is delayed to a later time, significant voluntary effort that includes contraction of the abdominal muscles and relaxation of the pelvic floor will be needed to push the stool into the anal canal and produce a bowel movement. If this sequence is difficult or cannot be produced effectively, constipation ensues.

PATHOGENESIS OF FUNCTIONAL CONSTIPATION

The pathophysiological mechanisms that underlie childhood functional constipation are multifactorial, and not understood well. In 90% to 95% of patients, no specific organic cause can be found.[9]

In some babies, an acute episode of constipation may occur associated with a change in diet. Passage of dry and hard stools may cause anal fissures and pain. Genetic predisposition may play a role, because constipation often dates back to the first months of life, and many patients have a positive family history of constipation.

The timing of toilet training is critical, because constipation may occur as a consequence of conflicts between the child and parents. Retentive posturing is probably the major cause for the development or persistence of constipation in toddlers.

Other causes of stool withholding behavior include the previous passage of large, hard, or painful stools; anal fissures; significant behavioral problems; lack of time for regular toileting; and distaste for toilets other than the child's own.[27]

When the retentive toddler experiences the urge to defecate, he or she assumes an erect posture and holds the legs stiffly together to forcefully contract the pelvic and gluteal muscles. Consequently, the rectum accommodates to its content, and the urge to defecate disappears. The retained stools become progressively more difficult to evacuate, leading to a vicious circle in which the rectum increasingly is distended by large fecal contents. Finally, chronic rectal distension may cause overflow incontinence, loss of rectal sensitivity, and in the end, loss of normal urge to defecate. This aberrant behavior may lead to the unconscious contraction of the external sphincter during defecation.[28,29] Furthermore, abnormalities in rectal function were felt to be responsible for persistent complaints and relapses. Increased compliance of the rectal wall has been proposed as a contributing mechanism for intractable pediatric constipation. A recent study demonstrated that recovered adolescents had a lower rectal compliance when compared with patients who had functional constipation. In almost half of the recovered patients, however, rectal compliance was above the normal range.[30]

FUNCTIONAL CONSTIPATION

The term functional constipation' describes all children in whom constipation does not have an organic etiology. Because functional constipation and functional fecal retention often overlap, the two disorders have been merged into one category termed functional constipation.

Approximately 40% of children who functional constipation develop symptoms during the first year of life, with a peak incidence during the time of toilet training, often between 2 and 4 years of age.[5,31]

A careful history needs to elicit the time after birth of the first bowel movement, the time of onset of the problem, characteristics of stools, the presence of associated symptoms (pain at defecation or fecal incontinence), stool withholding behavior, urinary problems, and neurologic deficits. Fecal incontinence may be mistaken for diarrhea by some parents. Urinary problems are also common in these children.

Onset of constipation frequently occurs during one of three periods: 1) when the infant switched from breast milk to either formula milk or introduction of solids, 2) when the toddler is acquiring toileting skills and finds defecation painful, and 3) when the child starts school (they tend to avoid defecation throughout the school day).

The physical examination includes assessment of the size of the rectal fecal mass, which often is estimated by calculating the height above the pelvic brim with bimanual palpation on either side of the rectus sheath and rectal examination after establishing a relationship with the patient and the family. When the history is typical for functional constipation, the perineum should be inspected, but a digital rectal examination may be delayed to facilitate bonding between the child and the clinician or until failure of a treatment trial. If the clinician plans a single consultation without follow-up, a rectal examination is necessary to evaluate the child for a rare obstructing mass or fecal impaction.

External examination of the perineum and perianal area should exclude signs of spinal dysraphism.

A plain radiograph of the abdomen can be useful for determining the presence of fecal retention in a child who is obese or refuses rectal examination.

Diagnosis

Childhood functional constipation is a clinical diagnosis that can be made in most cases on the basis of a typical history and an essentially normal physical examination. In the absence of red flags, testing is neither necessary nor desirable (**Box 1**).[4] In atypical cases or when conventional treatment fails, the primary care physician may choose diagnostic tests to diagnose an organic cause or to consult with a subspecialist.

The initial diagnostic workup includes serologic assays for celiac disease, evaluation of thyroid function in selected cases, and serum electrolytes, calcium level, allergic testing.[10] Manometric studies usually are not indicated in the evaluation of adolescents who have defecation disorders. They are useful only in a subset of

Box 1
Alarming features for childhood constipation

Onset of constipation <12 months of age

Delayed passage of meconium

No withholding

No fecal incontinence

Failure to thrive

Empty rectal ampulla

Pigmentary abnormalities

Heme-positive stools

Presence of extraintestinal symptoms

Bladder disease

No response to conventional treatment

patients who have constipation that is refractory to treatment.[32] The main indication for anorectal manometry is to demonstrate the presence of RAIR. The presence of RAIR excludes Hirschsprung's disease.[10] Other diagnostic tests such as colonic manometry, barium enema, colonic transit time, and rectal biopsy can be useful in selected cases.

Assessment of total and segmental colonic transit time (CTT) using radio-opaque markers provides accurate and reliable information about colorectal motor function in defecation disorders.[33] The marker technique is used to localize the delay in colonic transit and is particularly helpful if bowel history is unreliable. Studies in children who have constipation show different colonic transit patterns: normal transit time, dyssynergic defecation-delayed transit through the anorectal region, and slow transit constipation-prolonged transit through the entire colon. Normal CTTs are found in 39% to 58% of constipated children. The most common type of delayed CTT in children is outlet delay caused by dyssynergic defecation. The radio-opaque marker test is useful for differentiating children who have constipation from those who have functional nonretentive fecal incontinence.[22] Colonic transit abnormalities in both the left colon and rectum may be responsible for constipation in children who have severe brain damage.[34]

Colonic manometry can be used to discriminate between functional and the rare neuromuscular causes of severe and therapy-resistant constipation. The markers for normal motility are the presence of HAPCs and the presence of a gastrocolonic response to a meal. In most children who have constipation, colonic motility is normal, showing HAPCs and an increase in motility in response to a pharmacologic stimulus or administration of a meal. In those patients who have colonic neuropathies, contractions are often present but may be disorganized with absence or incomplete propagation of the HAPCs. In patients who have myopathies, colonic contractions are absent or very weak and are unable to propel stool.[26]

MANAGEMENT OF CHILDREN WITH FUNCTIONAL CONSTIPATION

The Childhood Constipation Working Group of the British Society of Pediatric Gastroenterology, Hepatology, and Nutrition recently reported that on the basis of a systematic review of available treatments, there was insufficient evidence to make any recommendations for practice, and that guidelines would need to be based on clinical experience, evidence, and consensus.[35] The general approach to the child who has functional constipation includes the following steps: education, disimpaction, prevention of reaccumulation of feces, and follow-up.[36]

A critical first step is to manage anxiety among parents and children. An important component of treatment includes behavior modification and regular toilet habits. The child may be fearful of painful defecation, and parents need to understand that coercive toilet training in this period of life will be ineffective. The child is instructed to attempt to defecate after meals three times daily for 5 minutes. The child is encouraged to strain actively while placing his or her feet on a footrest. In older children, fecal incontinence and its social consequences need a nonaccusatory management approach; it is essential to provide reassurance regarding the benign nature of this behavioral disorder.[10,13]

The objectives of treatment are to remove fecal impaction, to restore a normal bowel habit with soft stools that can be passed without discomfort, and to ensure self-toileting and passage of stools at appropriate places.[37] Disimpaction is indicated when a large fecal mass is present that is unlikely to be expelled without pain. This is accomplished best with oral medication or enemas. High doses of polyethylene glycol 3350 (1 to 1.5 g/kg/d for 3 days) have been shown to be effective.[38] The use of suppositories, enemas, and manual evacuation is more contentious, and a careful balancing of physical and psychologic benefits and harms is necessary. Once impaction has been removed, the treatment should focus on preventing a recurrence. This treatment consists of dietary interventions, behavioral modification, and laxatives to assure that bowel movements occur at normal intervals with easy evacuation.

The association between fiber intake and constipation is still controversial. Two case control studies in children have examined fiber intake in constipated children compared with healthy controls.[39,40] Discriminant analysis showed that only fiber intake was correlated independently with constipation.[39] On the other hand, it has been demonstrated that constipated children generally do not consume less fiber than healthy children, and treatment with increased fiber intake did not result in clinical improvement.[23] Two small double-blind placebo-controlled trials in 20 neurologically impaired constipated children and in 31 otherwise healthy constipated children showed beneficial effects on stool frequency, stool consistency, incontinence episodes, suppository use, and adverse effects for glucomannan, a fiber gel polysaccharide.[41,42] Although the authors recommended an increased fiber intake in children who have constipation, larger clinical trials are needed to confirm these studies.

The aim of a combination of behavioral treatment (toilet training in combination with a rewarding system, diminishing of toilet phobia), cognitive (psychotherapy, cognitive therapy and family therapy, or educational intervention) and laxative treatment is to lower the level of distress and develop or restore normal bowel habits by positive reinforcement, preservation of self-respect, and encouragement of the child and parents during the treatment.[43] In a large prospective randomized–controlled trial of 162 constipated children, a higher cure rate was found in children receiving behavioral intervention (toilet training, positive reinforcing scheme, and dietary advice) plus laxatives (polyethylene glycol, oral and rectal bisacodyl, followed by a long-term treatment of mineral oil plus phenolphthalein) compared with those receiving solely behavioral intervention at both 6 and 12 months of follow-up.[44] In a randomized– controlled trial of 87 constipated children (8.6 $\pm$ 2.0 years), enhanced toilet training (intensive medical treatment plus behavior management) was more effective than either intensive medical treatment or biofeedback training, although the difference was not statistically significant.[44]

Once disimpaction has been achieved, it is essential to begin an oral daily laxative immediately and continue treatment for several months to prevent reaccumulation of retained stools and recurrence of stool withholding behavior. Osmotic laxatives, stimulant laxatives, and prokinetics are recommended. Recently, polyethylene-glycol (PEG) has been suggested as a laxative in adults and children who have constipation. The correct dose is that which produces a daily evacuation of soft stool without adverse effects.

In children, uncontrolled, unblinded, and randomized–controlled studies have been performed to assess the effects of PEG. These studies have reported the effects of PEG at low doses, with mean effective doses ranging from 0.6 to 0.8 g/d.[23] A double-blind, randomized–controlled trial showed that both PEG and lactulose significantly increase stool frequency and decrease the frequency of incontinence. Abdominal pain, straining, and pain with defecation decreased significantly; however, more children on PEG complained about the bad taste.[45] Controlled studies of PEG in childhood constipation show that neither PEG 4000 (without added salts at 4 to 8 g) nor lactulose at 3.3 to 6.6 g induced any change in blood electrolytes, total protein, serum albumin, or vitamins A and D over a 3-month period. These studies confirm the efficacy and safety of PEG 4000 in childhood constipation.[46,47] In addition, a more recent randomized, double-blind crossover trial showed that PEG 3350 plus electrolytes is

Table 2
Medications for use in treatment of constipation

Medications	Treatment Adverse Effects and Comments	Quality of Evidence[10]
Oral administration		
Lubricant	*Softens stool and eases passage*	
Mineral oil: <1 year-old not recommended; disimpaction 15–30 mL/y of age, up to 240 mL daily for maintenance 1 to 3 mL/kg/d given once daily or in divided doses twice daily	Chill or give with juice; risk of lipoid pneumonia; adherence problems; leakage may occur if dose is too high or impaction is present.	In children: I
Osmotic laxatives	*Retain water in stool, which adds bulk and softness*	
Lactulose (concentration: 10 g/15 mL): 1 to 3 mL/kg/d given in divided doses twice daily	Abdominal cramping, flatus; lactulose is a synthetic disaccharide	In infants: III In children: I
Magnesium hydroxide (milk of magnesia; concentration: 400 mg/ 5 mL): 1 to 3 mL/kg/ d given in divided doses twice daily magnesium hydroxide (concentration: 800 mg/5 mL): 0.5 mL/kg/d given in divided doses twice daily	Infants are susceptible to magnesium poisoning; with overdose or renal insufficiency: risk of hyperrmagnesemia, hypophosphatemia, or secondary hypocalcemia	In children: I
PEG 3350 (17 g/240 mL of water or juice): disimpaction: 1–1.5 g/kg/d for 3 days PEG 3350–4000 maintenance: 0.26–0.84 g/kg/d	Solution may be prepared in advance for administration over one to two days. Excellent adherence	In children: III
Sorbitol: 1 to 3 mL/kg/d given in divided doses twice daily	Less costly than lactulose	In infants: III In children: I
Stimulants	*Short-term use only; improves effectiveness of colonic and rectal muscle contractions*	
Senna syrup (8.8 g sennoside per 5 mL) Age 2–6 years: 2.5–7.5 mL/d given in divided doses twice daily Age 6–12 years: 5–15 mL/d given in divided doses twice daily	Risk of idiosyncratic hepatitis, melanosis coli, hypertropic osteoarthropathy, analgesic nephropathy, abdominal cramping; melanosis coli improves after medication is stopped; tablets and granules are available	In children: II–I
Bisacodyl (5 mg tablets): one to three tablets given once or twice daily	Abdominal cramping, diarrhea, hypokalemia	In children: II–I
Rectal administration		
Glycerin suppository	No adverse effects	
Bisacodyl suppository (10 mg): one-half to one suppository administered once or twice daily	Abdominal cramping, diarrhea, hypokalemia	

significantly more effective than placebo for treating chronic constipation in children.[48] The doses of these medications are reported in **Table 2**. Discontinuation should be considered only when the child is having regular bowel movements and without difficulty.[23] Although 60% of all children referred to a tertiary medical center for chronic constipation were treated successfully at 1 year follow-up by intensive medical and behavioral treatment, however, one third of the children followed-up beyond puberty continued to have severe complaints of constipation.[49]

CONSTIPATION AND ATOPY

In several studies, chronic constipation in children has been reported as a clinical manifestation of cow's milk allergy (CMA).[50,51] Iacono and colleagues found that in children who had chronic constipation, 68% demonstrated improvement in their bowel habit when treated for 2 weeks with dietary elimination of cow's milk proteins. In these children, fecal retention was associated with pain on defecation, possibly related to allergic proctitis. Supporting this hypothesis was the presence of eosinophils in the lamina propria of 59% of these patients.[49] In another study, although an association between chronic constipation and CMA was reported, no correlation was found between the clinical response to elimination diet, specific IgE levels, or prick test for milk proteins.[52]

There are conflicting data on this association, however. Loening-Baucke reported that children who had chronic constipation and a history of cow's milk protein allergy or atopy did not improve on a 2-week elimination diet.[53] In contrast, a recent study by Simeone and colleagues[54] evaluated the prevalence of chronic constipation in unselected children, its association with atopy, and the efficacy of a cow's milk protein elimination diet on refractory constipation. In this study of 5000 pediatric subjects, prevalence of atopy among children who had chronic constipation was similar to that of the general population, and refractoriness to chronic constipation was not related to CMA.

NONRETENTIVE FECAL INCONTINENCE

Nonretentive fecal incontinence represents the repeated and inappropriate passage of stool at a place other than the toilet in a child older than 4 years who has no evidence of fecal retention.

According to the Rome III criteria, children who present with symptoms listed subsequently are considered to have functional nonretentive fecal incontinence (FNRFI). Diagnostic criteria (must be fulfilled for at least 2 months before diagnosis) for nonretentive fecal incontinence[4] must include all of the following in a child with developmental age of at least 4 years:

- Defecation into places inappropriate to the social context at least once per month
- No evidence of an inflammatory, anatomic, metabolic, or neoplastic process that explains the subject's symptoms
- No evidence of fecal retention

Children with FNRFI often have daily bowel movements in the toilet but additionally have nearly complete stool evacuation in their underwear more than once a week. They have neither palpable abdominal or rectal fecal mass on physical examination nor a fecal mass identified on abdominal radiographs. An abdominal radiograph may be required to diagnose occult fecal retention because of incomplete passage of stool.

Colonic radiopaque marker studies in these children reveal that they have normal CTTs. The frequency of daytime and nighttime enuresis is higher (40% to 45%) for children who have FNRFI compared with constipated children. Children who have FNRFI have significantly more behavioral problems and more externalizing or internalizing of psychosocial problems than controls.

Treatment for FNRFI is based on education, a nonaccusatory approach, regular toilet use with rewards, and referral to a mental health professional when appropriate. Successful resolution of symptoms may require prolonged treatment and follow-up.[8,55,56]

ORGANIC CONSTIPATION

Organic causes actually affect 5% to 10% of children presenting with constipation, and Hirschsprung's disease is an uncommon condition even in young infants.

Box 2 summarizes the most common organic conditions responsible for childhood constipation.

Hirschsprung's Disease

Epidemiology

Hirschsprung's disease occurs in approximately 1 of each 5000 live births and with a male predominance of 4:1. It is generally sporadic, although in 3%% to 7% of cases a genetic transmission has been reported. The risk for short-segment disease is 5% in brothers and 1% in sisters of index cases; for long-segment disease, the risk is 10%, regardless of sex.[57]

Etiology

Hirschsprung's disease is a heterogeneous genetic disorder, resulting from an anomaly of the enteric nervous system of neural crest cells origin, and characterized by the absence of parasympathetic intrinsic ganglion cells in the submucosal and myenteric plexuses. It is regarded as the consequence of the premature arrest of the craniocaudal migration of vagal neural crest cells in the hindgut, between the fifth and 12th week of gestation, to form the enteric nervous system. Therefore it is regarded as a neurocristopathy.[58] The aganglionic segment is contracted permanently, causing proximal dilatation.[59]

Hirschsprung's disease may be classified according to the length of the aganglionic segment. The classic form (short segment 70% to 75% of cases) is limited to the rectum and sigmoid colon; the long segment, or subtotal colonic disease (10% to 15%), generally involves the bowel up to the splenic flexure. Total colonic aganglionosis (TCA: 3% to 6%) may extend to involve a variable amount of the short bowel, and total intestinal aganglionosis sometimes is associated with intestinal malrotation or volvulus.[60] Ultrashort-segment aganglionosis is considered a functional alteration, without any detectable histologic finding. Although longer aganglionic segments tend to produce more dramatic symptoms, some patients with even short-segment disease deteriorate rapidly.[61]

Pathophysiology

The hallmark of diagnosis is the absence of ganglion cells from the myenteric and submucosal plexuses, as seen on a suction (mucosal–submucosal) biopsy of the rectum. Proximal contents fail to enter the unrelaxed, aganglionic segment. The lack of nonadrenergic–noncholinergic inhibitory innervation is responsible for a tonic contraction of the affected segment, with absence of peristalsis and dilatation of the gut proximally. Morphologically, ganglion cells are absent from the narrowed segment and

Box 2
Most common organic causes of constipation

Anatomic

- Abscess
- Anal fissures
- Skin tags
- Anal stenosis
- Imperforate anus
- Anteriorly displaced anus
- Acquired strictures from inflammatory bowel disease or necrotizing enterocolitis
- Metabolic
- Hypokalemia
- Hypomagnesemia
- Hypophosphatemia
- Hypercalcemia
- Cystic fibrosis
- Celiac disease

Endocrine

- Diabetes mellitus
- Multiple endocrine neoplasia (MEN) 2B
- Hypothyroidism
- Hyperparathyroidism

Neuropathic

- Cerebral palsy
- Spina bifida
- Myelomeningocele

Colonic neuropathies

- Hirschsprung's disease
- Intestinal neuronal dysplasia
- Pseudo-obstruction
- Others

Drugs

- Anticholinergics
- Antidepressants
- Antihypertensives
- Opiates
- Iron

for some distance (1 to 5 cm usually) into the dilated segment. The pattern of nerve fibers is abnormal also; they are hypertrophic with abundant, thickened bundles. Specific stains for acetylcholinesterase are used to highlight the abnormal morphology.[62] Furthermore, the lack of nitric oxide (NO)-producing nerve fibers in the aganglionic intestine probably contributes to the inability of the smooth muscle to relax, thereby causing lack of peristalsis in Hirschsprung's disease.[63] In addition, in the aganglionic segments, interstitial cells of Cajal are scarce, and their networks are disrupted.[64]

Hirschsprung's disease occurs as an isolated trait in 70% of cases. Associated congenital anomalies that are found in 18% of Hirschsprung's disease patients include GI malformation, cleft palate, polydactyly, cardiac septal defects, and craniofacial anomalies. The higher rate of associated anomalies in familial cases than in isolated cases (39% versus 21%) strongly suggests syndromic clinical presentations with Mendelian inheritance.[65] Consequently, assessment of all patients who have Hirschsprung's disease should include a careful clinical and genetic evaluation. Numerous chromosomal anomalies have been described in patients who have Hirschsprung's disease (12% of Hirschsprung's disease cases). Free trisomy 21 (Down's syndrome) is by far the most frequent, representing more than 90% of chromosomal disorders associated with Hirschsprung's disease and 2% to 10% of ascertained Hirschsprung's disease cases. Hirschsprung's disease has been reported associated with several syndromes: pleiotropic neurocristopathies (Waardenburg-Shah, Piebaldism, MEN2A, Riley-Day), syndromes with Hirschsprung's disease as a mandatory feature (Goldberg-Shprintzen, BRESHEK, Werner mesomelic dysplasia), and occasional association (Bardet-Biedl, Kauffman-McKusick, cartilage-hair hypoplasia, the Smith-Lemli-Opitz syndrome type 2).[66]

Ten genes are known to be involved in Hirschsprung's disease in people, namely the proto-oncogene RET (REarranged during Transfection), glial cell line-derived neurotrophic factor (GDNF), neurturin (NTN), endothelin B receptor (EDNRB), endothelin 3 (EDN3), endothelin-converting enzyme 1 (ECE1), SOX10, SIP1, paired-like homeobox 2B (PHOX2B), and T-cell factor 4 (TCF4) genes. Mutations of these genes give dominant, recessive, or polygenic patterns of inheritance. RET mutations account for 50% of Hirschsprung's disease cases. RET is a 1114 amino acid transmembrane receptor. Over 80 mutations have been identified, including large deletions of the RET gene, microdeletions and insertions, nonsense, missense, and splicing mutations.[67,68]

GDNF was shown to be the RET ligand. To activate RET, GDNF needs the presence of a novel glycosylphosphatidylinositol (GPI)-linked coreceptor (GFRA1).[69] Four related GPI linked coreceptors, GFRA1-4, and four related soluble growth factors ligands of RET have been identified, namely GDNF, NTN, persephin (PSPN), and artemin.[70] GDNF mutations have been identified in six patients with Hirschsprung's disease, and it can be regarded as a rare cause of Hirschsprung's disease (less than 15%). Moreover, GDNF mutations may not be sufficient to lead to Hirschsprung's disease, since four out of six patients have additional contributory factors such as RET mutations or trisomy 21. Similarly, an NTN mutation has been identified in one family, in conjunction with a RET mutation.[71,72] EDNRB and EDNRA are G protein- coupled heptahelical proteins that transduce signals through the endothelins (EDN1,2,3). Although EDN3 mutations seldom were found, EDNRB mutations were identified in approximately 5% of patients. The penetrance of EDN3 and of EDNRB heterozygous mutations is incomplete, and S-Hirschsprung's disease is largely predominant. Interstitial 13q22 deletions encompassing the EDNRB gene in patients who have Hirschsprung's disease make haploinsufficency the most likely mechanism for Hirschsprung's disease.[73,74]

The role of polymorphic mutations as genetic risk factors predisposing to Hirschsprung's disease is not clear. The PHOX2B A→G (1364) polymorphism is associated with Hirschsprung's disease.[75] Whether it directly contributes to disease susceptibility or represents a marker for a locus in LD with PHOX2B needs further investigation. The T-allele of the 561C/T polymorphism of EDNRB gene was over- represented in the Hirschsprung's disease/Down's syndrome patient group when compared with normal controls.[76]

CLINICAL SIGNS AND SYMPTOMS

In the newborn, symptoms may appear during the first hours of life with failure to pass meconium, or in the first week with a picture of functional intestinal obstruction. The delay in the passage of meconium, however, does not always occur and a percentage of children still present late or with complications despite a history of complications since birth. Enterocolitis, the most common complication, is always severe and is an important cause of mortality in these young patients.

In infants and children, the presentation is often less dramatic and may not mimic acute intestinal obstruction. Severe constipation and recurrent fecal impaction are more common. Physical examination reveals a distended abdomen and a contracted anal sphincter and rectum in most children. The rectum is devoid of stool except in cases of short-segment aganglionosis. As the finger is withdrawn, there may be an explosive discharge of foul-smelling liquid stools, with decompression of the proximal normal bowel. The classic clinical manifestations described for enterocolitis include abdominal distension, explosive diarrhea, vomiting, fever, lethargy, rectal bleeding, and shock.

Abdominal radiographs show intestinal cut-off signs in the rectosigmoid region with absence of air distally. Other common findings are small bowel dilatation in 74% of patients and multiple air-fluid levels.[77] Because of the risk of perforation, contrast enema should not be performed in the presence of clinical enterocolitis.

Rectal washout should be the initial approach, regardless of age, in patients who present with enterocolitis. Along with washouts, intravenous antibiotics or oral metronidazole (in mild cases) should be used. Should the disease process fail to improve, or the infant's condition deteriorates, the performance of a defunctioning colostomy should be considered.[78]

Diagnosis

The subject's history is very important in making a diagnosis for Hirschsprung's disease, and this includes the age of appearance of symptoms, the passage of meconium, or history of episodes of functional intestinal obstruction. In these children, it is important to exclude a functional (idiopathic) megacolon. When the history (early onset of constipation, absence of fecal incontinence) or the physical examination (empty rectal ampulla) suggest an organic cause, anorectal manometry should be performed.

When the rectal balloon is inflated, normally there is a reflex relaxation of the anal sphincter.[79] This RAIR is absent in patients who have Hirschsprung's disease; either there is no relaxation, or there may even be paradoxical contraction of the anal sphincter (**Fig. 1**). Anorectal manometry is particularly useful when the aganglionic segment is short, and results of radiologic or pathologic studies are equivocal.

Barium enema is helpful in assessing a transition zone between the aganglionic and ganglionic bowel, and in providing an estimate of the length of aganglionic segment. Demonstration of the transition zone is easier if no effort is made to cleanse the bowel (**Fig. 2**). In the newborn, dilatation of the proximal normal bowel may not have developed, and radiological diagnosis can be difficult. The sensitivity and specificity for recognition of a transition zone have been reported to be about 80% and 76%,

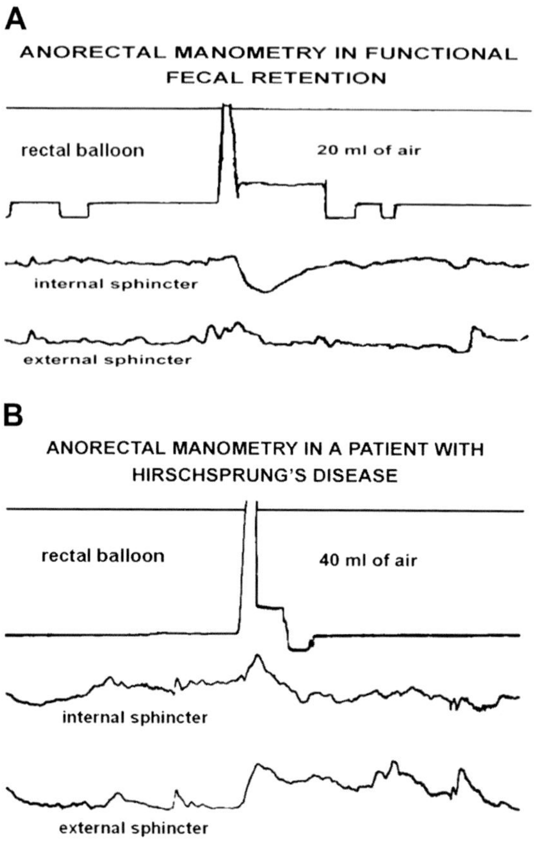

Fig. 1. (*A*) Anorectal manometry in a 2-month-old boy with functional constipation. Note that the distention of a rectal balloon with air for 1 second produces a decrease of anal pressure (rectosphincter reflex). (*B*) Anorectal manometry in a 3-month-old boy with Hirschsprung's disease. Distention of a rectal balloon with air for 1 second produces no decrease of anal pressure.

respectively.[80] The barium enema may not show a transition zone in cases of total colonic Hirschsprung's disease, or may be indistinguishable from cases of functional constipation when ultrashort-segment Hirschsprung's disease is present.

Nevertheless, the diagnosis is based on histologic evidence. Since the mid-1970s, demonstration of acetylcholinesterase activity in mucosal biopsies has allowed the noninvasive suction rectal biopsy technique to become the most reliable diagnostic method for aganglionosis.[81] The histologic diagnosis is based on the demonstration of the total absence of ganglion cells in the affected segment of the intestine with an overgrowth of large nerve trunks in the intermuscular and submucosal zone (**Fig. 3**). Two small samples of rectal mucosa and submucosa, taken using suction rectal biopsy technique, are sufficient for diagnosis. Two pieces must be taken not less then 2 cm above the dentate line, to avoid the physiologic hypoganglionic zone, and not more than 5 cm above the dentate line to avoid failure to diagnosis of short-segment disease. Acetylcholinesterase activity in the normal colon shows only few fibers in the lamina propria and muscularis mucosae. In Hirschsprung's disease there is an increase in thick, knotted acetylcholinesterase-positive nerve fibers in

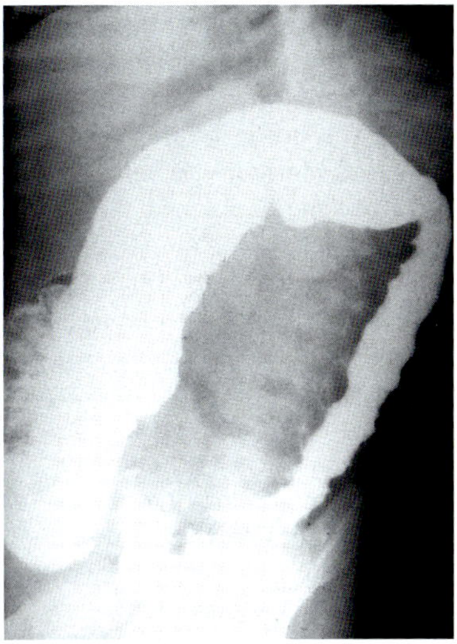

Fig. 2. Barium enema showing a long narrowed segment in a child with Hirschsprung's disease.

the muscularis mucosae and lamina propria, and hypertrophied nerve trunks in the submucosa.

Other causes of intestinal obstruction should be considered when abdominal distension and failure to pass meconium are observed in a newborn infant. These include:

Meconium ileus resulting from cystic fibrosis

Intestinal malformations such as lower ileal and colonic atresia which occasionally is associated with Hirschsprung's disease, intestinal malrotation, or duplication

Enteric nervous system anomalies grouped as chronic intestinal pseudo-obstruction syndromes

Functional intestinal obstruction resulting from maternal infection, maternal intoxication, or congenital hypothyroidism

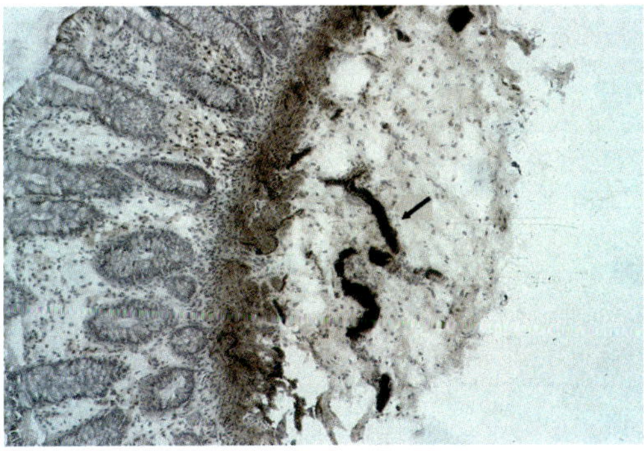

Fig. 3. Intense acetylcholinesterase activity in a patient with Hirschsprung's disease. Note the absence of neurones and the presence of increase in thick knotted nerve fibers in the muscularis mucosa and lamina propria. In addition, hypertrophied nerve trunks are visible in the submucosa (*arrow*).

Treatment Options

The treatment of Hirschsprung's disease is surgical. After careful preoperative management, the underlying principle is to correct the normal bowel to the anus and to release the tonic contraction of the internal anal sphincter. A one-stage procedure is possible when diagnosis is made early, before colonic dilatation, and in short-segment disease. For long-segment disease and total colonic aganglionosis, temporary enterostomy is often the first step in management before definitive surgery. Laparoscopic and transanal pull-through techniques have been proposed more recently in Hirschsprung's disease surgery. These techniques offer surgery without a scar, but comparative long-term results are pending.[82,83] Neuronal precursor cells isolated from the developing human enteric nervous system may open the route to cell therapy.[58]

Fistula nd stenosis of the anastomosis and enterocolitis are the main short-term complications. Long-term complications include chronic constipation (10% to 15%) and incontinence. Mortality has been below 6% since the 1980s and may be related to short-term complications or the associated malformations.[84] The treatment of children with TCA, however, remains hazardous.[85]

ANORECTAL MALFORMATIONS

Anorectal malformations (ARM) comprise a wide spectrum of disorders that affect boys and girls and involve the distal anus and rectum and the urinary and genital tracts. Defects range from those that are minor, easily treated, and with an excellent functional prognosis, to those that are complex, difficult to manage, often associated with other anomalies, and have a poor functional prognosis. Anorectal malformations are congenital anomalies that occur in approximately 1 in 5000 live births.

The classification presented here attempts to group together defects that have common diagnostic, therapeutic, and prognostic features:

Males: recto-perineal fistula, rectourethral-bulbar fistula, rectourethral-prostatic fistula, rectobladderneck fistula, imperforated anus without fistula, and complex and unusual defects.

Females: recto-perianal fistula, rectovestibular fistula, cloaca with short common channel (less than 3 cm), cloaca with long common channel (greater than 3 cm), and imperforated anus without fistula.

Complex and unusual defects: cloacal exstrophy, covered cloacal extraposterior cloaca associated with presacral mass, and rectal atresia.[86]

The etiology of ARM remains unclear and likely is multifactorial. There are, however, reasons to believe there is a genetic component. Mutations in specific genes encoding transcription factors have been described in patients having Townes-Broks syndrome, Currarino's syndrome, and Pallister-Hall syndrome, each of which have autosomal dominant modes of inheritance. In addition, it has been found that there is not only an increased incidence of ARM in patients who have trisomy 21, but that 95% of patients who have trisomy 21 and ARM have imperforate anus without fistula, compared with only 5% of all patients who have ARM. Based on this evidence, it is likely that the mutation of various genes can result in ARM, or that the etiology of ARM is multigenic.[87,88]

The radiologic evaluation of a newborn who has imperforate anus includes an abdominal ultrasound to evaluate for urologic anomalies. In the case of persistent cloaca, a distended vagina can be identified. Plain radiographs of the spine can show anomalies such as spina bifida and spinal hemivertebrae. Plain radiographs of the sacrum in the anterior–posterior and lateral projections can demonstrate sacral anomalies such as a hemisacrum and sacral hemivertebrae.

A spinal ultrasound and an MRI from the newborn period up to 3 months of age can be used to look for evidence of a tethered spinal cord and other spinal anomalies. A cross-table lateral radiograph can help show the air column in the distal rectum in the small percentage of patients for whom clinical evidence does not delineate in 16 to 24 hours the likely anorectal anomaly.[87]

The surgical approach to repairing these defects changed dramatically in 1980 with the introduction of the posterior sagittal approach, which allowed surgeons to view the anatomy of these defects clearly, to repair them under direct vision, and to learn about the complex anatomic arrangement of the junction of rectum and genitourinary tract. Fecal and urinary incontinence can occur even with an excellent anatomic repair, mainly because of associated problems such as a poorly developed sacrum, deficient nerve supply, and spinal cord anomalies. For these patients, an effective bowel management program, including enema and dietary restrictions, has been devised to improve their quality of life.[87,89]

CONSTIPATION IN NEUROLOGICALLY IMPAIRED CHILDREN

Chronic constipation is a frequent and distressing complaint in children who have neurologic diseases. Several mechanisms may be involved in the pathogenesis of chronic constipation in these patients, including a lack of conscious urge to defecate, immobilization, motor paralysis of the abdominal and perineal muscles, and disruption of the neural modulation of colonic motility. More than 90% of children with cerebral palsy have oral motor dysfunctions, which contribute to a reduced oral fiber intake. Chronic constipation in children who have severe brain damage primarily results from prolonged transit at the level of the colon and rectum. It is likely that these children have a predisposition to colonic motor dysfunction secondary to the brain damage and not necessarily to the low intake of dietary fiber.[90]

Spina bifida or myelomeningocele is a neural tube defect that occurs within the first 28 days of gestation and occurs in about 1 in 1000 live births. The child will have motor and sensory deficits to the lower extremities ranging from mild to complete neurologic dysfunction. Because the nerves that control the bladder and bowel are located in the sacral spinal cord, the child most likely will have deficits in these areas also. Bowel dysfunction occurs in children who have spina bifida, because the RAIR is maintained, but the defecation urge is not present.[91] When the internal sphincter relaxes, bowel accidents or fecal incontinence can occur. Constipation results from an increased CTT and a lack of sphincteric contraction with rectal distention. Colonic transit studies show that the CTT is prolonged, and the transit index is higher in children who have functional constipation and spina bifida occulta. This is suggestive of outlet obstruction. The total CTT in nonretentive fecal incontinence children who had spina bifida occulta was significantly more prolonged compared with those without spina bifida occulta. Children who have spina bifida may benefit from behavior modification techniques. The goal of the behavior modification program is to teach the child to self-initiate a bowel movement.[92]

REFERENCES

1. Corazziari E, Staiano A, Miele E, et al. Bowel frequency and defecatory patterns in children: a prospective nationwide survey. Clin Gastroenterol Hepatol 2005;3: 1101–6.
2. Loening-Baucke V. Constipation in children. N Engl J Med 1998;339(16):1155–6.

3. Benninga MA. Children with constipation: what happens to them when they grow up? Scand J Gastroenterol Suppl 2004;241:23–6.
4. Rasquin A, Di Lorenzo C, Forbes D, et al. Childhood functional gastrointestinal disorders: child/ adolescent. Gastroenterology 2006;130:1527–37.
5. Voshulijl WP, Heijmans J, Heijmans HS, et al. Use of Rome II criteria in childhood defecation disorders: applicability in clinical and research practice. J Pediatr 2004;145:213–7.
6. Benninga M, Candy D, Catto-Smith A, et al. The Paris consensus on childhood constipation terminology (PACCT) group. J Pediatr Gastroenterol Nutr 2005;40:273–5.
7. Boccia G, Manguso F, Coccorullo P, et al. Functional defecation disorders in children: PACCT criteria versus Rome II criteria. J Pediatr 2007;151:394–8.
8. Loening-Baucke V. Functional fecal retention with encopresis in childhood. J Pediatr Gastroenterol Nutr 2004;38:79–84.
9. van Diijk M, Benninga M, Grootenhuis M, et al. Chronic childhood constipation: a review of the literature and the introduction of a protocolized behavioral intervention program. Patient Educ Couns 2007;67:63–77.
10. Baker S, Di Lorenzo C, Liptak G, et al. Evaluation and the treatment of constipation in infants and children: recommendation of the North American Society for Pediatric Gastroenterology, Hepatology and Nutrition. J Pediatr Gastroenterol Nutr 2006;43:e1–13.
11. Nyhan WE. Stool frequency of normal infants in the first weeks of life. Pediatrics 1952;10:414–25.
12. Weaver LT, Steiner H. The bowel habits of young children. Arch Dis Child 1983; 59:649–52.
13. Loening-Baucke V. Chronic constipation in children. Gastroenterology 1993;105: 1557–64.
14. Miele E, Simeone D, Marino A, et al. Functional gastrointestinal disorders in children: an Italian prospective survey. Pediatrics 2004;114:73–8.
15. Loening-Baucke V. Prevalence, symptoms, and outcome of constipation in infants and toddlers. J Pediatr 2005;146:359–63.
16. Di Lorenzo C. Childhood constipation: finally some hard data about hard stools! J Pediatr 2000;136:4–7.
17. Loening-Baucke V. Prevalence rates for constipation and faecal and urinary incontinence. Arch Dis Child 2007;92:486–9.
18. Elawad MA, Sullivan PB. Management of constipation in children with disabilities. Dev Med Child Neurol 2001;43:829–32.
19. Afzal N, Murch S, Thirrupathy K, et al. Constipation with acquired megarectum in children with autism. Pediatrics 2003;112:939–42.
20. Cunningham C, Taylor HG, Minich NM, et al. Constipation in very low birth weight children at 10 to 14 years of age. J Pediatr Gastroenterol Nutr 2001;33:23–7.
21. Staiano AM, Andreotti MR, Perrotta V, et al. Prevalence of digital arches in children with abdominal pain and constipation. J Pediatr 1990;117:435–6.
22. Abrahamian FP, Lloyd-Still JD. Chronic constipation in childhood: a longitudinal study of 186 patients. J Pediatr Gastroenterol Nutr 1984;3:460–7.
23. Benninga MA, Voskuijl WP, Taminiau JA. Childhood constipation: is there new light in the tunnel? J Pediatr Gastroenterol Nutr 2004;39:448–64.
24. Bassotti G, Crowel MD, Whitehead WE. Contractile activity of the human colon: lessons from 24-hour studies. Gut 1993;34:129–33.
25. Narducci F, Bassotti G, Gaburri M, et al. Twenty-four hour manometric recording of colonic motor activity in healthy man. Gut 1987;28:17–25.

26. Pensabene L, Youssef NN, Griffiths JM, et al. Colonic manometry in children with defecatory disorders. Role in diagnosis and management. Am J Gastroenterol 2003;98(5):1052–7.
27. Borowitz SM, Cox DJ, Tam A, et al. Precipitants of constipation during early childhood. J Am Board Fam Pract 2003;16:213–8.
28. Van der Plas RN, Benninga MA, Buller HA, et al. Biofeedback training in treatment of childhood constipation: a randomised–controlled study. Lancet 1996;348:776–80.
29. Taubman B, Blum NJ, Nemeth N. Stool toileting refusal. Arch Pediatr Adolesc Med 2003;157:1193–6.
30. van den Berg MM, Voskuijl WP, Boeckxstaens GE, et al. Rectal compliance and rectal sensation in constipated adolescents, recovered adolescents, and healthy volunteers. Gut 2008;57:599–603.
31. Caplan A, Walker L, Rasquin A. Validation of the pediatric Rome II criteria for functional gastrointestinal disorders using the questionnaire on pediatric gastrointestinal symptoms. J Pediatr Gastroenterol Nutr 2005;41:305–16.
32. Youssef NN, Sanders L, Di Lorenzo C. Adolescent constipation: evaluation and management. Adolesc Med Clin 2004;15:37–52.
33. Zaslavsky C, da Silveira TR, Maguilnik I. Total and segmental colonic transit time with radio-opaque markers in adolescents with functional constipation. J Pediatr Gastroenterol Nutr 1998;27:138–42.
34. Staiano A, Del Giudice E. Colonic transit and anorectal manometry in children with severe brain damage. Pediatrics 1994;94:169–73.
35. Rubin G, Dale A. Chronic constipation in children. BMJ 2006;333:1051–5.
36. Baker SS, Liptak GS, Colletti RB, et al. Constipation in infants and children: evaluation and treatment. J Pediatr Gastroenterol Nutr 1999;29:612–26.
37. Clayden GS, Keshtgar AS, Carcani-Rathwell I, et al. The management of chronic constipation and related faecal incontinence in childhood. Arch Dis Child 2005; 90:58–67.
38. Youssef NN, Peters JM, Henderson W, et al. Dose response of PEG 3350 for the treatment of childhood fecal impaction. J Pediatr 2002;141:410–4.
39. Morais MB, Vitolo MR, Aguirre AN, et al. Measurement of low dietary fiber intake as a risk factor for chronic constipation in children. J Pediatr Gastroenterol Nutr 1999;29:132–5.
40. Roma E, Adamidis D, Nikolara R, et al. Diet and chronic constipation in children: the role of fiber. J Pediatr Gastroenterol Nutr 1999;28:169–74.
41. Staiano A, Simeone D, Del Giudice E, et al. Effect of the dietary fibre glucomannan on chronic constipation in neurologically impaired children. J Pediatr 2000;136:41–5.
42. Loening-Baucke V, Miele E, Staiano A. Fiber (glucomannan) is beneficial in the treatment of childhood constipation. Pediatrics 2004;113:e259–64.
43. McGrath ML, Mellon MW, Murphy L. Empirically supported treatments in paediatric psychology: constipation and encopresis. J Pediatr Psychol 2000;25:225–54.
44. Brazzelli M, Griffiths P. Behavioural and cognitive interventions with or without other treatments for the management of faecal incontinence in children. Cochrane Database Syst Rev 2006;(2):CD002240.
45. Voskuijl W, de Lorijn F, Verwijs W, et al. PEG 3350 (Transipeg) versus lactulose in the treatment of childhood functional constipation: a double-blind, randomised, controlled, multicentre trial. Gut 2004;53(11):1590–4.
46. Dupont C, Leluyer B, Amar F, et al. A dose determination study of polyethylene glycol 4000 in constipated children: factors influencing the maintenance dose. J Pediatr Gastroenterol Nutr 2006;42:178–85.

47. Dupont C, Leluyer B, Maamri N, et al. Double-blind randomized evaluation of clinical and biological tolerance of polyethylene glycol 4000 versus lactulose in constipated children. J Pediatr Gastroenterol Nutr 2005;41:625–33.
48. Thomson MA, Jenkins HR, Bisset WM, et al. Polyethylene glycol 3350 plus electrolytes for chronic constipation in children: a double-blind, placebo-controlled, crossover study. Arch Dis Child 2007;92:996–1000.
49. Van Ginkel R, Reitsma JB, Büller HA, et al. Childhood constipation: longitudinal follow-up beyond puberty. Gastroenterology 2003;125:357–63.
50. Iacono G, Cavataio F, Montalto G, et al. Intolerance of cow's milk and chronic constipation in children. N Engl J Med 1998;339:1100–4.
51. Shah NF, Goldani M, Louis D, et al. Abnormal oro-anal transit in atopic mediated refractory constipation. J Pediatr Gastroenterol Nutr 1999;28:570.
52. Daher S, Tahan S, Sole D, et al. Cow's milk protein intolerance and chronic constipation in children. Pediatr Allergy Immunol 2001;12:339–42.
53. Loening-Baucke V. Controversies in the management of chronic constipation. J Pediatr Gastroenterol Nutr 2001;32:S38–9.
54. Simeone D, Miele E, Boccia G, et al. Prevalence of atopy in children with chronic constipation. Arch Dis Child 2008, in press.
55. Bongers ME, Tabbers MM, Benninga MA. Functional nonretentive fecal incontinence in children. J Pediatr Gastroenterol Nutr 2007;44:5–13.
56. Benninga MA, Taminiau JA. Diagnosis and treatment efficacy of functional nonretentive fecal soiling in childhood. J Pediatr Gastroenterol Nutr 2001;32(Suppl 1): S42–3.
57. Amiel J, Sproat-Emison E, Garcia-Barcelo M, et al. Hirschsprung's disease, associated syndromes, and genetics: a review. J Med Genet 2008;45(1):1–14.
58. Heanue TA, Pachnis V. Enteric nervous system development and Hirschsprung's disease: advances in genetic and stem cell studies. Nat Rev Neurosci 2007;8: 466–79.
59. Gershon MD, Chalazonitis A, Rothman TP. From neural crest to bowel: development of the enteric nervous system. J Neurobiol 1993;24:199–214.
60. Badner JA, Sieber WK, Garver KL, et al. A genetic study of Hirschsprung's disease. Am J Hum Genet 1990;46:568–80.
61. Staiano A, Corazziari E, Andreotti MR, et al. Esophageal motility in children with Hirschsprungvs disease. Am J Dis Child 1991;145:310–3.
62. Romanska HM, Bishop AE, Brereton RJ, et al. Increased expression of muscular neural cell adhesion molecule in congenital aganglionosis. Gastroenterology 1993;105:1104–9.
63. Larsson LT, Shen Z, Ekbland E, et al. Lack of neuronal nitric oxide synthase in nerve fibers of aganglionic intestine : a clue to Hirschsprung's disease. J Pediatr Gastroenterol Nutr 1995;20:49–53.
64. Vanderwinden JM, Rumessen JJ, Liu H, et al. Interstitial cells of cajal in human colon and in Hirschsprung's disease. Gastroenterol 1996;111:901–10.
65. Brooks AS, Breuning MH, Meijers C. Spectrum of phenotypes associated with Hirschsprung's disease: an evaluation of 239 patients from a single institution. The Third International Meeting: Hirschsprung Disease and Related Neurocristopathies, Evian; January France 1998.
66. Amiel J, Lyonnet S. Hirschsprung disease, associated syndromes, and genetics: a review. J Med Genet 2001;38:729–39.
67. Amiel J, Sproat-Emison E, Garcia-Barcelo M, et al. Hirschsprung Disease Consortium. Hirschsprung's disease, associated syndromes, and genetics: a review. J Med Genet 2008;45(1):1–14.

68. Auricchio A, Griseri P, Carpentieri ML, et al. Double heterozygosity for a RET substitution interfering with spicing and an EDNRB missense mutation in Hirschsprung's disease. Am J Hum Genet 1999;64:1216–21.
69. Treanor JJ, Goodman L, de Sauvage F, et al. Characterization of a multicomponent receptor for GDNF. Nature 1996;382:80–3.
70. Baloh RH, Tansey MG, Lampe PA, et al. Artemin, a novel member of the GDNF ligand family, supports peripheraland central neurons and signals through the GFRalpha3-RET receptor complex. Neuron 1998;21:1291–302.
71. Angrist M, Bolk S, Thiel B, et al. Mutation analysis of the RET receptor tyrosine kinase in Hirshsprung's disease. Hum Mol Genet 1995;4:821–30.
72. Doray B, Salomon R, Amiel J, et al. Mutation of the RET ligand, neurturin, supports multigenic inheritance in Hirschsprung's disease. Hum Mol Genet 1998;7:1449–52.
73. Chakravarti A. Endothelin receptor-mediated signaling in Hirschsprung disease. Hum Mol Genet 1996;5:303–7.
74. Kusafuka T, Wang Y, Puri P. Novel mutation of the endothelin receptor gene in isolate patients with Hirshsprung's disease. Hum Mol Genet 1996;5:347–9.
75. Garcia-Barceló M, Sham MH, Lui VC, et al. Association study of PHOX2B as a candidate gene for Hirschsprung's disease. Gut 2003;52:563–7.
76. Zaahl MG, du Plessis L, Warnich L, et al. Significance of novel endothelin-B receptor gene polymorphisms in Hirschsprung's disease: predominance of a novel variant (561C/T) in patients with coexisting Down's syndrome. Mol Cell Probes 2003;17:49–54.
77. Elhalaby EA, Coran AG, Blane CE, et al. Enterocolitis associated with Hirschsprung's disease: a clinical–radiological characterization based on 168 patients. J Pediatr Surg 1995;30:1023–7.
78. Marty TL, Matlak ME, Hendrickson M, et al. Unexpected death from enterocolitis after surgery for Hirschsprung's disease. Pediatrics 1995;96:118–21.
79. Loening-Baucke V. Modulation of abnormal defecation dynamics by biofeedback treatment in chronically constipated children with encopresis. J Pediatr 1990;116:214–22.
80. Taxman TI, Yulish BS, Rothstein FC. How useful is barium enema in diagnosis of infantile Hirschsprung's disease? Am J Dis Child 1986;140:881–4.
81. Lake BD, Puri P, Nixon HH, et al. Hirschsprung's disease. An appraisal of histochemically demonstrated acetylcholinesterase activity in suction rectal biopsy specimens as an aid to diagnosis. Arch Pathol Lab Med 1978;26:288–91.
82. Langer JC, Durrant AC, de la Torre L, et al. One-stage transanal soave pull through for Hirschsprung's disease: a multicenter experience with 141 children. Ann Surg 2003;238:569–83.
83. El-Sawaf MI, Drongowski RA, Chamberlain JN, et al. Are the long-term results of the transanal pull-through equal to those of the transabdominal pull-through? A comparison of the 2 approaches for Hirschsprung's disease. J Pediatr Surg 2007;42:41–7.
84. Yanchar NL, Soucy P. Long term outcome after Hirschsprung' disease: patients' perspectives. J Pediatr Surg 1999;34:1152–60.
85. Miele E, Tozzi A, Staiano A, et al. Persistence of abnormal gastrointestinal motility operation for Hirschsprung' disease. Am J Gastroenterol 2000;95:1226–30.
86. Levitt MA, Peña A. Anorectal malformations. Orphanet J Rare Dis 2007;26(2):33.
87. Peña A, Levitt MA. Anorectal malformations. In: Stringer M, Oldham K, Mouriquadn PDE, editors. Pediatric surgery and urology: long-term outcomes. 2nd edition. Cambridge (UK): Cambridge University Press; 2007. p. 401–15.

88. Falcone RA Jr, Levitt MA, Peña A, et al. Increased heritability of certain types of anorectal malformations. J Pediatr Surg 2007;42(1):124–7.
89. Levitt M, falcone R, Pena A. Pediatric fecal incontinence. In: Ratto C, Doglietto GB, editors. Fecal incontinence: diagnosis and treatment. Heidelberg, Germany: Springer-Verlag; 2007. p. 341–50.
90. Staiano A, Simeone D, Del Giudice E, et al. Effect of the dietary fiber glucomannan on chronic constipation in neurologically impaired children. J Pediatr 2000;136(1):41–5.
91. Di Lorenzo C, Benninga MA. Pathophysiology of pediatric fecal incontinence. Gastroenterology 2004;126:S33–40.
92. Tobias N, Mason D, Lutkenhoff M, et al. Management principles of organic causes of childhood constipation. J Pediatr Health Care 2008;22:12–23.

Diagnosis and Management of Urinary Incontinence and Functional Fecal Incontinence (Encopresis) in Children

Rien J.M. Nijman, MD, PhD,

KEYWORD

• Urinary incontinence • Encopresis • Fecal incontinence

The ability to maintain normal continence for urine and stools is not achievable in all children by a certain age. Most children will be continent by the time they go to school, but in approximately 6% to 9% of children the ability to gain control of continence will be insufficient. Gaining control of urinary and fecal continence is a complex process, and not all steps and factors involved are fully understood. Normal development of anatomy and physiology are prerequisites to becoming fully continent. In contrast, anatomic abnormalities, such as bladder exstrophy, epispadias, ectopic ureters, and neurogenic disturbances that can usually be recognized at birth and cause incontinence will require specialist treatment, not only to restore continence but also to preserve renal function. Most forms of urinary incontinence are not caused by an anatomic or physiologic abnormality and, hence, are more difficult to diagnose and their management requires a sound knowledge of bladder and bowel function.

Most children become dry between the ages of 2 to 3 years: night-time continence will follow within a couple of weeks to months. The problem of nocturnal incontinence or enuresis is usually not associated with other symptoms, such as urinary tract infections, vesicoureteric reflux, or bladder dysfunction and will not be discussed in this article. Terminology and definitions used in this article are in accordance with the recommendations of the International Children's Continence Society.[1]

Department of Urology, University Medical Centre Groningen, Hanzeplein 1,9713 GZ Groningen, The Netherlands
E-mail address: j.m.nijman@uro.umcg.nl

Gastroenterol Clin N Am 37 (2008) 731–748
doi:10.1016/j.gtc.2008.06.007
gastro.theclinics.com
0889-8553/08/$ – see front matter

NORMAL DEVELOPMENT OF BLADDER AND SPHINCTER CONTROL

Normal bladder storage and voiding involve low-pressure and adequate bladder volume filling followed by a continuous detrusor contraction that results in bladder emptying, associated with adequate relaxation of the sphincter complex. This process requires normal sensation and normal bladder outlet resistance. The neurophysiologic mechanisms involved in normal bladder storage and evacuation include a complex integration of sympathetic, parasympathetic, and somatic innervation, which is ultimately controlled by a complex interaction between spinal cord, brain stem, midbrain, and higher cortical structures.[2]

Immediately after birth, voiding is very infrequent during the first few days of life. After the first week, frequency increases rapidly and peaks at the age of 2 to 4 weeks, to an average of once per hour. It then decreases and remains stable after 6 months to about 10 to 15 times per day. After the first year it decreases to 8 to 10 times per day, while voided volumes increase by three- to fourfold. Even in small infants micturition does not occur during sleep.[3]

In response to bladder distension during sleep, an infant nearly always exhibits clear electro-encephalographic evidence of cortical arousal, facial grimaces or limb movements, or actual awakening. Sleeping infants are always seen to wake up before the bladder contracts and voiding occurs. This arousal period may be transient and the infant may cry and move for a brief period before micturition, and then shortly afterward go back to sleep. The control of micturition involves complicated neural pathways and higher centers. A pronounced reorganization of pre-existing synaptic connections and neural pathways involved in bladder and bowel control occurs during the early postnatal period.

In newborns micturition occurs at frequent intervals and may have an intermittent pattern that will disappear with increasing age. They are thought to represent variations between individual infants in the maturation of detrusor and sphincteric coordination during the first 1 to 2 years of life. Voiding pressures are much higher than in adults, especially in boys.[4,5]

Between the age of 1 and 2, conscious sensation of bladder filling develops. The ability to void or inhibit voiding voluntarily at any degree of bladder filling commonly develops in the second and third years of life. Central inhibition is crucial to obtain continence.

During the second and third year of life, there is progressive development toward a socially conscious continence and a more voluntary type of micturition control develops. Through an active learning process, the child acquires the ability to voluntarily inhibit and delay voiding until a socially convenient time, then actively initiate urination, even when the bladder is not completely full, and allow urination to proceed to completion.

The final steps are usually achieved at the age of 3 to 4 years, when most children have developed the adult pattern of urinary control and are dry both day and night. The child has learned to inhibit a micturition reflex and postpone voiding and voluntarily initiate micturition at socially acceptable and convenient times and places. This development is also dependent on behavioral learning and can be influenced by toilet training, which in turn depends on cognitive perception of the maturing urinary tract.

It is understandable that this series of complex events is highly susceptible to the development of various types of dysfunction. Various functional derangements of the bladder-sphincter-perineal complex may occur during this sophisticated course of early development of normal micturition control mechanisms.

Fecal incontinence during childhood may be a symptom of delayed acquisition of toileting skills or may reflect serious underlying organic or functional pathology. There are considerable cultural differences in toilet training, and across the world children acquire bowel control at anytime between 1 year and 4 years of age.[6–8]

The pattern of bowel actions changes during early life from an average of three stools per day in the neonate to 1.7 stools per day at 1 year of age. Among preschool children in the United Kingdom, 97% will pass stool within the range three times per day to alternate days.[9]

PATHOPHYSIOLOGY AND CLASSIFICATION OF URINARY INCONTINENCE

Urinary incontinence in children may be caused by a congenital anatomic or neurologic abnormality, such as ectopic ureter, bladder exstrophy, or myelomeningocele. In many children, however, there is no obvious cause for the incontinence and they are referred to as having "functional incontinence."

On the basis of urodynamic studies, the functional dysfunctions can be termed "urge syndrome" (detrusor overactivity), "dysfunctional voiding" (detrusor-sphincter dyscoordination), "underactive bladder" and "non-neurogenic neurogenic bladder" (occult neurogenic bladder).[10] Functional urinary incontinence in children may be because of disturbances of the filling phase, the voiding phase, or a combination of both (**Table 1**).

Overactivity of the detrusor muscle may lead to disturbances in the filling phase, characterized by urgency, frequency, and at times urge incontinence, often associated with nocturia that is present in the absence of pathologic or metabolic factors that may cause or mimic these symptoms. Urge syndrome is best characterized by frequent episodes of an urgent need to void, countered by contraction of the pelvic floor muscles (guarding reflex) and hold maneuvers, such as squatting and the Vincent curtsey sign. The voiding phase is essentially normal, but detrusor contraction during voiding may be extremely powerful.

The etiology of the overactive bladder in children is unclear, but it appears to be related to a lack of ability to voluntarily inhibit the infant voiding reflex, a delay in central nervous system maturation. Girls present with symptoms of detrusor overactivity more often than boys. In addition to the urinary symptoms, children with functional urinary incontinence may also have recurrent urinary tract infections and constipation. Depending on fluid intake and urine production, the complaints of incontinence

Table 1
Symptoms in overactive bladder, dysfunctional voiding, and voiding postponement

Symptoms	Overactive Bladder/ Urge Syndrome	Dysfunctional Voiding	Voiding Postponement
Frequency	>7/day	Varying	<5/day
Urgency	Yes	Varying, decreases with age	Yes
Incontinence	± Urge incontinence	Varying, decreases with age	Urge incontinence
Uroflow	May be tower-shaped	Staccato/interrupted	Normal or staccato
PVR	Usually <20 mL	Increased (>20 mL)	Varying
Presenting symptoms	Frequency/urgency/ incontinence/holding maneuvers	Recurrent UTI/ incontinence	Incontinence, holding maneuvers

Abbreviations: PVR, Post-void residual; UTI, Urinary tract infection.

become worse toward the end of the day because of loss of concentration and fatigue and may also occur during the night. Children usually diminish their fluid intake to minimize wetting, and therefore incontinence may not be the main complaint or symptom. A careful history and a bladder diary will demonstrate that they often suffer from urinary frequency and urgency, their fluid intake is small, and their voided volumes are less than expected.[11]

Frequent voluntary contractions of the pelvic floor muscles may also lead to postponement of defecation. Constipation and fecal soiling are often found in children with overactive bladder.[12] The constipation is aggravated by the decreased fluid intake. Constipation contributes to an increased risk of UTIs and may exacerbate the detrusor overactivity.

Incomplete relaxation or tightening of the sphincteric mechanism and pelvic floor muscles during voiding results in an intermittent voiding pattern that may be associated with elevated post-void residuals. These children with dysfunctional voiding are also prone to constipation and recurrent UTIs.[13]

Bladder function during the filling phase in these children may be essentially normal, but detrusor overactivity may be present. The cause of dysfunctional voiding is unclear. It may be that an overactive bladder eventually leads to overactivity of the pelvic floor muscles, with subsequent insufficient relaxation during voiding.[14] Alternatively, poor relaxation of the pelvic floor muscles during voiding may be a learned condition during the toilet training years, adopted following episodes of dysuria or constipation, or occur secondary to sexual abuse.[15] Because no true structural obstruction can be identified, the intermittent incomplete pelvic floor relaxation that occurs during abnormal voiding is termed a functional disorder.

Urgency and incontinence of urine may result from detrusor overactivity and thus be seen in conjunction with increased urinary frequency. Alternatively, infrequent or poor bladder emptying may precipitate symptoms. Micturition is often achieved with significant abdominal activity and urodynamic investigations may show an interrupted or staccato flow pattern. Children with dysfunctional voiding have a higher rate of recurrent UTIs than children with no voiding abnormality and also demonstrate increased incidence of higher grades of vesicoureteral reflux (VUR).[16,17]

The child's environment, in particular toilet conditions and privacy issues, can trigger or exacerbate voiding anomalies.[18] Signs of dysfunctional voiding reflect initial compensatory overactivity of the detrusor along with poor emptying ability. They may include small bladder capacity, increased detrusor thickness, decreased detrusor contractility, impaired relaxation of the external urinary sphincter during voiding, weak or interrupted urinary stream, and large PVR volumes of urine. There may also be ultrasound abnormalities, secondary VUR, fecal soiling, or constipation.[16,19]

In children with an underactive detrusor, voiding occurs without detrusor contractions, and PVRs and incontinence are the main characteristics. Children with this condition void infrequently and usually present with UTIs and incontinence. A correct diagnosis can only be made by urodynamic evaluation. Long-standing overactivity of the pelvic floor may in some children be responsible for "decompensation" of the detrusor, leading to a noncontractile detrusor. However, no data are available to support this theory.

A non-neurogenic neurogenic bladder has been postulated to be the end-stage of dysfunctional voiding. It has been referred to as "occult neuropathic bladder." A neurologic etiology must be ruled out before determining that the child's voiding problems are consistent with the non-neurogenic neurogenic bladder. Urodynamically, non-neurogenic neurogenic bladder is characterized by diminished bladder volume and compliance. Detrusor overactivity is often present and there is contraction of the pelvic floor muscles during voiding. Videourodynamic studies or a voiding cystourethrogram (VCUG) usually show all the features of a true neurogenic bladder. These children are at risk for upper tract damage and must be fully evaluated and seen regularly.

Lettgen and colleagues.[20] introduced the term "voiding postponement." In this condition, children will postpone imminent micturition until overwhelmed by urgency, which makes them rush to the toilet; but often they are too late and incontinence occurs. Traditionally, this syndrome was thought to be an acquired disorder caused by detrusor overactivity and voluntary overactivity of the urethral sphincter until the bladder becomes filled.[21]

A recent study that compared children with typical urge syndrome to those with voiding postponement revealed a significantly higher frequency of clinically relevant behavioral symptoms in postponers than in children with urge syndrome, suggesting that voiding postponement is an acquired or behavioral disorder.[20] It remains to be determined whether or not voiding postponement can develop in the setting of a perfectly normal urinary tract or whether urge syndrome is a necessary precursor.

In some children giggling can trigger partial to complete bladder emptying well into their teenage years, and intermittently into adulthood.[22] This condition occurs in both boys and girls and is generally self-limiting. The etiology of "giggle incontinence" is not defined. Urodynamic studies fail to demonstrate any abnormalities, there is no anatomic dysfunction, the upper tracts appear normal on ultrasound, the urinalysis is normal, and there are no neurologic abnormalities.[23]

Urinary leakage that occurs in girls a short time after voiding to completion that is not associated with any strong desire to void may be the result of vesicovaginal entrapment.[24] Vesicovaginal reflux may occur because of labial adhesions, a funnel shaped hymen, or an inappropriate position on the toilet. Obesity may be an associated risk factor. Changes in voiding position and treatment of labial adhesions will lead to resolution of the urine leakage.

The genitourinary tract and the gastrointestinal system are interdependent, sharing the same embryologic origin, pelvic region, and sacral innervation. Although children with voiding disturbances often present with bowel dysfunction, until recently this coexistence was considered coincidental. However, it is now accepted that dysfunction of emptying of both systems, in the absence of anatomic abnormality or neurologic disease, is inter-related.

The common neural pathways or the mutual passage through the pelvic floor musculature may provide a theoretical basis for this relationship, as may the acquisition of environmental and developmental learning. The latter can be influenced by episodes of UTI, constipation, anal pain or trauma, childhood stressors, reluctance to toilet, and poor toilet facilities.[12,18,25]

The elimination syndrome is seen more frequently in girls than boys and is associated with the presence of both VUR and UTI.[26] Children with elimination syndrome commonly complain of urinary incontinence, nocturnal enuresis, recurrent UTIs, urgency to void, or exceptional urinary frequency, and on investigation are often noted to have poor voiding efficiency, VUR, constipation, soiling, no regular bowel routine, and infrequent toileting.[27]

EPIDEMIOLOGY OF URINARY INCONTINENCE

Several studies have reported the prevalence of daytime incontinence. Outcomes differ as the study designs were different and definitions varied. A Swedish study showed urinary incontinence during the day in 6% of the 7-year old girls and in 3.8% of the boys.[28] In Australia, urinary incontinence in 5- to 12-year-old children was reported in 5%.[29] In Belgium, the reported prevalence in children between 10 to 14 years old was 8%.[30] These studies included all forms of loss of urine during the day, from once a month to several times a day.

Urinary Incontinence and UTI

Recurrent UTIs occur in 11% of all children.[31] Of the children with daytime urinary incontinence, up to 50% have recurrent UTIs,[32] while in children with dysfunctional voiding or underactive detrusor, up to 89% have recurrent UTIs.[33,34] In a British cohort study, children with urinary incontinence suffered a UTI during the last year in 9.9% (girls) and 2.1% (boys) of children studied.[31]

Urinary Incontinence and Constipation

Epidemiologic data on fecal incontinence in the normal childhood population is variable. Bellman observed a prevalence of 1.5% among 7-year-old Swedish children, and Rutter in the UK reported a similar prevalence in 10-11 year olds.[35,36] It accounts for 3% of referrals to a medical clinic in Boston and 25% of referrals to specialist gastroenterology clinics.[37,38] Constipation in childhood occurs in 0.3% to 8% of children, depending on age, excluding children with spina bifida, Hirschsprung, and other such diseases.[39–41] In a systematic review of 18 studies, prevalence varied between 0.7% and 29.6%, with a median of 8.9%.[42] Good and reliable prevalence studies in children are sparse and the different definitions of constipation make them difficult to compare.

According to the Rome III criteria, functional constipation is present if during an 8-week period at least two of the following symptoms are present:

- Two stools or less per week
- Fecal incontinence at least once a week
- Prolonged postponement
- Painful or firm stools
- Presence of large mass of fecal impaction
- Giant stools obstructing the toilet (elephant stool)

In studies on constipation, UTI are reported in 10% and urinary incontinence during the day in 30% of children. Thus, there seems to be a clear correlation between urinary incontinence and constipation. The underlying pathophysiology has not been investigated. It might be that overactivity of the urinary sphincter to prevent urine leakage may cause a high activity of the pelvic floor muscles, with subsequent abnormal voiding and defecation patterns.[43] However, urinary incontinence may also be the result of continuous pressure on the bladder of impacted fecal mass.[44] It is now generally accepted that by far the most common cause for fecal incontinence in childhood is secondary to functional fecal retention or constipation. Several studies indicate that treatment of constipation also improves the urinary symptoms.

Urinary Incontinence and Behavioral Problems

Several studies have indicated that children with urinary incontinence often have psychologic problems; more complex forms of incontinence are associated with a higher prevalence of attention deficit hyperactivity disorder (ADHD) as well as externalizing problems.[45] In children who postpone voiding, more often externalizing problems are found (31% versus 8%).[46] Children diagnosed with ADHD had a higher incidence of incontinence, constipation, urge, irregular voiding, night-time incontinence, and dysuria, compared with children without ADHD.[47]

EVALUATION OF CHILDREN WITH DAYTIME INCONTINENCE AND CONSTIPATION

Even with clear definitions, the approach to history-taking and physical examination has to be structured. The child's complaints at presentation are not synonymous with the signs and symptoms that have to be checked to arrive at a diagnosis. In addition, sociocultural aspects and psychomotor development will distort the presentation. Validated questionnaires are very helpful in structuring the history-taking as they provide checklists.[48,49] The general history-taking should include questions relevant to familial disorders, neurologic and congenital abnormalities, and information on previous urinary infections, relevant surgery, and menstrual and sexual functions (in pubertal and older children). Information should be obtained on medication with known or possible effects on the lower urinary tract. History-taking should also include assessment of bowel function; a similar proactive process using a questionnaire should be followed for defecation and fecal soiling (**Fig. 1**).

At times it is helpful to more formally evaluate the child's psychosocial status and the family situation, for example by using validated question forms such as the Child Behavior Checklist or the Butler forms.[50,51] A suspicion of child abuse is often signaled by symptoms of vesico-urethral dysfunction.[52] A voiding diary is mandatory to determine the child's voiding frequency and volumes, as well as fluid intake and urine output over 24-hour periods. It gives objective information on the number of voidings, the distribution of day time and night time voids, the voided volumes and episodes of urgency and leakage or dribbling, and functional bladder capacity. In order to obtain a complete picture, defecation frequency or soiling is also recorded. Ideally the diary should cover 3 complete days.[53]

Detailed questioning of the parent's observation of the child's voiding habits is essential, as is direct observation of the voiding, if possible. Children may have their voiding dysfunction ameliorated or even eliminated by correcting anomalies of body position detected when observing the child's micturition. Children may void in awkward positions, such as with their legs crossed or balancing on the toilet without proper support of the legs, thereby activating the pelvic floor and obstructing the free flow of urine.[54]

Physical Examination

Apart from a general pediatric examination, the physical examination should include an assessment of perineal sensation, perineal reflexes supplied by the sacral segments S1 to S4 (standing on toes, bulbocavernosus), and anal sphincter tone and control. Special attention should be paid to inspect of the male or female genital region and the urethral meatus. Asymmetry of buttocks, legs or feet, as well as other signs of occult neurospinal dysraphism in the lumbosacral area (subcutaneous lipoma, skin discoloration, hair growth and abnormal gait) should be looked for specifically.

In examining the abdomen, the presence of a full bladder or full sigmoid or descending colon is a significant finding with a history of constipation. Many pediatricians advocate a rectal examination when there is a history of constipation.[55] In order to be comprehensive, physical examination should include urinalysis to identify any infection, hypercalciuria, and glycosuria.

Uroflowmetry

Approximately 1% of school children have a voiding that can be labeled "abnormal" with flattened or intermittent flow curves. The remaining 99% have a bell-shaped flow curve.[56] Flow recordings with a voided volume of less than 50% of the functional capacity are not consistent: they represent voiding on command, and many children will try to comply by using abdominal pressure. A helpful tool in this respect is the bladder scan: before micturition the bladder volume can be assessed.[57]

Urinary flow may be described in terms of rate and pattern and may be continuous, intermittent (in fractions), or staccato. An intermittent flow pattern shows an interrupted flow, whereas in staccato voiding the flow does not stop completely, but fluctuates because of incomplete relaxation of the sphincter. Patterns and rates should be consistent to allow for evaluation, and several recordings are needed for definitive diagnosis.[58]

With ultrasound, bladder filling is assessed and when the bladder capacity is equal to the functional or expected bladder capacity for age, the child is asked to void into the flowmeter. After recording the flow, PVR is assessed again. Alternatively, children can be asked to use a flowmeter at home with a special flowmeter has been designed for that purpose.[59] Because some children have difficulty voiding in a strange environment, this option can overcome this insecurity.

Assessment of Fecal Retention

For grading constipation, scoring a plain X-ray of the abdomen (Barr score) yields inconsistent results.[60] A better way to match clues from the medical history with signs and symptoms is the measurement of colonic transit time. As many children with non-neurogenic detrusor-sphincter dysfunction habitually use their pelvic floor as an "emergency brake," there is a high prevalence of abnormal defecation frequency and constipation in this group. Overt constipation should be dealt with before embarking on treatment of incontinence or detrusor-sphincter dysfunction.

Another way of determining fecal retention is a transabdominal ultrasound study of the rectum. In children with constipation the rectal diameter was greater than 3.5 cm, whereas in children without constipation the diameter ranged from 2.1 cm to 2.4 cm.[61,62]

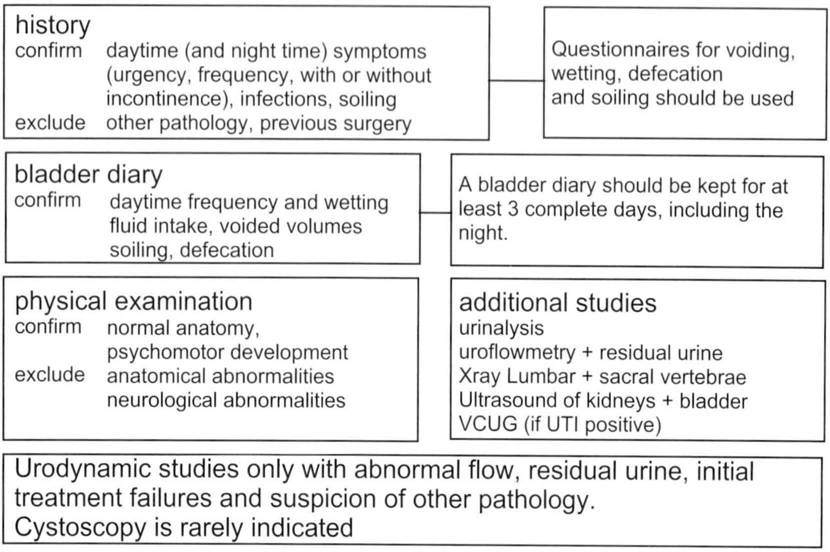

Fig. 1. Diagnostic work-up for functional incontinence.

Ultrasound

Upper tract abnormalities, such as duplex kidney, dilatation of the collecting system, and gross reflux nephropathy can be readily detected, but detection of the more subtle expressions of these abnormalities requires urologic expertise on the part of the ultrasound operator.[63] Lower urinary tract abnormalities are even more difficult to assess for the inexperienced, aside from bladder wall thickness: a bladder wall cross section of more than 3 mm to 4 mm, measured at 50% of expected bladder capacity, is suspicious of detrusor overactivity.[64,65]

URODYNAMIC STUDIES

In general urodynamic studies will only be done if the outcome will alter the management, or if there are possible treatments.[66] Indicators include voiding frequency of three or less per day, straining or manual expression during voiding, a weak urinary stream, previous febrile UTI, continuous dribbling incontinence or pronounced apparent stress incontinence, or previously identified dilating VUR. The finding of genitourinary abnormalities or signs of occult spinal dysraphism at physical examination also indicate the need for further tests.[67]

A clinically significant PVR on repeated occasions clearly points to incomplete bladder emptying. Invasive tests are indicated when the noninvasive program raises suspicion of neurogenic detrusor-sphincter dysfunction (occult spinal dysraphism), obstruction (especially posterior urethral valves), genitourinary abnormalities (eg, epispadias), advanced non-neurogenic detrusor-sphincter dysfunction (as in children with dilating VUR or febrile UTIs), or significant PVRs.[68]

A VCUG is an invasive procedure and should only be done if the outcome will influence the management. It is indicated in children with recurrent UTIs to detect reflux and in children with an abnormal flow pattern to detect bladder outlet abnormalities (such as valves, strictures or a syringocele). Women often recall their experience with VCUG during childhood as bordering on abuse. The use of VCUG in children should be limited to those situations when it is absolutely necessary.

When ultrasound imaging of kidneys and bladder, are performed together with the recording of urinary flow, and measurement of PVR and history and physical examination, the clinical entities caused by non-neurogenic detrusor-sphincter dysfunction can be diagnosed accurately in the majority of cases. A high level of suspicion can be maintained towards incomplete bladder emptying in both neurogenic detrusor-sphincter dysfunction and structural causes of incontinence. In a minority of incontinent children, this noninvasive assessment yields equivocal results, or results suggesting gross deviations from normal function. Only in these situations is there an indication for invasive investigations, such as VCUG, invasive urodynamic studies, and cystourethroscopy.

The upper urinary tract should be evaluated in children with recurrent infections and dysfunctional voiding. Uroflowmetry can be combined with pelvic floor electromyography to demonstrate overactivity of the pelvic floor muscles.[69] Urodynamic studies are usually reserved for patients with dysfunctional voiding and those not responding to treatment.[70]

NONPHARMACOLOGICAL TREATMENTS OF URINARY INCONTINENCE

The main objectives of treatment are to normalize the micturition pattern, normalize bladder and pelvic floor overactivity and cure the incontinence, infections, and constipation.

Many of the signs and symptoms of urge syndrome and other forms of functional urinary incontinence are the result of faulty perception of signals from the bladder and habitual nonphysiologic responses to the signals.[71] Children with urge syndrome need to learn to recognize the first sensation of bladder filling and learn how to suppress this by normal central inhibition instead of resorting to emergency procedures like urethral compression. Children with dysfunctional voiding need to learn how to void with a completely relaxed pelvic floor and to void with a detrusor contraction rather than the use of abdominal pressure.

There are several key components to the nonpharmacologic approach to the management of urge syndrome and dysfunctional voiding. The main points include:

- Education regarding the function of the bladder and sphincter mechanism
- Instructions on a voiding regimen, promoting regular voiding habits and proper positioning; those children with elevated PVRs are placed on double voiding regimens in addition to timed voiding regimens
- Bladder diaries
- Treatment of underlying constipation
- Treatment of concomitant urinary tract infections and antibiotic prophylaxis in those with recurrent UTIs

The initial treatment of daytime urinary incontinence involves a behavioral and cognitive approach. The child and parents or caregivers are educated about normal bladder function and responses to urgency, learning to recognize the desire to void and eradication of holding maneuvers (ie, immediate voiding without postponement). Micturition charts and diaries and voiding regimens are helpful in ensuring regular voiding. Voiding regimens and dietary changes may be instituted as needed. Treatment of UTIs and constipation are also essential. More active treatment involves pharmacotherapy, pelvic floor muscle relaxation techniques, and biofeedback, either alone or in combination.

The treatment of urge syndrome involves a multimodal approach. Behavioral modification is important and in some children may be all that is necessary. Others will require the addition of antimuscarinic medication. In some children, the addition of biofeedback is useful.

Treatment of dysfunction voiding is aimed at optimizing bladder emptying and inducing full relaxation of the urinary sphincter or pelvic floor before and during voiding. Specific goals are: consistent relaxation of the pelvic floor throughout voiding, a normal flow pattern, no residual urine, and resolution of voiding symptoms.

Strategies to achieve these goals include pelvic floor muscle awareness and timing training, repeated sessions of biofeedback visualization of pelvic floor activity and relaxation, clean intermittent self-catheterization for large PVR volumes of urine, and antimuscarinic drug therapy if detrusor overactivity is present. If the bladder neck is implicated in increased resistance to voiding, alpha-blocker drugs may be introduced. Recurrent urinary infections and constipation should be treated and prevented during the treatment period.

More active conventional management involves a combination of cognitive, behavioral, physical, and pharmacologic therapy methods. Common modes of treatment include parent and child reassurance, bladder retraining (including timed toileting), pharmacotherapy, pelvic floor muscle relaxation (physiotherapy), and the use of biofeedback to inhibit rises in detrusor pressure associated with urinary incontinence.[72,73] Rehabilitation of bladder and pelvic floor muscles using different modalities, such as explanation and instructions in combination with medical treatment of constipation and infections, physiotherapy, and biofeedback, plays a major role in the treatment of children with bladder and sphincter dysfunctions.[74] A combination of bladder training programs and pharmacologic treatment aimed specifically at reducing detrusor contractions is often useful and sometimes necessary.

In children with an underactive detrusor, bladder emptying can be achieved with timed and double voiding. If this does not provide adequate results, clean intermittent self-catheterization may be tried in combination with treatment of infections and constipation (which may be extreme in these patients).[75]

Neuromodulation has been used in adults for a variety of lower urinary tract symptoms. However, the invasive nature of the procedure makes it less attractive, particularly for children.

The use of transcutaneous stimulation of the sacral root (S3) using surface electrodes has shown promising results, but further studies are needed.[76] Several frequencies have been tried but stimulation at 2 Hz seems to be optimal.

Alarm therapy has traditionally been used for the treatment of nocturnal enuresis and has rarely been used for daytime wetting. In a randomized clinical trial, Halliday and colleagues[77] compared a contingent alarm (which sounded when the child wets) with a noncontingent alarm system (which sounded at intermittent intervals to remind the child to void). Although the risk of persistent wetting with the contingent alarm was 67% of the risk of persistent wetting with the noncontingent alarm, the difference in the reduction in wetting between the groups was not significant (risk ratio 0.67, 95% confidence interval 0.29–1.56).

Physiotherapy and biofeedback both focus on the pelvic floor. Relaxation of the pelvic floor during voiding is essential for normal voiding and most of these patients are unable to relax their pelvic floor muscles. Biofeedback is important for showing the children the effect of their efforts.

In children with a suspected bladder outlet obstruction, endoscopic investigations should be performed. Most often the abnormality can be treated at the same time. In girls, a meatal web may cause a deflection of the stream upwards (causing stimulation of the clitoris and bulbocavernosus reflex). A meatotomy may cure this problem, though no information on the long-term effects is available.[78]

PHARMACOLOGIC THERAPY OF URINARY INCONTINENCE

Antimuscarinic therapy remains one of the common forms of therapy for the overactive bladder. Its use is predicated on the concept that parasympathetic mediated stimulation of muscarinic receptors in the bladder causes detrusor overactivity, which is responsible for the symptoms of overactive bladder. Antimuscarinic agents have been demonstrated to increase bladder capacity, increase bladder compliance, and decrease detrusor contractions in neurogenic detrusor overactivity. More commonly, pharmacotherapy is instituted when behavioral therapy has failed to achieve a satisfactory outcome. The outcome of pharmacologic therapy for daytime urinary incontinence is unpredictable and inconsistent and there are few randomized studies available to assess drug safety and efficacy.

Currently the pharmacologic therapy most widely used in children with detrusor overactivity is oxybutynin.[79] Oxbutynin-XL, has been approved by the Food and Drug Administration for use in children.[80] Oxybutynin use has been limited by its adverse effect profile, with such side effects as dry mouth, constipation, facial flushing, and central nervous system effects. The incidence of side effects seems to be dose-related, both for oral and intravesical administration.[81] The central nervous system effects are related to the ability for oxybutynin to cross the blood brain barrier. Oxybutynin-XL uses a novel delivery system, bypassing the first pass metabolism in the liver, resulting in a more favorable tolerability profile. The delivery system requires an intact tablet and thus it cannot be cut or crushed to facilitate swallowing.

Other drugs are tolterodine, trospium, propiverine, and solifenacine.[82,83] None of these drugs have a pediatric indication and can only be prescribed off-label. The first three have all been studied prospectively in children, but only tolterodine was subjected to a placebo controlled, randomized trial and did not show a significant difference between placebo and study medication. Tolterodine was shown to have good safety profile. The chemical nature of tolterodine makes it less likely to penetrate the blood brain barrier, which is supported by EEG studies.[82] Efficacy seems to be comparable for oxybutynin and tolterodine.[84–86]

Botulinum toxin A is currently being used in children, mainly with neurogenic detrusor overactivity. Initial results seem promising, but more studies need to be done. In children 100 to 200 Units are injected in 20 to 30 spots.[87] Injection is also possible into the external sphincter, but the results are more variable and last only 3 to 4 months.[88]

Treatment of the overactive pelvic floor and sphincter is much more difficult. Treatment with α-adrenergic blockade produces variable results.[89,90]

FUNCTIONAL FECAL RETENTION AND FUNCTIONAL RETENTIVE SOILING

Of the children who soil, 95% have no inherent bowel or neurologic abnormality but are incontinent as a result of functional constipation. There has been considerable debate as to the relative influences of psychologic, behavioral, and physical factors in the development of constipation, but the cause of severe constipation is probably multifactorial.

Parents may describe maneuvers and postures adopted by the child that almost certainly represent avoidance of defecation. Such behavior is reinforced by episodes of painful defecation, as with anal fissure. In older children, reluctance to use toilet facilities at nursery and school may also precipitate stool holding and subsequent constipation.

Assessment of these children requires a detailed history and examination to exclude any organic cause. Few, if any, initial investigations are necessary, provided no other potential condition is discovered on assessment. The key to management following initial clear out remains a combination of a toilet training behavioral program with laxatives to keep the bowel clear. Increasing clear fluids and attention to diet to increase fiber content and reduce milk intake if necessary is also important. Over the last few years osmotic laxative treatment with macrogols (polyethylene glycol variations, with and without electrolytes) have been shown to be effective and safe both in large doses for initial clear out (this may take up to 5 days) and smaller doses for maintenance.[91,92]

If hospital admission for clearout is necessary, oral treatment for disimpaction using Kleen Prep by nasogastric tube is usually effective and avoids the use of rectal enemas or suppositories that can upset younger children. Although macrogols are effective for maintenance, some children will not be completely controlled and require additional stimulant laxatives, such as Senna or Sodium Picosulfate, the latter being more effective and better tolerated than the former.

FUNCTIONAL NONRETENTIVE SOILING

Children over 4 years who do not have underlying constipation and have no organic or anatomic abnormality but present with stool leakage are defined as having “nonretentive soiling.” They often pass normal stools and at normal stool frequency but into their clothing. Day and night-time urinary incontinence is commonly associated. Attention to signs of toilet training readiness is important, with specialist help in devising tailor-made programs to encourage continence for both urine and stools.

Soiling may result from loose stools in some children. Care needs to be taken to ensure that this is not overflow soiling, and to identify any underlying inflammatory bowel disease. Antidiarrheals may help to achieve continence.

Primary and involuntary soiling may be because of delayed toilet training. Children with neuro-developmental disorders, such as autism, ADHD, and developmental coordination disorder are more likely to have problems with constipation. They are more likely to have difficulties with establishing normal toilet training routines because of problems with poor attention, motivation, fine motor skills, and sequencing.[93]

Secondary or voluntary soiling is more likely to have an underlying psychologic cause, especially when it is related to specific and identifiable triggers. Children with a history of abuse or neglect often have continence problems with soiling in 26% of cases.[94]

TREATMENT OF FECAL INCONTINENCE

All treatment programs are based on explanation, demystification, and behavioral modification, including a regular toileting program. In general, stool softeners or laxatives such as lactulose or high dietary fiber are best avoided, as soft stools are more difficult to evacuate.

It is crucial that parents, caregivers, and the child understand the reason(s) for the soiling. The child is likely to have little or no perception of soiling episodes. Acknowledging this is a relief for the child who previously has been misunderstood, although it may cause some guilt for the parents.

Establishing a normal and regular pattern of bowel evacuation is central for the success in children with soiling from any cause. Star charts and reward systems can be used to reinforce this behavior. Externalization of the bowel problem, by using ideas such as goal scoring charts or beating that "sneaky poo" can be helpful. Behavioral programs like these on their own have been shown to be of benefit, but are even more successful when used in conjunction with appropriate laxative medication.[95,96] Continuing follow up and support to maintain motivation is important. A well-balanced diet with a reasonable fiber intake is likely to be helpful. Experimental studies have shown that increasing fiber results in shorter bowel transit times and stool greater volume and water content.[97]

There is general consensus that the child with constipation and overflow soiling requires laxative treatment with the aim of evacuating the retained stool and maintaining regular bowel actions thereafter.[98,99] Once retained stool is cleared, soiling will dramatically reduce. Various approaches have been used to maintain regular bowel actions: the mainstay being laxative treatment with behavioral approaches designed to establish a regular toileting routine, enhance compliance, and maintain motivation.

REFERENCES

1. Nevéus T, Von Gontard A, Hoebeke P, et al. The standardization of terminology of lower urinary tract function in children and adolescents: report from the Standardisation Committee of the International Children's Continence Society. J Urol 2006; 176:314–24.
2. Steers WD, et al. Physiology and pharmacology of the bladder and urethra. In: Walsh PC, Retol AB, Vaughan ED, et al, editors. Campbell's Urology. 7th edition. Philadelphia: WB Saunders; 1997. p. 870–916.
3. Ohel G, Haddad S, Samueloff A. Fetal urine production and micturition and fetal behavioral state. Am J Perinatol 1995;12:91–2.

4. Yeung CK, Godley ML, Dhillon HK, et al. Urodynamic patterns in infants with normal lower urinary tracts or primary vesico-ureteric reflux. Br J Urol 1998;81: 461–7.
5. Bachelard M, Sillen U, Hansson S, et al. Urodynamic pattern in asymptomatic infants: siblings of children with vesico-ureteric reflux. J Urol 1999;162:1733–7.
6. De Vries MW, de Vries MR. Cultural relativity of toilet training readiness: a perspective from East Africa. Pediatrics 1977;60:170–7.
7. Largo RH, Stutzle W. Longitudinal study of bowel and bladder control by day and at night in the first six years of life. I: epidemiology and interrelations between bowel and bladder control. Dev Med Child Neurol 1977;19:598–606.
8. Largo RH, Stutzle W. Longitudinal study of bowel and bladder control by day and at night in the first six years of life. II: the role of potty training and the child's initiative. Dev Med Child Neurol 1977;19:607–13.
9. Weaver LT, Steiner H. The bowel habit of young children. Arch Dis Child 1984;59: 694–702.
10. Nørgaard JP, van Gool JD, Hjälmås K, et al. Standardization and definitions in lower urinary tract dysfunction in children. Br J Urol 1998;81:1–16.
11. Bauer SB. Special considerations of the overactive bladder in children. Urology 2002;60(5 Suppl 1):43–8.
12. Loening-Baucke V. Urinary incontinence and urinary tract infection and their resolution with treatment of chronic constipation of childhood. Pediatrics 1997; 100:228–32.
13. Hjälmås K, Hoebeke PB, de Paepe H. Lower urinary tract dysfunction and urodynamics in children. Eur Urol 2000;38:655–65.
14. Abidari JM, Shortliffe LM. Urinary incontinence in girls. Urol Clin North Am. 2002; 29:661–75.
15. Ellsworth PI, Merguerian PA, Copening ME. Sexual abuse: another causative factor in dysfunctional voiding. J Urol 1995;153:773–6.
16. Hoebeke P, Laecke van E, Camp van C, et al. One thousand video-urodynamic studies in children with non-neurogenic sphincter dysfunction. BJU Int 2001;87: 575–80.
17. Benoit RM, Wise BV, Naslund MJ, et al. The effect of dysfunctional voiding on the costs of treating vesicoureteral reflux: a computer model. J Urol 2002;168: 2173–6.
18. Cooper CS, Abousally CT, Austin JC, et al. Do public schools teach voiding dysfunction? Results of an elementary school teacher survey. J Urol 2003;170: 956–8.
19. Mazzola BL, von Vigier RO, Marchand S, et al. Behavioral and functional abnormalities linked with recurrent urinary tract infections in girls. J Nephrol 2003;16: 133–8.
20. Lettgen B, von Gontard A, Olbing H, et al. Urge incontinence and voiding postponement in children: somatic and psychosocial factors. Acta Paediatr 2002;91: 978–84.
21. Hjalmas K. Urge incontinence and voiding postponement in children: somatic and psychoscocial factors. Acta Paediatr 2002;91:895–6.
22. Maizels M, Ghandi K, Keating B, et al. Diagnosis and treatment for children who cannot control urination. Curr Probl Pediatr 1993;402–50.
23. Chandra M, Saharia R, Shi Q, et al. Giggle incontinence in children: a manifestation of detrusor instability. J Urol 2002;168:2184–7.
24. Mattsson S, Gladh G. Urethrovaginal reflux—a common cause of daytime incontinence in girls. Pediatrics 2003;111:136–9.

25. Chase JW, Homsy Y, Siggaard C, et al. Functional constipation in children. J Urol 2004;171:2641–3.
26. Chen JJ, Mao W, Homayoon K, et al. A multivariate analysis of dysfunctional elimination syndrome, and its relationships with gender, urinary tract infection and vesicoureteral reflux in children. J Urol 2004;171:1907–10.
27. Bower WF, Yip SK, Yeung CK. Dysfunctional elimination symptoms in childhood and adulthood. J Urol. 2005;174(4 Pt 2):1623–7 [discussion: 1627–8] [erratum in: J Urol 2005;74:2428].
28. Hellström AL, Hanson E, Hansson S, et al. Micturition habits and incontinence in 7-year-old Swedish school entrants. Eur J Paediatr 1990;149:434–7.
29. Sureshkumar P, Craig J, Roy LP, et al. Daytime urinary incontinence in primary school children: a population-based survey. J Pediatr 2000;137:814–8.
30. Bakker E, Van Sprundel M, Van der Auwera JC, et al. Voiding habits and wetting in a population of 4,332 Belgian school children aged between 10 and 14 years. Scand J Urol Nephrol 2002;36:354–62.
31. Heron J, Joinson CJ. Symptoms of daytime wetting in a cohort of 7–8 year olds. The ALSPAC study. In: Proceedings International Children's Continence Society meeting, Antalya, Turkey, 2006.
32. Hansen A, Hansen B, Dahm TL. Urinary tract infection, day wetting and other voiding symptoms in seven-to eight-year old Danish children. Acta Paediatr Scand 1997;86:1345–9.
33. Bruegelmans A, Wyndaele JJ. Urodynamic findings in patients below 12 years old with different clinical kinds of enuresis. Acta Urol Belg 1992;60:65–71.
34. Van Gool J, Tanagho EA. External sphincter activity and recurrent urinary tract infection in girls. Urology 1977;10:348–53.
35. Bellman M. Studies on encopresis. Acta Paediatr Scand Suppl 1966;170:1–151.
36. Rutter M. Helping Troubled Children. Harmons-Worth (England): Penguin Education; 1995.
37. Levine MD. Children with encopresis: a descriptive analysis. Pediatrics 1975;56: 412–6.
38. Rasquin A, Di Lorenzo C, Forbes D, et al. Childhood functional gastrointestinal disorders: child/adolescent. Gastroenterology 2006;130:1370–90.
39. Hyman PE, Milla PJ, Benninga MA, et al. Childhood functional gastrointestinal disorders: neonate/toddler. Gastroenterology 2006;130:1519–26.
40. Loening-Baucke V. Prevalence, symptoms and outcome of constipation in infants and toddlers. J Pediatr 2005;146:359–63
41. Drossman DA. The functional gastrointestinal disorders and the Rome III process. Introduction. Gastroenterology 2006;130:1377–90.
42. Van den Berg MM, Benninga MA, Di Lorenzo C. Epidemiology of childhood constipation: a systematic review. Am J gastroenterol 2006;101:2401–9.
43. De Paepe H, Hoebeke P, Renson C, et al. Pelvic-floor therapy in girls with recurrent urinary tract infections and dysfunctional voiding. Br J Urol 1998; 81(Suppl 3):109–13.
44. Di Lorenzo C, Benninga MA. Pathophysiology of peditrac fecal incontinence. Gastroenterology 2004;126(130 Suppl 1):S33–40.
45. Baeyens D, Roeyers H, Vande Walle J, et al. Behavioural problems and attention-deficit hyperactivity disorder in children with enuresis: a literature review. Eur J Pediatr 2005;164:665–72.
46. Von Gontard A, Lettgen B, Olbing H, et al. Behavioral problems in children with urge incontinence and voiding postponement: a comparison of a pediatric and child psychiatric sample. Br J Urol 1998;81(Suppl 3):100–6.

47. Duel BP, Steinberg-Epstein R, Hill M, et al. A survey of voiding dysfunction in children with attention deficit-hyperactivity disorder. J Urol 2003;170:1521–4.
48. Sureshkumar P, Craig JC, Roy LP, et al. A reproducible pediatric daytime urinary incontinence questionnaire. J Urol 2001;165:569–73.
49. Sureshkumar P, Bower W, Craig JC, et al. Treatment of daytime urinary incontinence in children (protocol). The Cochrane Library 2005;3:1–6.
50. Butler RJ. Establishment of working definitions in nocturnal enuresis. Arch Dis Child 1991;66:267–71.
51. Achenbach TM. Manual for the Child Behavior Checklist 4–18 and 1991 profile. Burlington (VT): University of Vermont; 1991.
52. Bloom DA. Sexual abuse and voiding dysfunction [editorial]. J Urol 1995;153:777.
53. Bower WF, Moore KH, Adams RD, et al. Frequency-volume chart data from incontinent children. Br J Urol 1997;80:658–62.
54. Wennergren HM, Öberg BE, Sandstedt P. The importance of leg support for relaxation of the pelvic floor muscles. A surface electromyography study in healthy girls. Scand J Urol Nephrol 1991;25:205–13.
55. Biggs WS, Dery WH. Evaluation and treatment of constipation in infants and children. Am Fam physician 2006;7:469–77.
56. Mattson S, Spangberg A. Urinary flow in healthy school children. Neurourol Urodyn 1994;13:281–96.
57. Dudley NJ, Kirkland M, Lovett J, et al. Clinical agreement between automated and calculated ultrasound measurements of bladder volume. Br J Radiol 2003; 76:832–4.
58. Hannson S, Hellström A-L, Hermansson G, et al. Standardisation of urinary flow patterns in children. In: Nørgaard JP, Djurhuus JC, Hjälmås K, editors. Proceedings of the Third International Children's Continence Symposium. Royal Tunbridge Wells (UK): Wells Medical; 1996. p. 159–61.
59. Yang SS, Wang CC, Chen YT. Home uroflowmetry for the evaluation of boys with urinary incontinence. J Urol 2003;169:1505–7.
60. van den Bosch M, Graafmans D, Nievelstein R, et al. Systematic assessment of constipation on plain abdominal radiographs in children. Pediatr Radiol 2006;36: 224–6.
61. Singh SJ, Gibbons NJ, Vincent MV, et al. Use of pelvic ultrasound in the diagnosis of megarectum in children with constipation. J Pediatr Surg 2005;40:1941–4.
62. Klijn AJ, Asselman M, Vijverberg MA, et al. The diameter of the rectum on ultrasonography as a diagnostic tool for constipation in children with dysfunctional voiding. J Urol 2004;172:1986–8.
63. Kuzmic AC, Brkljacic B. Color Doppler ultrasonography in the assessment of vesicoureteric reflux in children with bladder dysfunction. Pediatr Surg Int 2002;18:135–9.
64. Müller L, Bergström T, Hellström AL, et al. Standardised ultrasound method for assessing detrusor muscle thickness in children. J Urol 2000;164:134–8.
65. Cvitkovic-Kuzmic A, Brkljacic B, Ivankovic D, et al. Ultrasound assessment of detrusor muscle thickness in children with non-neuropathic bladder/sphincter dysfunction. Eur Urol 2002;41:214–8.
66. Szabo L, Lombay B, Borbas E, et al. Videourodynamics in the diagnosis of urinary tract abnormalities in a single center. Pediatr Nephrol 2004;19:326–31.
67. Bauer SB. Pediatric urodynamics: lower tract. In: O'Donnell B, Koff SA, editors. Pediatric urology. Oxford (UK): Butterworth–Heineman; 1998. p. 125–51.
68. Chin-Peuckert L, Komlos M, Rennick JE, et al. What is the variability between 2 consecutive cystometries in the same child? J Urol 2003;170:1614–7.

69. Pfister C, Dacher JN, Gaucher S, et al. The usefulness of a minimal urodynamic evaluation and pelvic floor biofeedback in children with chronic voiding dysfunction. BJU Int 1999;84:1054–7.
70. Soygur T, Arikan N, Tokatli Z, et al. The role of video-urodynamic studies in managing non-neurogenic voiding dysfunction in children. BJU Int 2004;93:841–3.
71. Van Gool JD, de Jonge DA. Urge Syndrome and urge incontinence. Arch Dis Child 1989;64:1629–34.
72. Hellström A-L, Hjälmås K, Jodal U. Rehabilitation of the dysfunctional bladder in children: method and three year follow up. J Urol 1987;38:847–9.
73. Allen HA, Austin JC, Boyt MA, et al. Initial trial of timed voiding is warranted for all children with daytime incontinence. Urology 2007;69:962–5.
74. de Jong TP, Klijn AJ, Vijverberg MA, et al. Effect of biofeedback training on paradoxical pelvic floor movement in children with dysfunctional voiding. Urology 2007;70:790–3.
75. Pohl HG, Bauer SB, Borer JG, et al. The outcome of voiding dysfunction managed with clean intermittent catheterization in neurologically and anatomically normal children. BJU Int 2002;89:923–7.
76. Klingler HC, Pycha A, Schmidbauer J, et al. Use of peripheral neuromodulation of the S3 region for treatment of detrusor overactivity: a urodynamic-basic study. Urol 2000;56:766–71.
77. Halliday S, Meadow SR, Berg I. Successful management of daytime enuresis using alarm procedures: a randomly controlled trial. Arch Dis Child 1987;62: 132–7.
78. Hoebeke P, van Laecke E, Raes A, et al. Anomalies of the external urethral meatus in girls with non-neurogenic bladder sphincter dysfunction. BJU Int 1999;83:294–8.
79. Dikno AI, Lapides J. A new drug with analgesic and anticholinergic properties. J Urol 1972;108:307–10.
80. Youdim K, Kogan BA. Preliminary study of the safety and efficacy of extended-release oxybutynin in children. Urology 2002;59:428–32.
81. Kaplinsky R, Greenfield S, Wan J, et al. Expanded follow up on intravesical oxybutynin chloride used in children with neurogenic bladder. J Urol 1996;156: 753–6.
82. Todorova A, Vonderheid-Guth B, Dimpfel W. Effects of tolterodine, trospium chloride, and oxybutynin on the central nervous system. J Clin Pharmacol 2001;41: 636–44.
83. Lopez Pereira P, Miguelez C, Caffarati J, et al. Trospium chloride for the treatment of detrusor instability in children. J Urol 2003;170:1978–81.
84. Bolduc S, Upadhyay J, Payton J, et al. The use of tolterodine in children after oxybutynin failure. BJU Int 2003;91:398–401.
85. Munding M, Wessells H, Thornberry B, et al. Use of tolterodine in children with dysfunctional voiding: an initial report. J Urol 2001;165:926–8.
86. Reinberg Y, Crocker J, Wolpert J, et al. Therapeutic efficacy of extended release oxybutynin chloride, and immediate release and long acting tolterodine tartrate in children with diurnal urinary incontinence. J Urol 2003;169:317–9.
87. Hoebeke P, De Caestecker K, Vande Walle J, et al. The effect of botulium-A toxin in incontinent children with therapy resistant overactive detrusor. J Urol 2006;176: 328–30.
88. Mokhless I, Gaafar S, Fouda K, et al. Botulinum A toxin urethral sphincter injection in children with nonneurogenic neurogenic bladder. J Urol 2006;176:1767–8.

89. Cain MP, Wu SD, Austin PF, et al. Alpha blocker therapy for children with dysfunctional voiding and urinary retention. J Urol 2003;170:1514–5.
90. Yang SS, Wang CC, Chen YT. Effectiveness of alpha1-adrenergic blockers in boys with low urinary flow rate and urinary incontinence. J Formos Med Assoc 2003;102:551–5.
91. Loening-Baucke V. Polyethylene glycol without electrolytes for children with constipation and encopresis. J Pediatr Gastroenterol Nutr 2002;34:374–7.
92. Pashankar DS, Bishop WP. Efficiency and optimal dose of daily polyethylene glycol 3350 for treatment of constipation and encopresis in children. J Pediatr 2001;139:428–32.
93. Johnston BD, Wright JA. Attentional dysfunction in children with encopresis. J Dev Behav Pediatr 1993;14:381–5.
94. Gohlke BC, Khadilkar VV, Skuse D, et al. Recognition of children with psychosocial short stature: a spectrum of presentation. J Pediatr Endocrinol Metab 1998; 11:509–17.
95. Poenaru D, Roblin N, Bird M, et al. The pediatric bowel management clinic: initial results of a multidisciplinary approach to functional constipation in children. J Pediatr Surg 1997;32:843–8.
96. Nolan T, Debelle G, Oberklaid F, et al. Randomised trail of laxatives in treatment of childhood encopresis. Lancet 1991;338:523–7.
97. Taitz LS, Wales JKW, Urwin OM. Factors associated with outcome in management of defaecation disorders. Arch Dis Child 1986;61:472–6.
98. Loening-Baucke V. Encopresis and soiling. Pediatr Clin North Am 1996;43: 279–98.
99. Ramkumar D, Rao SS. Efficacy and safety of traditional medical therapies for chronic constipation: systematic review. Am J Gastroenterol 2005;100:936–71.

Index

Note: Page numbers of article titles are in **bold face** type.

A

Abdominal rectopexy, for rectal prolapse, 648, 652
Abscess, after restorative proctocolectomy, 671–672
Aganglionosis (Hirschsprung's disease), 718–724
Alarm therapy, for urinary incontinence, 741
Allergy, constipation and, 717
Altmeier procedure, for rectal prolapse, 650
Amitriptyline, for fecal incontinence, 592
Anal canal, functional length of, 514–515
Anal canal pressure, 502–503
Anal dilatation, for anal fissure, 637
Anal endosonography, 555–558, 646
Anal fissure, 634–638
  classification of, 634
  pathogenesis of, 634
  physiologic aspects of, 634–635
  treatment of, 635–638
Anal resting pressure, measurement of, 515
Anal sphincters
  anatomy of, 495–496
  artificial, 616–617
  bulking agents for, 617–618
  division of, for anal fissure, 637–638
  dysfunction of, 505, 676–677
  evaluation of, 514–516
  function of, 634–635, 712–713
  neurophysiologic evaluation of, 527–531
  new, creation of, 616–617
  repair of, 614
  ultrasonography of, 555–558
Anal squeeze pressure, measurement of, 515–516
Anorectal malformations, 724–725
Anorectal pain, functional, 686–689
Anorectal sensation modification, for fecal incontinence, 593
Anterograde colonic enema, for constipation, 610–611
Antibiotics, for prostatitis, 692
Antidepressants
  for painful bladder syndrome, 690
  for prostatitis, 692
Antimuscarinic agents, for urinary incontinence, 740–741
Anus, imperforate, 724–725
Artificial anal sphincter, for fecal incontinence, 616–617

Gastroenterol Clin N Am 37 (2008) 749–762
doi:10.1016/S0889-8553(08)00064-2
0889-8553/08/$ – see front matter
gastro.theclinics.com

Atopy, constipation and, 717
Attention deficit hyperactivity disorder, urinary incontinence and, 736–737
Autonomic nervous system
 of anal sphincters, 495
 of bladder, 540

B

Bacillus Calmette-Guérin vaccine, for painful bladder syndrome, 691
Baden-Walker system, for pelvic organ prolapse, 659
Balloon, in biofeedback training, for fecal incontinence, 593–594
Balloon distention test, 521–524, 574–575
Balloon expulsion test, 519
Band ligation, for hemorrhoids, 630
Barium studies
 in Hirschsprung's disease, 721
 in rectocele, 659–660
 in solitary rectal ulcer, 657
Barostat studies, 512, 520–527
Behavioral problems, urinary incontinence and, 736–737
Behavioral treatment
 for constipation, 714–715
 for fecal incontinence, 743
 for urinary incontinence, 699–701, 740
Bile salt malabsorption, after restorative proctocolectomy, 679
Biofeedback therapy
 for corrected rectal prolapse, 653
 for dyssynergic defecation, 579–582
 for fecal incontinence, 592–599
  anorectal sensation modification in, 593
  clinical trials of, 596–599
  coordination training in, 593–594
  efficacy of, 594
  electrical stimulation in, 594–595
  failure of, 595
  voluntary squeeze measures, 593
 for intussusception, 654–655
 for levator ani syndrome, 687–688
 for solitary rectal ulcer syndrome, 657–658
 for urinary incontinence, 740–741
Biopsy, in Hirschsprung's disease, 721–722
Bisacodyl, for constipation, 716
Bladder
 development of, 732–733
 incontinence related to. *See* Urinary incontinence.
 non-neurogenic neurogenic, 734–735
 overactive, 549–550, 690, 733–734, 740–741
 pain in, 689–691
 urodynamic evaluation of, **539–552**
Botulinum toxin
 for anal fissure, 636

for dyssynergic defecation, 582
for urinary incontinence, 742
Bowel habit, for fecal incontinence, 590–591
Bran, for dyssynergic defecation, 576–577
Broad ligaments, anatomy of, 493
Budesonide, for pouchitis, 678

C

Calcium channel blockers, for anal fissure, 635–636
Cardinal ligaments, anatomy of, 493
Chloride channel activators, for dyssynergic defecation, 578
Chronic pain disorders. *See* Pain disorders.
Ciprofloxacin, for pouchitis, 678
Cloacal malformations, 724–725
Clonidine, for proctalgia fugax, 689
Coagulation, for hemorrhoids, 630–631
Coccygeus muscle, anatomy of, 497–498
Codeine, for fecal incontinence, 592
Cognitive therapy
for constipation, 715
for urinary incontinence, 740
Colchicine, for dyssynergic defecation, 578–579
Colectomy, for constipation, 607–610
Colon, resection of, for constipation, 607–610
Colonic transit time, in constipation, 714
Colostomy
for constipation, 611
for Hirschsprung's disease, 721, 723–724
Colporrhaphy, posterior, for rectocele, 660–661
Compliance
bladder, 542–544
rectal, 524–527
Compound muscle action potentials, in pudendal nerve evaluation, 527–528
Computed tomography
in pelvic floor disorders, 498–499
interventional, 562–563
Congenital anomalies, anorectal, 724–725
Conjoint tendon, anatomy of, 495
Constipation. *See also* Dyssynergic defecation.
atopy and, 717
definition of, 710
diagnosis of, 713–714
epidemiology of, 710–711
evaluation of, **511–538**
fecal incontinence in, 702–703
functional, 711–717
genetic factors in, 712
in neurologic impairment, 725
in pediatric patients, **709–730**
in pelvic floor muscle dysfunction, 505–506

Constipation (*continued*)
in rectal prolapse, 646
nonsurgical treatment of, 703, 714–717
organic, 718–724
outlet obstruction type, 505
pathogenesis of, 711
physiologic considerations in, 712–713
red flags in, 713
slow-transit, 505
surgical treatment of, 606–613
anterograde colonic enema, 610–611
colonic resection, 607–610
historical, 606–607
options for, 606
sacral nerve stimulation, 611–612
stapled transanal rectal resection, 612–613
stoma, 611
urinary incontinence and, 736–739
versus normal defecation, 710
Continence, problems with. *See* Fecal incontinence; Urinary incontinence.
Corticosteroids, for pouchitis, 678
Cow's milk allergy, constipation and, 717
Cryotherapy, for hemorrhoids, 631
Cystitis, interstitial, 689–691
Cystometry, 540–544, 548–549
Cystoscopy, painful bladder syndrome, 690

D

Defecation
balloon expulsion test for, 519
dyssynergic. *See* Dyssynergic defecation.
in intussusception, 654
in solitary rectal ulcer, 657
normal, in pediatric patients, 710
physiology of, 712–713
rectoanal pressure evaluation during, 517–518
Defecography, 553–555
in dyssynergic defecation, 575
in rectal prolapse, 646
in rectocele, 659–660
MRI, 559–562
Delorme procedure, for rectal prolapse, 650
Dementia
fecal incontinence in, 701
urinary incontinence in, 698–699
Detrusor muscle, dysfunction of, 733–735, 740–741
Diapers, for fecal incontinence, 595
Diarrhea, fecal incontinence in, 703
Diet
for fecal incontinence, 591

for solitary rectal ulcer syndrome, 657
Digital rectal examination, in dyssynergic defecation, 572–573
Dilatation, of anus, for anal fissure, 637
Diltiazem, for anal fissure, 636
Dimethyl sulfoxide, for painful bladder syndrome, 690–691
Diphenoxylate, for fecal incontinence, 592
Docusates, for dyssynergic defecation, 578
Doppler-guided hemorrhoidal artery ligation, 631
Dyssynergic defecation, 505–506, **569–586**
clinical features of, 571–572
diagnosis of, 572–575
differential diagnosis of, 572
economic impact of, 570
epidemiology of, 569–570
etiology of, 570–571
pathophysiology of, 571
quality of life with, 570
rectoanal pressure relationships in, 517–518
treatment of, 575–582

E

Electrical stimulation
for fecal incontinence, 594–595, 616
for levator ani syndrome, 687–688
Electrocoagulation, for hemorrhoids, 631
Electrodes, in anal sensation evaluation, 520
Electromyography
in anal evaluation, 528–530
in bladder evaluation, 545–547
in rectal prolapse, 646–648
Electrosensitivity test, in anal sensation evaluation, 520–521, 523–524
Elimination syndrome, 735
Endometriosis, of bladder, 690
Endoscopic band ligation, for hemorrhoids, 630
Endosonography, anal, 555–558
Endothelin B receptor defects, Hirschsprung's disease in, 720
Endothelin box 2B defects, Hirschsprung's disease in, 720
Endothelin-converting enzyme defects, Hirschsprung's disease in, 720
Endovaginal ultrasonography, 559
Enema, anterograde, for constipation, 610–611
Enterocele, 650, 653, 661–662
Evacuation proctography. *See* Defecography.
Exercise
for fecal incontinence, 592
for solitary rectal ulcer syndrome, 657
for urinary incontinence, 740

F

Fecal impaction, incontinence in, 702–703
Fecal incontinence, **587–604**

Laxatives (*continued*)
for dyssynergic defecation, 577–578
Levator ani muscles
anatomy of, 497–498
neurophysiologic evaluation of, 528–530
Levator ani syndrome, 686–688
Lifestyle modifications
for fecal incontinence, 590–591
for hemorrhoids, 629
Ligation, for hemorrhoids, 630–631
Linaclotide, for dyssynergic defecation, 579
Loperamide, for fecal incontinence, 592
Lubiprostone, for dyssynergic defecation, 578

M

Magnesium hydroxide, for constipation, 716
Magnetic resonance imaging, in pelvic floor disorders, 499, 559–562
Malformations, anorectal, 724–725
Manometry, anorectal, 513–519
ambulatory, 519
balloon expulsion test, 519
equipment for, 513
high-resolution, 516
in constipation, 714
in defecation, 517–518
in dyssynergic defecation, 573–574
in rectal prolapse, 646–647
in rectoanal reflex activity measurement, 516–517
in sphincter function evaluation, 514–516
limitations of, 513–514
patient preparation for, 514
Massage, for painful bladder syndrome, 691
Megacolon, surgical treatment of, 610
Metronidazole, for pouchitis, 678
Milligan-Morgan hemorrhoidectomy, 631–632
Mineral oil, for constipation, 716
Myelomeningocele, constipation in, 725
Myenteric plexus, anatomy of, 495

N

Neosphincter, for fecal incontinence, 616–617
Neurologic disorders, constipation in, 725
Neurturin defects, Hirschsprung's disease in, 720
Nifedipine, for anal fissure, 636
Nitroglycerin, for anal fissure, 635
Nonretentive fecal incontinence, in pediatric patients, 717–718, 742–743
Nonsteroidal anti-inflammatory drugs, pouchitis due to, 678
Nortriptyline, for prostatitis, 692
Nursing homes, incontinence in, **697–707**
fecal, 701–704
urinary, 697–701

O

Obesity, fecal incontinence in, 591
Osmotic laxatives
  for constipation, 716
  for dyssynergic defecation, 578
Overactive bladder, 549–550, 690, 733–734, 740–741
Oxybutynin, for urinary incontinence, 741

P

Pain disorders, **685–696**
  anorectal, 686–689
  bladder, 689–691
  cardinal features of, 685–686
  classification of, 685
  interstitial cystitis, 689–691
  prostatitis, 691–692
Parasympathetic nervous system
  of anal sphincters, 495
  of bladder, 540
Pediatric patients
  anorectal malformations in, 724–725
  constipation in, **709–730**
    atopy and, 717
    definition of, 710
    diagnosis of, 713–714
    epidemiology of, 710–711
    functional, 711–717
    in neurologic impairment, 725
    organic, 718–724
    pathogenesis of, 711
    physiologic considerations in, 712–713
    red flags in, 713
    treatment of, 714–717
    versus normal defecation, 710
  fecal incontinence in, 717–718, 743
  fecal retention in, 738, 742–743
  urinary incontinence in, **731–748**
    behavioral problems and, 736–737
    classification of, 733
    constipation and, 736–739
    epidemiology of, 735–737
    evaluation of, 737–739
    pathophysiology of, 733–735
    treatment of, 739–742
    urinary tract infections and, 736
    versus normal bladder development and control, 732–733
Pelvic diaphragm, anatomy of, 493, 497–498
Pelvic floor disorders
  anal fissures, 634–638

Pelvic (*continued*)
anatomy of, 493–498
anorectal malformations, 724–725
constipation. *See* Constipation.
dyssynergic defecation. *See* Dyssynergic defecation.
enterocele, 650, 653, 661–662
evaluation of, **511–538**
anorectal sensation, 512
barostat studies, 512, 520–527
colonic transit studies, 512
diagnostic tests for, 512
manometric, 512–519, 646–647, 714
neurophysiologic, 512, 527–531
radiologic, 498–500, **553–567**
sensorimotor, 512, 520–527
ultrasonography in. *See* Ultrasonography.
urodynamic, **539–551**
functional pain, **685–696**
hemorrhoids, 627–633
ileal pouch dysfunction, **669–683**
in pediatric patients. *See* Pediatric patients.
incontinence in. *See also* Fecal incontinence; Urinary incontinence.
pelvic floor repair in, 613
physiology of, 500–506
rectal intussusception, 653–655
rectal prolapse, 645–653
rectocele, 658–661
solitary rectal ulcer syndrome, 655–658
treatment of
biofeedback therapy in. *See* Biofeedback therapy.
surgical, **605–625**
Pelvic nerves, anatomy of, 495
Pelvic tension myalgia (levator ani syndrome), 686–688
Pelvis, bony, anatomy of, 493
Pentosan polysulfate, for painful bladder syndrome, 690
Perineal proctosigmoidectomy, for rectal prolapse, 650, 652
Phenol sclerotherapy, for hemorrhoids, 629–630
PHOX2B gene mutations, Hirschsprung's disease in, 720
Physiotherapy
for levator ani syndrome, 687–688
for prostatitis, 692
for solitary rectal ulcer syndrome, 657–658
for urinary incontinence, 741
Plug, anal, for fecal incontinence, 595
Polyethylene glycol
for constipation, 714–716, 742
for dyssynergic defecation, 578
Pouchitis, after restorative proctocolectomy, 677–678
Pressure flow studies, in bladder function, 545
Probiotics, for pouchitis, 678
Procidentia, internal (intussusception), 653–655

Proctalgia fugax, 688–689
Proctocolectomy, restorative, ileal pouch dysfunction. *See* Ileal pouch dysfunction.
Proctography, evacuation. *See* Defecography.
Proctoscopy, in hemorrhoids, 628
Proctosigmoidectomy, perineal, for rectal prolapse, 650
Prolapse
  pelvic organ, 659
  rectal, 645–653
Prostatitis, chronic, 691–692
Psychologic issues, in dyssynergic defecation, 570, 572
Psyllium, for dyssynergic defecation, 576–577
Pubococcygeus muscle
  anatomy of, 497–498
  function of, 501–502
Puboperineal muscles, anatomy of, 498
Puborectalis muscles
  anatomy of, 495–498
  dysfunction of, 505
  function of, 501–506
  in defecation, 712
Puborectalis syndrome (levator ani syndrome), 686–688
Pubovisceral muscles, anatomy of, 498
Pudendal nerves
  function of, 498
  terminal motor latency test of, 527–528
Pyriformis syndrome (levator ani syndrome), 686–688

Q

Quality of life, in dyssynergic defecation, 570

R

Rectal augmentation procedure, for fecal incontinence, 618–619
Rectal reservoir dysfunction, fecal incontinence in, 618–619
Rectoanal reflex activity, evaluation of, 516–517
Rectocele, 658–661
Rectopexy
  for intussusception, 655
  for rectal prolapse, 648–653
  for solitary rectal ulcer syndrome, 658
Rectum
  atresia of, 724–725
  congenital fistulas of, 724–725
  intussusception of, 653–655
  irrigation of, for fecal incontinence, 595
  pain syndromes of, 686–689
  prolapse of, 645–653
    definition of, 645–646
    diagnosis of, 646–648
    etiology of, 646

Rectum (*continued*)
        occult (intussusception), 653–655
        pathogenesis of, 646
        symptoms of, 646
        treatment of, 648–653
    retained, in ileorectal anastomosis, 675–676
    solitary ulcer of, 655–658
Reflex activity, rectoanal
    evaluation of, 516–517
    in defecation, 712–713
Restorative proctocolectomy, ileal pouch dysfunction. *See* Ileal pouch dysfunction.
RET gene mutations, Hirschsprung's disease in, 720
Retroperitoneal fascia, anatomy of, 493
Ripstein procedure, for rectal prolapse, 648–650
Rubber-band ligation, for hemorrhoids, 630

S

Sacral nerves
    function of, 498
    stimulation of
        for constipation, 611–612
        for fecal incontinence, 614–616
        for painful bladder syndrome, 691
        for urinary incontinence, 741
Salbutamol, for proctalgia fugax, 689
Sclerotherapy, for hemorrhoids, 629–630
Senna, for constipation, 716
Sensorimotor evaluation, 512, 520–527
    anal, 520–521
    bladder, 541
    rectal, 521–527
        compliance, 524–527
        equipment for, 521–522
        patient preparation for, 522
        sensation, 522–524
        tone, 525–527
Sensory function, of anorectum, 500
Sepsis, after restorative proctocolectomy, 670–672
Sexual abuse, dyssynergic defecation and, 570
Sigmoidoscopy, in solitary rectal ulcer, 655
SIP1 gene mutations, Hirschsprung's disease in, 720
Skin care, in incontinence, 703–704
Small intestine, in enterocele, 650, 653, 661–662
Soiling, fecal, 742–743
Solitary rectal ulcer syndrome, 655–658
Somatosensory evoked potentials, 530–531
Sorbitol, for constipation, 716
SOX10 gene mutations, Hirschsprung's disease in, 720
Spasm, levator, 686–688
Sphincter(s)

anal. *See* Anal sphincters.
bladder, development of, 732–733
Sphincterotomy, of anus, 637–638
Spina bifida, constipation in, 725
Spinal nerves, anatomy of, 495
Stapled hemorrhoidopexy, 632
Stapled transanal rectal resection, 612–613
STARR (stapled transanal rectal resection), 612–613
Stimulant laxatives
for constipation, 716
for dyssynergic defecation, 578
Stoma
for constipation, 611
for fecal incontinence, 617
Stool softeners
for anal fissure, 635
for dyssynergic defecation, 578
Suppositories, for constipation, 716
Sympathetic nervous system
of anal sphincters, 495
of bladder, 540

T

T-cell factor 4 defects, Hirschsprung's disease in, 720
Thermoprobes, in anal sensation evaluation, 520
Thiele's technique, for painful bladder syndrome, 691
Thrombosis, of hemorrhoids, 628, 632
Tolterodine, for urinary incontinence, 742
Tone, rectal, evaluation of, 525–527
Transperineal ultrasonography, 559
Triangular ligament, anatomy of, 493

U

Ulcer, rectal, solitary, 655–658
Ultrasonography, 555–559
endovaginal, 559
in pelvic floor disorders, 499–500
in rectal prolapse, 646
in solitary rectal ulcer, 657
in urinary incontinence, 739
transperineal, 559
Urothra, muscle action on, 501
Urge resistance training, for fecal incontinence, 591
Urge syndrome, 733–735, 740
Urinary incontinence
behavioral problems and, 736–737
classification of, 733
constipation and, 736–739
epidemiology of, 735–737

Urinary (*continued*)
evaluation of, 548–549, 737–739
in nursing homes, 697–701
in pediatric patients, **731–748**
incomplete emptying, 700–701
pathophysiology of, 697–698, 733–735
skin care in, 703–704
stress, 548–549, 699–701
treatment of, 699–701, 739–742
urge, 699–701
urinary tract infections and, 736
versus normal bladder development and control, 732–733
Urinary tract infections, incontinence and, 736
Urodynamic evaluation, **539–552,** 548
anatomic considerations in, 540
components of, 540–547
cystometry in, 540–544, 548–549
electromyography in, 545–547
in neurologic disorders, 550
in overactive bladder, 549–550
in pediatric patients, 739
in pelvic organ prolapse, 548–549
in stress incontinence, 548–549
indications for, 547–550
neurologic pathways and, 540
pressure flow studies in, 545
uroflowmetry in, 544–545
video, 547
Uroflowmetry, 544–545, 737–738
Urogenital diaphragm, anatomy of, 493
Uterosacral ligaments, anatomy of, 494

V

Vagina
muscle action on, 501–504
rectocele in, 658–661
Vaginal high-pressure zone, 502, 504
Ventral(colpo)pexy, 650, 653
Vesicovaginal reflux, incontinence in, 735
Video urodynamics, 547
Voiding
development of, 732
dysfunctional, 733–734, 740. *See also* Urinary incontinence.
postponement of, 733, 735
Voiding cystourethrography, in urinary incontinence, 739
Voluntary squeeze measures, for fecal incontinence, 593
von Frey hairs, in anal sensation evaluation, 520
VSL #3 probiotic, for pouchitis, 678